Long COVID and Society

Deborah Lupton
Editor

Long COVID and Society

International Perspectives

palgrave
macmillan

Editor
Deborah Lupton
Vitalities Lab, Centre for Social Research
in Health and Social Policy Research
Centre
UNSW Sydney
Sydney, NSW, Australia

ISBN 978-981-96-9167-8 ISBN 978-981-96-9168-5 (eBook)
https://doi.org/10.1007/978-981-96-9168-5

This work was supported by University of New South Wales.

Cover illustration: Albert Shakirov/Alamy Stock Photo

This Palgrave Macmillan imprint is published by the registered company Springer Nature Singapore Pte Ltd.
The registered company address is: 152 Beach Road, #21-01/04 Gateway East, Singapore 189721, Singapore

This book is dedicated to the memory of my friend and UNSW Sydney colleague Gemma Carey. In addition to her world-leading research on social policy, disability and public health, Gemma was a fierce advocate for people with Long COVID and other chronic health conditions. Gemma had planned to contribute a chapter to this volume with her husband Ben O'Mara, but she died before she was able to start work on it. In this chapter's stead, Ben has written a personal essay about caring for Gemma during her illness and life with their young son following her death, which I have placed as a coda to the book. Gemma is greatly missed by her colleagues and friends.

Contents

Part I Introduction

1 **The Social Aspects and Impacts of Long COVID** 3
Deborah Lupton

Part II Knowledge-Making

2 **Long COVID: The Critical Role of Patient Advocacy-Research in Disease Recognition** 35
Elisa Perego

3 **Long COVID Times: An X/Twitter-Informed Rhythmanalysis of Pacing** 59
Sam Martin and Emma Uprichard

Part III Medical Responses

4 'Just Because You Didn't Detect It, Doesn't Mean It's Not There': Long COVID, ME/CFS and the Social Dynamics of Biomedical Knowledge Production 85
Kathy S. Anderson

5 Long COVID Services Between Medical Clinics and Healing Rituals: A Case Study in Switzerland 105
Marjolaine Viret and Francesco Panese

Part IV Biopolitics and Social Determinants

6 Long COVID and the Biopolitics of Pandemic Timings and Endings 131
Mark D. M. Davis

7 The Profound Societal Impacts of Long COVID and Pandemic Non-interventionism 151
Pantea Javidan

8 Equity Amidst Uncertainty: A Comparative Critique of Multiple Stakeholder Perspectives About Health Equity for People with Long COVID 181
Danielle Hitch, Sam Wills, Sara Holton, Rebecca Corva, and Krishna Vakil

Part V Lived Experience

9 We Will Not Be Silent: The Australia Long COVID Community Speak Out About the Role of Epistemic Injustice in Erasing Evidence of Long COVID in Australia 205
Robin Austin, Kirsty Yeates, Su Mon Kyaw-Myint, Ruth Newport, and Pippa Yeoman

10 Living with the Virus: An Autoethnography of Long COVID as Multilayered Traumatisation 227
Vivienne Matthies-Boon

11 **The Double Bind: Gaslighting, Cultural Violence and the Post COVID Experience** 249
Mary Zournazi

Part VI Specific Social Groups

12 **'I Have Disappeared': Long COVID, ME/CFS and Inclusion in Church Communities** 267
Penny Pullan

13 **The Debilitating Discourses of Long COVID: The Public Pedagogies of Sporting Bodies** 289
Matt Ventresca and Mary McDonald

14 **Long COVID in Children, Young People and Families** 311
Alice MacLean, Cervantée Wild, Sarah Nettleton, Sue Ziebland, and Kate Hunt

Part VII Coda

15 **My Strange Revelations from Grief and Long COVID: How Caring for My Wife Showed Me the Horror and Beauty of Loss from Disease** 331
Ben O'Mara

Index 341

Contributors

Kathy S. Anderson Sydney Centre for Healthy Societies, University of Sydney, Sydney, NSW, Australia

Robin Austin Australia Long COVID Community, Melbourne, VIC, Australia

Rebecca Corva The Institute for Mental and Physical Health and Clinical Translation (IMPACT), Deakin University, Melbourne, VIC, Australia

Mark D. M. Davis School of Social Sciences, Faculty of Arts, Monash University, Melbourne, Australia

Danielle Hitch School of Health and Social Development and Institute of Health Transformation, Deakin University, Melbourne, VIC, Australia

Sara Holton School of Public Health and Preventive Medicine, Monash University, Melbourne, VIC, Australia

Kate Hunt Institute for Social Marketing and Health, University of Stirling, Stirling, UK

Pantea Javidan Department of Psychiatry and Behavioral Sciences, School of Medicine, Stanford University, Stanford, CA, USA

Su Mon Kyaw-Myint Australia Long COVID Community, Melbourne, VIC, Australia

Deborah Lupton Vitalities Lab, Centre for Social Research in Health and Social Policy Research Centre, UNSW, Sydney, NSW, Australia

Alice MacLean Institute for Social Marketing and Health, University of Stirling, Stirling, UK

Sam Martin Rapid Research Evaluation and Appraisal Lab (RREAL), Department of Targeted Intervention, University College London (UCL), London, UK;
Oxford Vaccine Group, University of Oxford, Oxford, UK

Vivienne Matthies-Boon Department of Ethics and Political Philosophy, Faculty of Philosophy, Theology and Religious Studies, Radboud University, Nijmegen, The Netherlands

Mary McDonald School of History and Sociology, Georgia Institute of Technology, Atlanta, GA, USA

Sarah Nettleton Department of Sociology, University of York, York, UK

Ruth Newport Australia Long COVID Community, Melbourne, VIC, Australia

Ben O'Mara School of Social Sciences, Media, Film and Education, Faculty of Health, Arts and Design, Swinburne University, Hawthorn, VIC, Australia

Francesco Panese Faculty of Social and Political Sciences, Institute of Social Sciences, University of Lausanne, Lausanne, Switzerland;
Faculty of Biology & Medicine, Institute of Humanities in Medicine, University of Lausanne, Lausanne, Switzerland

Elisa Perego Institute of Archaeology, University College London, London, UK

Penny Pullan St Hild College, Sheffield, UK

Emma Uprichard Centre for Interdisciplinary Methodologies, University of Warwick, Coventry, UK

Krishna Vakil School of Medicine, Deakin University, Melbourne, VIC, Australia

Matt Ventresca School of History and Sociology, Georgia Institute of Technology, Atlanta, GA, USA

Marjolaine Viret Faculty of Law, Criminal Sciences and Public Administration, Centre of Comparative, European & International Law, University of Lausanne, Lausanne, Switzerland

Cervantée Wild Nuffield Department of Primary Care Health Sciences, University of Oxford, Oxford, UK;
Faculty of Medical and Health Sciences, Department of Paediatrics: Child and Youth Health, School of Medicine, University of Auckland, Auckland, New Zealand

Sam Wills Department of Allied Health, Western Health, Footscray, VIC, Australia

Kirsty Yeates Australia Long COVID Community, Melbourne, VIC, Australia;
Research School of Biology, College of Science and Medicine, The Australian National University, Canberra, ACT, Australia

Pippa Yeoman Australia Long COVID Community, Melbourne, VIC, Australia;
The University of Sydney, Camperdown, NSW, Australia

Sue Ziebland Nuffield Department of Primary Care Health Sciences, University of Oxford, Oxford, UK

Mary Zournazi School of Humanities, Creative Industries and Social Sciences, University of Newcastle, Callaghan, NSW, Australia

List of Tables

Table 5.1 Example of activity pacing from a Long COVID service 115
Table 9.1 Ranking of the top 12 most severe symptoms reported and the overall prevalence of these symptoms (n varies from 570 to 594) 210
Table 9.2 Treatments tried, with corresponding reports of improvement (n varies from 375 to 401) 214
Table 9.3 Ranking of the Australian Government's high-level COVID-19 pandemic response (n varies from 595 to 607) 215
Table 9.4 2023 survey responses related to government health messaging and support services (n varies from 539 to 614) 216

Part I

Introduction

1

The Social Aspects and Impacts of Long COVID

Deborah Lupton

Introduction: The Shadow Pandemic

Long COVID is a new health condition, caused by infections with the novel coronavirus SARS-CoV-2 and the resulting disease COVID-19. There are varying definitions, but the term 'Long COVID' (also referred to in the medical literature as 'post-acute sequelae of COVID-19' or 'post-COVID-19 condition') is most commonly used to refer to prolonged or new symptoms for which there is no alternative explanation following an initial acute COVID infection. After the first cases of COVID were identified at the end of 2019, the virus began to spread quickly around the world. By 11 March 2020, the World Health Organization had declared COVID to be a pandemic (World Health Organization, 2020). Since then, COVID infections have caused millions of deaths globally (World Health Organization, 2025), as well as reducing

D. Lupton (✉)
Vitalities Lab, Centre for Social Research in Health, Social Policy Research Centre, UNSW, Sydney, NSW, Australia
e-mail: d.lupton@unsw.edu.au

D. Lupton (ed.), *Long COVID and Society*,
https://doi.org/10.1007/978-981-96-9168-5_1

life expectancy and increasing premature mortality rates due to both the direct and indirect impacts of the disease (for example, disruptions to healthcare services) (Ahmadi-Abhari et al., 2025). As the pandemic is continuing unabated, the number of people developing Long COVID is also increasing. While many governments now urge their citizens to learn to 'live with COVID' (Stokoe et al., 2022), people with Long COVID are facing an uncertain future with a disabling chronic illness for which there is currently no cure. Long COVID has therefore been described as the 'shadow pandemic' (World Health Organization, 2023).

There is lack of agreement in the medical literature about how long symptoms should linger to be defined as contributing to 'long' or 'post-acute' COVID rather than acute COVID. To some extent, this inconsistency in definition is understandable, as Long COVID is still a new condition, with much yet to learn about why some people infected with the novel coronavirus have not fully recovered and how best to diagnose the condition (da Silva et al., 2024). However, the World Health Organization's definition using 12 weeks/three months post-infection is the most common in current medical definitions and diagnoses of Long COVID (Gutzeit et al., 2025).

A large body of medical research studies has identified the impacts of Long COVID on the human body, demonstrating that COVID infection can affect all organs and blood vessels. Some people who had their first COVID infection from the ancestral variant of SARS-CoV-2 very early in the pandemic (early 2020) are still disabled or dealing with illness with little sign of recovery. Other people's symptoms are more recent, caused by later variants or sub-variants, or by reinfections. Each COVID infection carries a cumulative risk of Long COVID, or of experiencing worsening symptoms if an individual already has Long COVID (Al-Aly & Topol, 2024; Sawano et al., 2025). A range of symptoms are associated with Long COVID, including but not limited to fatigue that does not improve with rest, heart palpitations, joint or muscle pain, cognitive impairment, disordered sleep, tinnitus, shortness of breath, exercise intolerance and post-exertional malaise, postural orthostatic tachycardia syndrome, myocardial inflammation and renal, dermatological, dental and digestive tract symptoms. Some definitions of Long COVID incorporate medical problems that may emerge in the future following even a 'mild' infection, such as immune dysregulation, metabolic disorders, inflammation and damage to blood vessels and the organ systems of the body (Al-Aly et al., 2024; Greenhalgh et al., 2024). As well as neurological disorders, psychiatric conditions such as anxiety and depressive mood have been identified in Long COVID patients (Gutzeit et al., 2025).

The prevalence of Long COVID is also difficult to ascertain, as many nations do not collect data on the condition or even on COVID infections, deaths or hospitalisations. This is particularly the case for countries in the Global South, as most data collection about COVID and medical and public health research on Long COVID is focused on high-income countries (Gmanyami et al., 2024). A further difficulty in finding accurate data on Long COVID is that given the lack of public education about Long COVID, people may be uncertain about whether they have it. For example, in a 2023 study, of over 750,000 patients registered with a general practitioner, 4.8% reported Long COVID, but a further 9.1% were unsure (Woodrow et al., 2025). However, a systematic review of studies published up to April 2024 involving a meta-analysis of data from 48 studies provided sobering statistics. Of the studies included, 21 were from European countries, 14 studies were from the American region, 10 were from Asia, two were from Australia and one study was from the African continent. The meta-analysis identified the pooled prevalence of Long COVID as 45% after three months following acute infection (Sk Abd Razak et al., 2024). The latest research also suggests that full recovery from Long COVID is difficult to achieve. In a prospective multi-site study following up people in the USA who had verified COVID over a period of up to three years following infection, almost 30% of respondents reported Long COVID symptoms, with a mean duration of two years. Less than 2 per cent had resolved symptoms (Gottlieb et al., 2025).

This edited collection focuses on the social aspects and impacts of Long COVID from an international perspective, bringing social and political theory together with the insights offered from lived experience. From the beginning, Long COVID, like COVID itself (Lupton, 2022), has been a social and political as well as a medical phenomenon. Long COVID can have serious effects on individuals' opportunities to fully participate in society, including in education, employment, leisure activities and social relationships. Many people with Long COVID are facing the major impacts of mental distress, lack of access to healthcare and social marginalisation caused by contestations over whether the condition is 'real', 'serious' or 'psychosomatic'. They are confronting ableism, social stigma, exclusion and shunning. To many others, the plight of people with Long COVID is invisible. All these topics and issues are examined and held up to the light in this collection.

Following this introductory chapter are a further 15 chapters contributed by researchers in the UK, Italy, Switzerland, the Netherlands. USA and Australia that address this important area of social research. Crucially, most of the authors are themselves living with or caring for someone with Long COVID or work closely with Long COVID patient communities and others with lived experience. The book highlights how Long COVID affects people's identities, social relationships, life opportunities and inclusion in society. It also throws a spotlight on the struggles over the legitimacy of lay expertise versus medical authority and addresses how people with lived experience of Long COVID are supporting and learning from each other and engaging in activism and advocacy initiatives. Methods of social inquiry employed in the book include textual analysis of social media, news media, medical, policy and government inquiry documents; reflections on the authors' own experiences of Long COVID; surveys; epidemiological data and qualitative methods such as interviews with people with Long COVID, their family members and clinicians. Concepts and perspectives from social, philosophical and political theory used to add depth to the analyses include rhythmanalysis; epistemic injustice; political economy and social determinants of health perspectives; biopolitical theory; the sociology and anthropology of knowledge, suffering, medical power, diagnosis, disability, stigma and temporality; trauma studies; social justice studies; narrative theory and psychosocial perspectives.

Prior to the outbreak of the COVID pandemic and the emergence of the condition of Long COVID, an extensive body of literature in health sociology and medical anthropology had already addressed relevant topics of the lived experience of illness and healthcare, the social structuring of medicine, medical dominance and authority, patient expertise and activism, social stigma related to certain illnesses and diseases, the responsibilisation of personal health, and the biopolitics of contested and psychologised health conditions. There are now numerous studies published on the social dimensions of Long COVID. The remainder of this introductory chapter provides an overview of key insights from these literatures, interweaving the new findings from the contributors to this volume to site them in this previous scholarship.

Social Inequalities and Biopolitics

Since the 1970s, an extensive body of literature has been published on the biopolitical dimensions of medicine and healthcare. This scholarship, initially based in political economy critiques of medical authority and power in capitalist societies, identifies the ways that members of the medical profession have institutionalised their claim to expert knowledge, rewarded with high income and status. From this perspective, health states are sites of struggle and contestation between those with power and high socioeconomic status and those without. The symbolic power held by medical professionals and the lack of recognition of the contribution of socioeconomic disadvantage and social marginalisation to poor health has meant that some social groups have not been well served when seeking healthcare (Doyal & Pennell, 1979; Freidson, 1970). Critical public health scholars identified 'the social determinants of health' as affecting people's opportunities to achieve good health, including poverty, poor housing, lack of access to nutritious food, racism, dangerous employment conditions and the withdrawal of the state from offering economic supports and social services (Marmot & Wilkinson, 2005; Navarro, 2009).

The growth of neoliberalism in most healthcare systems since the 1980s has also contributed to a focus on individual responsibility for health, ignoring the role of socioeconomic factors in people's health and illness states (Schrecker, 2016). In other words, people are blamed for becoming ill, with moral judgements and othering typically used to portray them as weak even when they are dealing with entrenched social structural conditions of poverty, poor housing or lack of access to affordable, high-quality healthcare (Crawford, 1994; Navarro, 2009). Drawing on the theory of Michel Foucault (1988, 2008), scholars in health sociology and anthropology (Ayo, 2012; Clarke & Shim, 2011; Lupton, 1995, 2012) have noted how biopolitics, or the political dimensions of managing and governing human bodies, directs attention to individuals' role in promoting their health and wellbeing. Those who do not conform to norms and expectations set by governing agencies about managing their own health are routinely positioned as lacking knowledge, willingness or strength of character, and subjected to moral judgements. As writers contributing to critical disability studies or crip theory (Hsu, 2024; Rodgers et al., 2023) have pointed out, neoliberalism pathologises bodily differences such as disability and chronic health conditions, as these are viewed as detracting from people's contributions to the economy. Disabilities and illnesses are portrayed as individual problems that require individual rather than structural changes to accommodate (Rodgers et al., 2023). Gender, sexual identity and ethnicity/cultural background intersect with the stigma, discrimination, ableist violence and neglect experienced by disabled or chronically ill people (Hsu, 2024).

In the COVID era, these inequalities continue to exist across global health systems. Biases and social discrimination due to ethnicity/cultural background, age and gender, combined with entrenched socioeconomic inequalities, existing chronic illnesses or disabilities and social stigma mean COVID affects already marginalised and disadvantaged communities and populations far more than privileged groups and regions. This is the case for both COVID infections and deaths (Ahmadi-Abhari et al., 2025; Islam et al., 2021; Levin et al., 2022) and Long COVID morbidity (Mkoma et al., 2024; Nguyen et al., 2024; Woodrow et al., 2025). Following the outbreak of COVID, Archille Mbembe (2021) built on his concept of necropolitics to argue that people of colour have been routinely subjected to violence and loss of autonomy during the pandemic as their health and lives are treated as less important than that of White people. There are other social groups who are subjected to necropolitics. As Hsu (2024) points out, when government and public health agencies decided to loosen or drop COVID mitigations, it was usually claimed that the rationale was a decline in death rates. This involved an assessment of a 'tolerable deaths' threshold. Those people whose deaths were viewed as tolerable were disproportionately not only people of colour but also LGBTQIA+, older, fat and disabled people. The continuing politicisation of face mask wearing (Lupton et al., 2021), including the widespread discarding of these protective items by medical and other healthcare professionals when treating patients, speaks to the lack of care mainstream society and even healthcare workers have for those who are immunocompromised, chronically ill or disabled.

The biopolitical dimensions and social determinants of Long COVID are explored by several contributors to this volume. For Mark Davis, Long COVID is viewed as a distinctive turning point in pandemic biopolitics, taken form and force through appropriating and resisting virological, immunological, epidemiological and other knowledges of pandemics and combining them with lived experience. Analysing government, public health and news media texts, Davis documents efforts to end the pandemic through the procurement of 'COVID normal' conditions that obscure and marginalise Long COVID. In her chapter, Pantea Javidan synthesises the now extensive body of epidemiological and public health literature detailing how social groups in the USA experiencing socioeconomic inequities in the contexts of the workplace and educational settings are further disadvantaged by the impacts of Long COVID. As she points outs, expectations that workers ignore the impacts of continual exposure to COVID infections is leading to decreased participation in the workforce due to constant or prolonged illness and disability from the very virus that they are expected to 'live with'.

The analysis of submissions to Australia's COVID and Long COVID inquiries conducted by Danielle Hitch and colleagues also highlights socioeconomic inequalities and health equity issues. Engaging with the Health Equity Framework, Hitch and colleagues found that in their submissions, Australians with Long COVID expressed deep mistrust in Australia's political leadership and frustration with political inaction or poor responses to Long COVID, including inadequate healthcare resourcing, with disadvantaged social groups most badly affected. As Robin Austin and colleagues' surveys of Australians living with Long COVID identified, cultural, geographic and resource barriers are faced by those who are already in disadvantaged social groups. Their findings illuminate the social impact on families and communities, the economic challenges of maintaining employment and accessing government benefits and the increased burden of navigating health systems ill-equipped to address chronic complex conditions.

Given the continual messaging from governments, public health agencies and the news media that it is only certain categories of people who are particularly 'vulnerable' to severe or long-lasting impacts of COVID (most often described as older people, disabled people and those with pre-existing health conditions), those who are outside these categories are frequently dismissed. As shown in Alice MacLean and colleagues' chapter, British children and young people with Long COVID and their parents attempting to advocate for them have been particularly subjected to medical ignorance, stigmatisation and silencing. Even highly privileged people's status and life opportunities can be stymied by Long COVID. As Matt Ventresca and Mary McDonald demonstrate (this volume), while North American elite athletes with Long COVID can receive the best medical attention, they struggle with 'fighting' the condition while attempting to meet expectations of the superior sporting performer. Ableist norms and discourses refuse to accept that these young, supremely fit and physically talented people can be laid low by a chronic illness. Athletes who fail to recover from injuries or illnesses are deemed to be 'unproductive' and expendable. There is simply no space allowed for the concept of an elite athlete who is also disabled or chronically ill.

Contested Illnesses, Epistemic Injustice and Patient-Generated Knowledge

Scholars in the sociology and anthropology of health and illness have demonstrated the immense suffering experienced by people who are living with contested conditions and the failures of the medical profession to acknowledge their experiences. Contested illnesses are health conditions where the aetiology is difficult to identify or are complex or poorly understood and are therefore subject to differing claims concerning their legitimacy as illnesses. Medical experts differ about how best to diagnose or treat these conditions—or even whether they should be considered an illness at all, instead characterising them as psychiatric or psychosomatic (Dumit, 2006; Moss & Teghtsoonian, 2008). Examples of such illnesses include myalgic encephalomyelitis/chronic fatigue syndrome (ME/CFS), fibromyalgia, irritable bowel syndrome—and now Long COVID.

In the contemporary era, contested illnesses are debated in an environment in which 'empowered' patients are expected to take more control in the medical encounter yet are continually faced with medical authority in relation to diagnosis and treatment which is very difficult to challenge (Lupton, 2012). The sociology of diagnosis has shown that diagnosis, as a gate-keeping practice that is highly regulated and credentialled by members of the medical profession, can be a particularly contested phenomenon (Jeske et al., 2024; Jutel, 2014). People with unrecognised conditions often long for a diagnosis so that they can give a label to their suffering that can legitimise it in the eyes of others and potentially find a pathway for treatments. When this diagnosis is not forthcoming from the medical professionals from whom they seek help, feelings of frustration, grief and hopelessness are frequently the outcomes. This situation creates 'fragile disease identities'—those that are continually open to contestation and doubt from others (Roth & Gadebusch-Bondio, 2022).

The struggles of people living with contested, chronic, rare, stigmatised or invisible illnesses have been described as an example of 'epistemic injustice' (Blease et al., 2017; de Boer, 2021): a concept which describes inequalities in the generation of and access to knowledge. As outlined by philosopher Miranda Fricker in her foundational book *Epistemic Injustice: Power and the Ethics of Knowing* (2007) epistemic injustice is a distinctive mode of the operation of power and the entrenchment of injustice, involving 'a wrong done to someone specifically in their capacity as a knower' (Fricker, 2007, p. 2). Knowledge is epistemic privilege, which can be founded on expert training and education or on lived experience. There is often asymmetry in epistemic privilege, with expert knowledge frequently having greater authority than lived experience. Fricker specifies two forms of epistemic injustice. The first is testimonial injustice, occurring when prejudice against a speaker results in their words being discredited and losing authority. The second form is hermeneutical injustice, caused by a gap in collective interpretive resources, with the consequence that some individuals or social groups are placed at an unfair disadvantage when attempting to understand their experiences.

In the domain of medicine and healthcare, epistemic injustice is evident in the ways that only those with medical authority have the power to legitimise and acknowledge people's suffering, discounting or even rejecting the lay expertise that has accumulated. From this perspective, both the medical profession and patients have a right to epistemic privilege and authority, but due to the high status and professional accreditation of medical practitioners, the knowledge that lay people and patients derive from their and others' lived experiences is treated as irrelevant or inferior. Particularly if the medical condition is rare or novel, or a physiological cause cannot be identified, people often find themselves battling to find recognition of their suffering from medical practitioners in the context of asymmetry of power between the medical profession and patients (Blease et al., 2017; Carel & Kidd, 2017; de Boer, 2021).

In recent times, digital devices and platforms have provided unprecedented opportunities for patients to gather and share information about contested, new or rare conditions (Lupton, 2017). In the case of Long COVID, digital communities have made a crucial contribution to the generation and distribution of epistemic authority for lay people. From the early days of the COVID pandemic, the use of social media and other digital platforms have been central to the definition of Long COVID and the sharing of information and support. Online communities have provided significant validation and social support for people with Long COVID, who have used these groups to share information about the condition. The contribution of medical professionals and researchers who are themselves living with Long COVID has blurred the boundaries between expert and lay epistemic privilege and what is considered 'clinical evidence' (Mullard et al., 2023; Roth & Gadebusch-Bondio, 2022; Russell et al., 2022; Yeoman, 2024).

The initial discussions of what came to be known as 'Long Haul COVID' or 'Long COVID' began early in the pandemic, when some of the first people to have been infected by the novel coronavirus began to recognise that their symptoms were not improving weeks or months after the initial acute infection (Callard & Perego, 2021; Perego et al., 2020; Rushforth et al., 2021). In this book, Elisa Perego, one of the first contributors to the development of defining Long COVID and establishing patient communities, provides a detailed history recounting how people across the world became involved in the grassroots development of Long COVID patient communities on X/Twitter. As she notes, these major patient-led contributions to building Long COVID knowledge has not been sufficiently acknowledged in the medical literature or news media reporting. Perego traces the emergence of hashtag activism involving hashtags such as #longhaulers, #apresJ20, #CountLongCovid, #TreatLongCovid and #LongCovid and the individuals and groups who drew attention to the persistence of symptoms following acute COVID and defined the condition as a multi-system disease entity.

Another method of generating patient expertise and new knowledge about health and illness is lay people's use of digital self-tracking technologies such as apps and wearable devices to monitor and quantify aspects of their bodily functions. This practice can provide people with better self-knowledge about a health condition. Further, because digital tools and the data they generate are often viewed as more 'accurate' and less 'subjective' than people's explanations of how their bodies feel, medical professionals can more readily accept this information as evidence (Lupton, 2016, 2019). Unsurprisingly, therefore, research has shown that some people with Long COVID are using self-tracking to create new forms of knowledge and to some extent challenge the power differentials and fraught sociopolitical climate of the pandemic.

Self-tracking can be a valuable tool to gain insight into Long COVID symptoms and evaluate interventions. It provides people with a sense of empowerment, control, encouragement, and, very importantly, validation (Homewood, 2023; Homewood et al., 2024; Jayadeva & Lupton, 2025). These forms of self-generated information can then be shared online so that others can benefit from what people have learned about Long COVID, as forms of self-care and care for community (Jayadeva & Lupton, 2025). Sam Martin and Emma Uprichard (this volume) show how tweets about self-tracking provided others with advice about the best way to accomplish epistemic authority. These activities, by enhancing individual and collective knowledge, thereby challenge both testimonial and hermeneutical injustice. However, as is the case for other people self-tracking chronic illnesses (Lupton, 2016, 2019), the constant monitoring and tracking of Long COVID symptoms can serve as an unwelcome reminder of illness and can exacerbate feelings of frustration and loss of control if symptoms appearing to be worsening (Martin and Uprichard, this volume; Jayadeva & Lupton, 2025).

The chapters by Kathy Anderson and Marjolaine Viret and Francesco Panese demonstrate how people with Long COVID are expected to engage in 'partnerships' with healthcare providers to work together to generate information about the condition, even as their attempts to contribute to medical knowledge are often spurned. With reference to testimonial and hermeneutical justice, Mark Davis considers how Long COVID disrupts established knowledge and assumptions about pandemic timings and endings and augurs for more equitable and just post-COVID politics and related science and practice. Where biomedicine is failing to provide effective treatments, as demonstrated by Viret and Panese, Long COVID services appear willing to promote strategies such as pacing and even alternative therapies as last resorts, which themselves demand sustained work from patients so that they can learn to effectively 'cure' themselves. They analyse this situation through the lens of healing rituals, which influence patients' experiences, reshape their identities, impact on their social environments and help them to cope with their chronic condition but also force them to adapt to it.

Focusing on the sociology of knowledge in relation to contested illnesses, Kathy Anderson's chapter in this volume draws on interviews with 20 clinicians, researchers and advocates in ME/CFS and Long COVID knowledge production. Using the concepts of 'thought styles' and 'thought collectives' developed by Ludwik Fleck, Anderson examines the development of clinical guidelines and biomedical classifications for these conditions. She shows that although patient-led expertise has to some extent challenged the epistemic authority of clinicians, there is still a long way to go. While the importance of 'lived experience' and 'patient inclusion' in knowledge production is frequently championed, members of the medical profession are often still resistant to relinquishing some epistemic ground to their patients.

These analyses demonstrate the emphasis placed by the medical profession and patients themselves on the importance of taking up the role of the responsibilised patient who engages in self-help and the 'healing rituals' they are offered in the face of lack of effective treatments provided by scientific medicine. As Viret and Panese argue, patients must negotiate the fine line between empowerment and resignation to uncertainty and the possibility of delayed recovery: offering 'partnership' in knowledge production when it is requested of them but being careful not to take things too far by being overly demanding of their healthcare providers or challenging of their epistemic authority.

Phenomenology, Cultures and Narratives of Illness

Social inquiry has provided in-depth insights into the phenomenology of illness, exploring what it feels like to be ill and how everyday life and identity are affected (Lupton, 2012). Sociologists of health and illness often refer to the concept of 'biographical disruption' that occurs when chronic health conditions prevent people from going through the usual life stages (Bury, 1982). References to 'crip time' in the crip theory literature (Rodgers et al., 2023) acknowledge that disabled and chronically ill people often experience temporalities differently from others, including non-linear recovery. Examinations of social stigma in medicine and healthcare have pointed to the continuing practices of shaming, blaming and othering to which people with some health conditions or disabilities are subjected (Chapple et al., 2004; Crawford, 1994) and what Goldberg (2017, p. 475) refers to as the 'corrosive harm' to those who are stigmatised.

Social research has shown that Long COVID can cause serious biographical disruptions in people's life course, as they attempt to cope with the debilitating effects of Long COVID in a context in which long-term illness or disability remains misunderstood, stigmatised or ignored

(Callan et al., 2022; Ghai & Tenneti, 2024; Hunt et al., 2024; Rushforth et al., 2021; Spence et al., 2023). Many people with Long COVID have spoken of feeling 'left behind' as governments and health agencies apparently want to move on from the COVID pandemic, posing major challenges to their mental health and wellbeing, including feelings of hopelessness and isolation (Aughterson et al., 2022; Kennelly et al., 2023). People often describe the temporal dimensions of Long COVID. These include not just the extended symptoms beyond the initial acute COVID infection to which 'long' refers, but also relapses in recovery, difficulty with meeting scheduled obligations or memory lapses that mean people may not be able to remember details of past experiences (Cheston et al., 2023; Howell, 2022).

Many analyses presented in this volume identify accounts of biographical disruption, social exclusion and challenges to people's sense of temporality, belonging and identity. The research by Danielle Hitch and colleagues and that by Robin Austin and colleagues on the experiences of people with Long COVID in Australia highlight the multiple serious disruptions they have experienced to their lives. These authors also demonstrate how the sheer fatigue and other impairing symptoms experienced by people with Long COVID, as well as their desire to prevent further exposure to infections, prevent many from being able to be involved in civic and social participation, further contributing to feelings of abandonment, isolation and invisibility. They conclude that despite the two Australian government inquiries into COVID and Long COVID, which consumed so much time and effort from those who wrote submissions, there has been little evidence of improved provision of medical, financial and practical support for people living with Long COVID.

In their chapter, Matt Ventresca and Mary McDonald show how elite North American athletes' careers have been effectively ended by Long COVID. The research by Alice MacLean and colleagues demonstrates that young adults with Long COVID have found that the temporalities of the usual life course have been upended by their illness, making them feel that they have 'regressed' to the dependence of childhood. MacLean and colleagues use the term 'biographical retrogression' to describe this process: a revision of the 'biographical disruption' concept. Sam Martin and Emma Uprichard's contribution to this book draw on the temporal concept of rhythmanalysis, based on the foundational theory of Henri Lefebvre, to examine the phenomenological experiences of time and temporality that are part of the lives of people with Long COVID. This is a form of biographical disruption that focuses attention not only on events across the life course but also how everyday life is affected. Based on an analysis of posts on the X/Twitter platform, Martin and Uprichard show that the rhythms of quotidian life are profoundly disrupted by Long COVID. They propose the concept of 'complex multi-dimensional polyrhythms' to encapsulate these temporal disruptions.

Social research on Long COVID has identified aspects of the social stigma, ableism and othering to which people are subjected, and the distress this causes (Byrne, 2022; Samper-Pardo et al., 2023; Scholz et al., 2023). Despite major successes in fighting for making Long COVID visible, multiple studies have demonstrated that people with Long COVID still report discrimination, dismissal, ignorance of the science, lack of validation and stigma when they seek medical care. People with Long COVID find it difficult to obtain diagnoses and treatment (Maclean et al., 2023; Mullard et al., 2024) and may therefore experience self-doubt about the nature and severity of their illness (Clutterbuck et al., 2024). They are therefore still struggling for epistemic justice, with women, people of colour and other marginalised groups particularly affected (Aghaei et al., 2022; Au et al., 2022; Baz et al., 2023; Bergmans et al., 2024; Callan et al., 2022; Clutterbuck et al., 2024; Miller & de Klerk, 2024; Mullard et al., 2024; Samper-Pardo et al., 2023). Furthermore, people with Long COVID are dealing with this disabling condition in a fraught sociopolitical climate in which COVID risks are frequently minimised or denied by governments and public health authorities (Feldman & Bassett, 2024; Morris, 2024) and there are regular public debates over whether Long COVID is a 'real' condition (Kaplan & Mendenhall, 2024; Lokugamage et al., 2021).

In this volume, Penny Pullan's research with Church of England community members living with Long COVID and other invisible conditions surfaces the ways that people can be shut out of communities when they can no longer meet expectations and norms of membership. Even in a context in which there is an overtly expressed discourse of inclusion for all by the church, together with the longstanding Christian ideal of supporting marginalised groups and offering them succour and compassion, people with Long COVID have felt excluded and that they are not 'real' or 'dedicated' Christians. Robin Austin and colleagues' survey findings from the Australia Long COVID community, of which they are all a part, demonstrate the profound feelings of feeling invisible, shunned and silenced by mainstream society and the healthcare system. By detailing the effects of epistemic injustice in their lives, they speak out against the structural silencing to which they have been subjected. As Alice MacLean and colleagues found in their research, children and young people are 'doubly invisible' among the ranks of those living with Long COVID who are already fighting apathy and scepticism about their condition, because there had been so many statements made by medical and public health experts that children were not badly affected by COVID and were not at risk of Long COVID (see also Wild et al., 2024).

There is strong evidence of continuing medical and societal discounting of the existence and severity of Long COVID, and even a backlash against the considerable body of patient epistemic authority that has been established largely online. For example, in 2024, two clinicians, one from Norway, the other from the UK, published a commentary in the *Journal of Clinical Evaluation of Practice*. In this commentary, the clinicians claimed that members of the public were being exposed to too much information from medical practitioners and the news media about post-acute effects of COVID. According to these authors, an 'infodemic' about Long COVID is leading to more people to think that they have the condition by instigating 'fear' and 'augmenting people's stress response': in other words, they were positioning Long COVID as predominantly a psychosomatic condition. These authors therefore conclude that the general public should be protected from information about Long COVID, as such exposure is a 'public health problem in itself' (Vogt & Garner, 2024, p. 838). Another such perspective is illustrated by the opinion of three New Zealand psychiatrists, who described Long COVID as akin to 'hysteria' (Little et al., 2024). Other medical professionals and government agencies have made the decision to replace the term Long COVID with medicalised terms such as 'post-acute sequelae of COVID' (Parotto et al., 2023): thereby denying the patient-made and preferred terminology for their own condition. As Kathy Anderson (this volume) demonstrates in her interviews with clinicians, these attitudes can be traced back to the ways the medical profession has treated patients with ME/CFS for decades.

Several autoethnographic accounts of Long COVID have been published in which academic researchers have portrayed their own lived experiences and drawn on social theory to make sense of what they are going through (Ghai & Tenneti, 2024; Homewood, 2023; Yeoman, 2024). A well-known exponent of this approach is medical anthropologist Arthur Frank, who has written about cancer with a focus on the narratives of illness, healthcare and recovery that dominate his and others' experiences of this disease. In his book *The Wounded Storyteller* (2013), Frank emphasises the importance of autobiographical and other modes of storytelling to give a voice to ill people.

Three chapters in this volume are by wounded storytellers who recount their personal experiences of either living with Long COVID or caring for a loved one. The term 'gaslighting' is frequently used by patients to describe what they view as the abusive experience of having their sense of reality deliberately undermined by health professionals and others in their lives (Au et al., 2022; Karra et al., 2023; Plastina, 2025; Russell et al., 2022). Drawing on her experience of Long COVID, Mary Zournazi's chapter in this volume provides the background to the gaslighting term, bringing in theorists Rene Girard and Gregory Bateson to define what she sees as the cultural violence to which people with Long COVID are exposed when their lived reality is doubted or challenged by experts and loved ones. Zournazi notes that in the context of Long COVID, gaslighting can manifest when different forms of authority, whether medical, judicial, organisational or interpersonal, take hold of the pervading narrative of what constitutes a sick or well body, leaving the patient experience abandoned or ignored. When this happens, people may feel as they are 'going crazy', and they begin to feel unsafe about bearing witness to their own suffering.

In her autoethnography, Vivienne Matthies-Boon also references trauma and violence in relation to the betrayal and injustice experienced by people with Long COVID. For Matthies-Boon, an injustice becomes traumatic when the capacity to speak back to the inflicted injustice is destroyed. She argues that Long COVID entails a multilayered traumatic abandonment, entailing bodily incapacitation, medical neglect and psychologisation and social isolation as well as political neglect. Patients are faced with denial, indifference and even aggression that compounds the traumatic burden of their physical illness. She views such traumatisation not as a psychological disorder, but instead as traumatic status subordination, entailing a fundamental betrayal of the counterfactual presupposition of being treated as an equal human being in relation to another. Violence is also inflicted on people with Long COVID by the typical therapies offered them, such as cognitive behavioural therapy and graded exercise therapy, which cause further harm, mental distress and physical deterioration.

A short personal essay by Ben O'Mara constitutes a coda for this book. He writes about the Long COVID-related illness and death of his wife Gemma Carey, his care for her while she was ill and suffering, and how he is rebuilding his life with their young son. O'Mara adopts a literary memoir style drawing on the genre of 'weird fiction' to express the coexisting feelings of 'beauty' and 'horror' that he encountered during this time.

Conclusion: Slow Death

Throughout this book, narratives of lived experience demonstrate the sheer devastation—physical, psychological and emotional—that is integral to life with Long COVID in a society in which the condition is neglected, ignored, contested and stigmatised—not only for people who are socioeconomically disadvantaged but also those who are otherwise are from privileged backgrounds. These sociocultural and political conditions cannot be understood without a wider perspective on how the COVID pandemic has been mismanaged across the world, and the increasing tendency for governments and health agencies, both regional and global, to ignore its continuing threats. COVID has been politicised from the beginning of the pandemic, with straightforward and time-honoured strategies for containing viral spread, such as testing and tracing systems, quarantine, border closures, respirator mask wearing and lockdowns frequently met with challenges from vested interests who prioritised the economy and profit over public health (Lupton, 2022, 2023; Lupton et al., 2021). Those already living with Long COVID are the victims of widespread apathy, complacency and ignorance about the continuing risks of COVID. Meanwhile, the lack of mitigations and protections for reducing further COVID infections is leading to the ranks of people with Long COVID swelling as people become reinfected with the novel coronavirus.

Importantly, it is not only people living with Long COVID who these days are challenged about their grasp on reality. Others who continue to advocate for strong COVID mitigations and protections are also frequently labelled as having unrealistic beliefs or are simply ignored in a context in which most people want to believe that no further risks from COVID exist (Feldman & Bassett, 2024; Galvão, 2023; Gunter, 2024; Lupton, 2023; Murdoch & Caulfield, 2023). In both COVID prevention efforts and Long COVID lived experiences, gaslighting operates as a potent form of silencing, erasure and social control in response to the inconvenient truths that COVID still poses an enormous threat to people's health and quality of life. In the broader context of an apparent desire for governments and citizens across the worlds to want to 'forget' the COVID pandemic and claim that it is 'over', people with Long COVID, whether they are the earliest or the latest survivors of the novel coronavirus, are tangible reminders of the continuing suffering it causes.

Writing about the relationship of capitalism with illness well before the outbreak of COVID, Lauren Berlant (2007, p. 754) refers to 'slow death' or 'the physical wearing out of a population and the deterioration of people in that population that is very nearly a defining condition of their experience and historical existence'. The condition of slow death differs from discrete time-framed phenomena such as emergencies and health crises, as its temporality is extended into the foreseeable future. Slow death is ordinary rather than extraordinary. Using this notion of slow death, we can view both the continuing COVID pandemic and the shadow pandemic of Long COVID as examples of slow deaths. The very notion of 'living with COVID' encapsulates a desire to move on from the crisis phase of COVID, to include it as part of everyday life rather than seek to implement strong control measures to contain it, as many nations did in the first two years of the pandemic. People are still dying from COVID, even though these deaths are rarely mentioned by government and health agencies or in the news media. People are still becoming very ill, hospitalised, or left with prolonged symptoms. Their bodies are being sacrificed for the illusion of 'normality' and governments' attempts to ensure that 'the economy' is bolstered.

References

Aghaei, A., Zhang, R., Taylor, S., Tam, C.-C., Yang, C.-H., Li, X., & Qiao, S. (2022). Social life of females with persistent COVID-19 symptoms: A qualitative study. *International Journal of Environmental Research and Public Health, 19*(15). https://www.mdpi.com/1660-4601/19/15/9076

Ahmadi-Abhari, S., Bandosz, P., Shipley, M. J., Lindbohm, J. V., Dehghan, A., Elliott, P., & Kivimaki, M. (2025). Direct and indirect impacts of the COVID-19 pandemic on life expectancy and person-years of life lost with and without disability: A systematic analysis for 18 European countries, 2020–2022. *PLOS Medicine, 22*(3). https://doi.org/10.1371/journal.pmed.1004541

Al-Aly, Z., Davis, H., McCorkell, L., Soares, L., Wulf-Hanson, S., Iwasaki, A., & Topol, E. J. (2024). Long COVID science, research and policy. *Nature Medicine*. https://doi.org/10.1038/s41591-024-03173-6

Al-Aly, Z., & Topol, E. (2024). Solving the puzzle of Long COVID. *Science, 383*(6685), 830–832. https://doi.org/10.1126/science.adl0867

Au, L., Capotescu, C., Eyal, G., & Finestone, G. (2022). Long COVID and medical gaslighting: Dismissal, delayed diagnosis, and deferred treatment. *SSM - Qualitative Research in Health, 2*. https://www.sciencedirect.com/science/article/pii/S2667321522001299

Aughterson, H., Burton, A., Fancourt, D., & Philip, K. E. J. (2022). Factors shaping the mental health and well-being of people experiencing persistent COVID-19 symptoms or 'long COVID': Qualitative study. *BJPsych Open, 8*(2). https://www.cambridge.org/core/product/0D8086DFB26FFA876655B051BB75B407

Ayo, N. (2012). Understanding health promotion in a neoliberal climate and the making of health conscious citizens. *Critical Public Health, 22*(1), 99–105. https://doi.org/10.1080/09581596.2010.520692

Baz, S. A., Fang, C., Carpentieri, J., & Sheard, L. (2023). 'I don't know what to do or where to go'. Experiences of accessing healthcare support from the perspectives of people living with Long COVID and healthcare professionals: A qualitative study in Bradford, UK. *Health Expectations, 26*(1), 542–554. https://doi.org/10.1111/hex.13687

Bergmans, R. S., Chambers-Peeple, K., Yu, C., Xiao, L. Z., Wegryn-Jones, R., Martin, A., Dell'Imperio, S., Aboul-Hassan, D., Williams, D. A., Clauw, D. J., & DeJonckheere, M. (2024). 'I'm still here, I'm alive and breathing': The experience of Black Americans with long COVID. *Journal of Clinical Nursing, 33*(1), 162–177. https://doi.org/10.1111/jocn.16733

Berlant, L. (2007). Slow death (sovereignty, obesity, lateral agency). *Critical Inquiry, 33*(4), 754–780. https://doi.org/10.1086/521568

Blease, C., Carel, H., & Geraghty, K. (2017). Epistemic injustice in healthcare encounters: Evidence from chronic fatigue syndrome. *Journal of Medical Ethics, 43*(8), 549–557. https://doi.org/10.1136/medethics-2016-103691

Bury, M. (1982). Chronic illness as biographical disruption. *Sociology of Health & Illness, 4*(2), 167–182. https://doi.org/10.1111/1467-9566.ep11339939

Byrne, E. A. (2022) Understanding Long Covid: Nosology, social attitudes and stigma. *Brain, Behavior, and Immunity, 99*, 17–24. https://doi.org/10.1016/j.bbi.2021.09.012

Callan, C., Ladds, E., Husain, L., Pattinson, K., & Greenhalgh, T. (2022). 'I can't cope with multiple inputs': A qualitative study of the lived experience of 'brain fog'after COVID-19. *BMJ Open, 12*(2). https://bmjopen.bmj.com/content/12/2/e056366.abstract

Callard, F., & Perego, E. (2021). How and why patients made Long COVID. *Social Science & Medicine, 268*. https://www.sciencedirect.com/science/article/pii/S0277953620306456

Carel, H., & Kidd, I. J. (2017). Epistemic injustice in medicine and healthcare. In I.J. Kidd, J. Medina, & G. Pohlhaus (Eds.), *The Routledge handbook of epistemic injustice* (pp. 336–346). Routledge.

Chapple, A., Ziebland, S., & McPherson, A. (2004). Stigma, shame, and blame experienced by patients with lung cancer: qualitative study. *British Medical Journal, 328*(7454). https://doi.org/10.1136/bmj.38111.639734.7C

Cheston, K., Cenedese, M.-L., & Woods, A. (2023). The long or the post of it? Temporality, suffering, and uncertainty in narratives following COVID-19.

Journal of Medical Humanities, 46, 3–20. https://doi.org/10.1007/s10912-023-09824-y
Clarke, A. E., & Shim, J. (2011). Medicalization and biomedicalization revisited: Technoscience and transformations of health, illness and American medicine. In B. Pescosolido, J. Martin, J. McLeod, & A. Rogers (Eds.), *Handbook of the sociology of health, illness, and healing* (pp. 173–199). Springer.
Clutterbuck, D., Ramasawmy, M., Pantelic, M., Hayer, J., Begum, F., Faghy, M., Nasir, N., Causer, B., Heightman, M., & Allsopp, G. (2024). Barriers to healthcare access: Findings from a co-produced Long COVID case-finding study. *medRxiv*. https://www.medrxiv.org/content/,https://doi.org/10.1101/2024.01.03.24300767v1
Crawford, R. (1994). The boundaries of the self and the unhealthy other: Reflections on health, culture and AIDS. *Social Science & Medicine, 38*(10), 1347–1365. https://doi.org/10.1016/0277-9536(94)90273-9
da Silva, R., Vallinoto, A. C. R., & Dos Santos, E. J. M. (2024). The silent syndrome of Long COVID and gaps in scientific knowledge: A narrative review. *Viruses, 16*(8). https://doi.org/10.3390/v16081256
de Boer, M. L. (2021). Epistemic in/justice in patient participation. A discourse analysis of the Dutch ME/CFS Health Council advisory process. *Sociology of Health & Illness, 43*(6), 1335–1354. https://doi.org/10.1111/1467-9566.13301
Doyal, L., & Pennell, I. (1979). *The political economy of health*. Pluto Press.
Dumit, J. (2006). Illnesses you have to fight to get: Facts as forces in uncertain, emergent illnesses. *Social Science & Medicine, 62*(3), 577–590. https://doi.org/10.1016/j.socscimed.2005.06.018
Feldman, J. M., & Bassett, M. T. (2024). US public health after COVID-19: Learning from the failures of the hollow state and racial capitalism. *British Medical Journal, 384*. http://www.bmj.com/content/384/bmj-2023-076969.abstract
Foucault, M. (1988). Technologies of the self. In L. Martin, H. Gutman, & P. Hutton (Eds.), *Technologies of the self: A seminar with Michel Foucault* (pp. 16–49). Tavistock.
Foucault, M. (2008). *The birth of biopolitics: Lectures at the Collège de France, 1978–79* (G. Burchell, Trans.). Palgrave Macmillan.
Frank, A. W. (2013). *The wounded storyteller: Body, illness, and ethics* (2nd ed.). University of Chicago Press.
Freidson, E. (1970). *Professional dominance: The social structure of medical care*. Transaction Publishers.

Fricker, M. (2007). *Epistemic injustice: Power and the ethics of knowing*. Oxford University Press.

Galvão, J. (2023). COVID-19: Forgetting a pandemic that is not over. *The Lancet, 401*, 1422–1423. https://doi.org/10.1016/S0140-6736(23)00637-2

Ghai, A., & Tenneti, S. (2024). An autoethnographic reflection of COVID-19 and/as biographical disruption. *Indian Journal of Gender Studies, 31*(1), 43–60. https://doi.org/10.1177/09715215231210537

Gmanyami, J. M., Quentin, W., Lambert, O., Jarynowski, A., Belik, V., & Amuasi, J. H. (2024). Excess mortality during the COVID-19 pandemic in low-and lower-middle-income countries: a systematic review and meta-analysis. *BMC Public Health, 24*(1). https://doi.org/10.1186/s12889-024-19154-w

Goldberg, D. S. (2017). On stigma & health. *The Journal of Law, Medicine & Ethics, 45*(4), 475–483. https://doi.org/10.1177/1073110517750581

Gottlieb, M., Yu, H., Chen, J., Spatz, E. S., Gentile, N. L., Geyer, R. E., Santangelo, M., Malicki, C., Gatling, K., Saydah, S., O'Laughlin, K. N., Stephens, K. A., Elmore, J. G., Wisk, L. E., L'Hommedieu, M., Rodriguez, R. M., Montoy, J. C. C., Wang, R. C., Rising, K. L. … Weinstein, R. A. (2025). Differences in Long COVID severity by duration of illness, symptom evolution, and vaccination: A longitudinal cohort study from the INSPIRE group. *The Lancet Regional Health—Americas, 44*. https://doi.org/10.1016/j.lana.2025.101026

Greenhalgh, T., Sivan, M., Perlowski, A., & Nikolich, J. Ž. (2024). Long COVID: A clinical update. *The Lancet, 404*(10453), 707–724. https://doi.org/10.1016/S0140-6736(24)01136-X

Gunter, J. (2024). The vacuum of information about COVID's prevalence puts me at risk—Bring back better data collection. *British Medical Journal, 386*. https://doi.org/10.1136/bmj.q1905

Gutzeit, J., Weiß, M., Nürnberger, C., Lemhöfer, C., Appel, K. S., Pracht, E., Reese, J. P., Lehmann, C., Polidori, M. C., Hein, G., & Deckert, J. (2025). Definitions and symptoms of the post-COVID syndrome: An updated systematic umbrella review. *European Archives of Psychiatry and Clinical Neuroscience, 275*(1), 129–140. https://doi.org/10.1007/s00406-024-01868-y

Homewood, S. (2023). Self-tracking to do less: An autoethnography of long COVID that informs the design of pacing technologies. *Proceedings of the 2023 CHI Conference on Human Factors in Computing Systems*. https://doi.org/10.1145/3544548.3581505

Homewood, S., Just, K. O., & Johansson, O. B. (2024). The unanticipated use of fitness tracking technologies during post-COVID syndrome. *Proceedings of the Designing Interactive Systems Conference (DIS '24)*. https://doi.org/10.1145/3643834.3661617

Howell, J. (2022). COVID-19 narratives and layered temporality. *Medical Humanities, 48*(2). http://mh.bmj.com/content/48/2/211.abstract

Hsu, V. J. (2024). Dispatches from a body on fire: Slow death at the intersections of race, gender, and disability. *Quarterly Journal of Speech, 110*(3), 460–469. https://doi.org/10.1080/00335630.2024.2334389

Hunt, K., MacLean, A., Locock, L., O'Dwyer, C., Nettleton, S., Ziebland, S., & Wild, C. (2024). Young adults' experiences of biographical retrogression whilst living with long COVID. *Sociology of Health & Illness, 46*(8) 1526–1546. https://doi.org/10.1111/1467-9566.13798

Islam, N., Lacey, B., Shabnam, S., Erzurumluoglu, A. M., Dambha-Miller, H., Chowell, G., Kawachi, I., & Marmot, M. (2021). Social inequality and the syndemic of chronic disease and COVID-19: County-level analysis in the USA. *Journal of Epidemiology and Community Health, 75*(6), 496–500. https://doi.org/10.1136/jech-2020-215626

Jayadeva, S., & Lupton, D. (2025). 'A gift and a curse': The benefits and limitations of self-tracking Long COVID. *Information, Communication & Society, Online First.* https://doi.org/10.1080/1369118X.2025.2483834

Jeske, M., James, J., & Joyce, K. (2024). Diagnosis and the practices of patienthood: How diagnostic journeys shape illness experiences. *Sociology of Health & Illness, 46*(S1). https://doi.org/10.1111/1467-9566.13614

Jutel, A. (2014). *Putting a name to it: Diagnosis in contemporary society*. John Hopkins University Press.

Kaplan, K., & Mendenhall, E. (2024). Framing Long COVID through patient activism in the United States: Patient, provider, academic, and policymaker views. *Social Science & Medicine, 350.* https://www.sciencedirect.com/science/article/pii/S0277953624003459

Karra, A. R., Jaiswal, R., & Dey, S. (2023). Fishing for validation: Understanding promises and challenges of a private social media group for COVID-19 long-hauler patients. Proceedings of the ACM on Human Computer Interaction. https://doi-org.wwwproxy1.library.unsw.edu.au/, https://doi.org/10.1145/3579487

Kennelly, C. E., Nguyen, A. T., Sheikhan, N. Y., Strudwick, G., Ski, C. F., Thompson, D. R., Bartram, M., Soklaridis, S., Rossell, S. L., & Castle, D. (2023). The lived experience of Long COVID: A qualitative study of mental health, quality of life, and coping. *PLOS One, 18*(10). https://journals.plos.org/plosone/article?id=, https://doi.org/10.1371/journal.pone.0292630

Levin, A. T., Owusu-Boaitey, N., Pugh, S., Fosdick, B. K., Zwi, A. B., Malani, A., Soman, S., Besançon, L., Kashnitsky, I., & Ganesh, S. (2022). Assessing the burden of COVID-19 in developing countries: systematic review, meta-analysis and public policy implications. *BMJ Global Health, 7*(5). https://doi.org/10.1136/bmjgh-2022-008477

Little, J., Higgins, M., & Palepu, R. (2024). Long COVID—Can we deny a diagnosis without denying a person's reality? *Australasian Psychiatry, 32*(1), 44–46. https://doi.org/10.1177/10398562231222809

Lokugamage, A., Simpson, F., & Chew-Graham, C. (2021). Patient commentary: How power imbalances in the narratives, research, and publications around Long COVID can harm patients. *British Medical Journal, 373*. http://www.bmj.com/content/373/bmj.n1579.abstract

Lupton, D. (1995). *The imperative of health: Public health and the regulated body*. Sage.

Lupton, D. (2012). *Medicine as culture: Illness, disease and the body* (3rd ed.). Sage.

Lupton, D. (2016). *The quantified self: A sociology of self-tracking*. Polity Press.

Lupton, D. (2017). *Digital health: Critical and cross-disciplinary perspectives*. Routledge.

Lupton, D. (2019). *Data selves: More-than-human perspectives*. Polity Press.

Lupton, D. (2022). *COVID societies: Theorising the coronavirus crisis*. Routledge.

Lupton, D. (2023). *Risk* (3rd ed.). Routledge.

Lupton, D., Southerton, C., Clark, M., & Watson, A. (2021). *The face mask in COVID times: A sociomaterial analysis*. de Gruyter.

MacLean, A., Hunt, K., Brown, A., Evered, J. A., Dowrick, A., Fokkens, A., Grob, R., Law, S., Locock, L., Marcinow, M., Smith, L., Urbanowicz, A., Verheij, N., & Wild, C. (2023). Negotiation of collective and individual candidacy for Long COVID healthcare in the early phases of the Covid-19 pandemic: Validated, diverted and rejected candidacy. *SSM—Qualitative Research in Health, 3*. https://www.sciencedirect.com/science/article/pii/S266732152200169X

Marmot, M., & Wilkinson, R. (Eds.). (2005). *Social determinants of health* (2nd ed.). Oxford University Press.

Mbembe, A. (2021). The universal right to breathe. *Critical Inquiry, 47*(S2), S58–S62. https://doi.org/10.1086/711437

Miller, T., & de Klerk, J. (2024). An uncertain recovery: The physical toll of COVID-19 infection on liberal arts and sciences students in the Netherlands. *Global Public Health, 19*(1). https://doi.org/10.1080/17441692.2024.2372788

Mkoma, G. F., Agyemang, C., Benfield, T., Rostila, M., Cederström, A., Petersen, J. H., & Norredam, M. (2024). Risk of long COVID and associated symptoms after acute SARS-COV-2 infection in ethnic minorities: A nationwide register-linked cohort study in Denmark. *PLOS Medicine, 21*(2). https://doi.org/10.1371/journal.pmed.1004280

Morris, R. D. (2024). How denialist amplification spread COVID misinformation and undermined the credibility of public health science. *Journal of Public Health Policy, 45*(1), 114–125. https://doi.org/10.1057/s41271-023-00451-4

Moss, P., & Teghtsoonian, K. (Eds.). (2008). *Contesting illness: Process and practices.* University of Toronto Press.

Mullard, J., Kawalek, J., Parkin, A., Rayner, C., Mir, G., Sivan, M., & Greenhalgh, T. (2023). Towards evidence-based and inclusive models of peer support for long covid: A hermeneutic systematic review. *Social Science & Medicine, 320.* https://www.sciencedirect.com/science/article/pii/S0277953623000242

Mullard, J., Mir, G., Herbert, C., Evans, S., & Consortium, L. (2024). 'You're just a guinea pig': Exploring the barriers and impacts of living with Long COVID-19: A view from the undiagnosed. *Sociology of Health & Illness, 46*(8), 1602–1625. https://doi.org/10.1111/1467-9566.13795

Murdoch, B., & Caulfield, T. (2023). COVID-19 lockdown revisionism. *CMAJ, 195*(15), E552–E554. https://doi.org/10.1503/cmaj.221543

Navarro, V. (2009). What we mean by social determinants of health. *Global Health Promotion, 16*(1), 5–16. https://doi.org/10.1177/1757975908100746

Nguyen, K. H., Bao, Y., Mortazavi, J., Allen, J. D., Chocano-Bedoya, P. O., & Corlin, L. (2024). Prevalence and factors sssociated with Long COVID symptoms among U.S. Adults, 2022. *Vaccines, 12*(1). https://www.mdpi.com/2076-393X/12/1/99

Parotto, M., Gyöngyösi, M., Howe, K., Myatra, S. N., Ranzani, O., Shankar-Hari, M., & Herridge, M. S. (2023). Post-acute sequelae of COVID-19: Understanding and addressing the burden of multisystem manifestations. *The Lancet Respiratory Medicine, 11*(8), 739–754. https://doi.org/10.1016/S2213-2600(23)00239-4

Perego, E., Callard, F., Stras, L., Melville-Jóhannesson, B., Pope, R., & Alwan, N. (2020). Why we need to keep using the patient made term "Long COVID". *The BMJ Opinion.* https://blogs.bmj.com/bmj/2020/10/01/why-we-need-to-keep-using-the-patient-made-term-long-covid/

Plastina, A. F. (2025, April 1). Long COVID patients' reconstruction of medical gaslighting discourse in online epistemic communities. *Patient Education and Counseling, 134*. https://doi.org/10.1016/j.pec.2025.108665

Rodgers, J., Thorneycroft, R., Cook, P. S., Humphrys, E., Asquith, N. L., Yaghi, S. A., & Foulstone, A. (2023). Ableism in higher education: The negation of crip temporalities within the neoliberal academy. *Higher Education Research & Development, 42*(6), 1482–1495. https://doi.org/10.1080/07294360.2022.2138277

Roth, P. H., & Gadebusch-Bondio, M. (2022). The contested meaning of "Long COVID"—Patients, doctors, and the politics of subjective evidence. *Social Science & Medicine, 292*. https://www.sciencedirect.com/science/article/pii/S0277953621009515

Rushforth, A., Ladds, E., Wieringa, S., Taylor, S., Husain, L., & Greenhalgh, T. (2021). Long COVID—The illness narratives. *Social Science & Medicine, 286*. https://doi.org/10.1016/j.socscimed.2021.114326

Russell, D., Spence, N. J., Chase, J.-A. D., Schwartz, T., Tumminello, C. M., & Bouldin, E. (2022). Support amid uncertainty: Long COVID illness experiences and the role of online communities. *SSM - Qualitative Research in Health, 2*. https://www.sciencedirect.com/science/article/pii/S2667321522001391

Samper-Pardo, M., Oliván-Blázquez, B., Magallón-Botaya, R., Méndez-López, F., Bartolomé-Moreno, C., & León-Herrera, S. (2023). The emotional well-being of Long COVID patients in relation to their symptoms, social support and stigmatization in social and health services: A qualitative study. *BMC Psychiatry, 23*(1). https://doi.org/10.1186/s12888-022-04497-8

Sawano, M., Wu, Y., Shah, R. M., Zhou, T., Arun, A. S., Khosla, P., Kaleem, S., Vashist, A., Bhattacharjee, B., Ding, Q., Lu, Y., Caraballo, C., Warner, F., Huang, C., Herrin, J., Putrino, D., Michelsen, T., Fisher, L., Adinig, C., Iwasaki, A., & Krumholz, H. M. (2025). Long COVID characteristics and experience: A descriptive study from the Yale LISTEN Research Cohort. *The American Journal of Medicine, 138*(4). https://doi.org/10.1016/j.amjmed.2024.04.015

Scholz, U., Bierbauer, W., & Lüscher, J. (2023). Social stigma, mental health, stress, and health-related quality of life in people with Long COVID. *International Journal of Environmental Research and Public Health, 20*(5). https://www.mdpi.com/1660-4601/20/5/3927

Schrecker, T. (2016). Neoliberalism and health: The linkages and the dangers. *Sociology Compass, 10*(10), 952–971. https://doi.org/10.1111/soc4.12408

Sk Abd Razak, R., Ismail, A., Abdul Aziz, A. F., Suddin, L. S., Azzeri, A., & Sha'ari, N. I. (2024). Post-COVID syndrome prevalence: A systematic review and meta-analysis. *BMC Public Health, 24*(1). https://doi.org/10.1186/s12889-024-19264-5

Spence, N. J., Russell, D., Bouldin, E. D., Tumminello, C. M., & Schwartz, T. (2023). Getting back to normal? Identity and role disruptions among adults with Long COVID. *Sociology of Health & Illness, 45*(4), 914–934. https://doi.org/10.1111/1467-9566.13628

Stokoe, E., Simons, S., Drury, J., Michie, S., Parker, M., Phoenix, A., Reicher, S., Wardlaw, B., & West, R. (2022). What can we learn from the language of "living with COVID"? *British Medical Journal, 376*. http://www.bmj.com/content/376/bmj.o575.abstract

Vogt, H., & Garner, P. (2024). 'Long COVID' and how medical information is causing illness: A philosophical issue affecting public health. *Journal of Evaluation in Clinical Practice, 30*(5), 838–841. https://doi.org/10.1111/jep.13934

Wild, C., MacLean, A., Nettleton, S., Hunt, K., & Ziebland, S. (2024). The double invisibility of Long COVID in children. *Social Science & Medicine, 347*. https://www.sciencedirect.com/science/article/pii/S0277953624002144

Woodrow, M., Ziauddeen, N., Smith, D., & Alwan, N. A. (2025). Exploring long COVID prevalence and patient uncertainty by sociodemographic characteristics using GP patient survey data. *Health Expectations, 28*(2).https://doi.org/10.1111/hex.70202

World Health Organization. (2020, March 11). WHO Director-General's opening remarks at the media briefing on COVID-19. https://www.who.int/director-general/speeches/detail/who-director-general-s-opening-remarks-at-the-media-briefing-on-covid-19---11-march-2020

World Health Organization. (2023). Knocked back by COVID-19 reinfection—The experience of Abbie, a British nurse living with long COVID. https://www.who.int/europe/news-room/feature-stories/item/knocked-back-by-covid-19-reinfection---the-experience-of-abbie--a-british-nurse-living-with-long-covid

World Health Organization. (2025). *WHO Coronavirus (COVID-19) Dashboard*. https://data.who.int/dashboards/covid19/deaths?n=c

Yeoman, P. (2024). Knowledge, knowing, and the knower: A postdigital autoethnography of learning to live with Long COVID. In J. Lamb & L. Carvalho (Eds.), *Postdigital learning spaces: Towards convivial, equitable, and sustainable spaces for learning* (pp. 139–154). Springer Nature Switzerland. https://doi.org/10.1007/978-3-031-59691-9_8

Part II

Knowledge-Making

2

Long COVID: The Critical Role of Patient Advocacy-Research in Disease Recognition

Elisa Perego

Introduction

Long COVID has been called the first illness identified, named and defined by patients finding one other on social media like X/Twitter (Callard & Perego, 2021) and an advocacy-research movement that changed the arc of medical history (Al Aly, 2021). As a patient-made term and disease entity, Long COVID carries a unique potential to elevate the patient voice in biomedicine and society at large, highlighting the knowledge and power that lie within patient communities. The first research on, and accounts of, persistent COVID symptoms and sequelae, with particular regard to non-hospitalised patients, were produced and disseminated by people directly affected by SARS-CoV-2 infection (Callard & Perego, 2021). This often happened through means outside the formal channels of biomedical research, such as X/Twitter threads, polls and conversations; posts on other social media platforms;

E. Perego (✉)
Institute of Archaeology, University College London, London, UK
e-mail: elisaperego78@yahoo.it; e.perego@ucl.ac.uk

D. Lupton (ed.), *Long COVID and Society*,
https://doi.org/10.1007/978-981-96-9168-5_2

surveys developed within support groups; blogs; exchanges on WhatsApp and other messaging app groups; and interviews to the press and other outlets (Perego & Callard, 2021; Perego, 2023a; Turner et al., 2023). This dense process of collective knowledge building spanned multiple countries in just a few months and led to recognition of Long COVID by the World Health Organization (WHO) as early as 2020 (Callard & Perego, 2021; Perego, 2023a; Turner et al., 2023).

However, this aspect of the COVID pandemic's history is not sufficiently addressed in venues such as biomedical papers and the press. The consequences of this partial erasure for disability activism and patient empowerment cannot be underestimated (Perego, 2023a).

By discussing patient-driven contributions to knowledge that have never been fully addressed before, therefore, in this chapter I provide new insights into how Long COVID was defined as a multi-system disease entity by patients in the early phase of the pandemic. The research presented here builds on my own lived experience as a patient and researcher, who endured COVID in the early epicentre of Lombardy, Italy, and participated actively in the grassroots, collective, international movement that first brought Long COVID into the spotlight in 2020–2021.

This chapter complements my ongoing work on Long COVID as a disease entity and an advocacy-research patient movement. I offer snapshots into instances of patient-led knowledge building, often in the forms of interview quotes, threads and especially tweets, which have been critical for the emergence and consolidation of Long COVID (Ng et al., 2024). The very same nature and structure of X/Twitter allowed the free flow of critical information on COVID across the pandemic (Perego & Callard, 2021). This makes the platform a vital source of information on Long COVID patient-led advocacy-research: albeit one under threat in view of changes to the platform state, exodus of users and the ephemeral nature of digital data.

Long COVID and Social Media Advocacy

Long COVID is the patient-made term for the long-term symptoms, signs and sequelae of SARS-CoV-2 infection (Perego et al., 2020a). Broadly speaking, the term addresses the prolonged disease process triggered and potentially driven by SARS-CoV-2 infection. It is also used as an umbrella term for the broad range of COVID sequelae. As a term, Long COVID emerged on X/Twitter and gained consistency on social media to draw attention to the prolonged disease course that COVID survivors were experiencing in early 2020. This disease experience was longer, more torturous and often more severe than suggested by early guidelines, which posited recovery from SARS-CoV-2 infection in 2 to 6 weeks (Callard & Perego, 2021). 'Young and healthy' people were supposed to rebound from infection quickly: COVID survivors and their carers, however, found this to be already incorrect by early 2020 (Callard, 2020). Long COVID also addressed and corrected early descriptions of COVID as a self-contained respiratory illness, which was deemed especially dangerous and fatal only, or mostly, for 'the old and frail'. Rather, COVID/Long COVID was a multi-system, 'multi-phasic' disease entity with 'multiple sequelae' even in younger survivors, with 'Long' emphasising the prolonged nature of the condition (Callard & Perego, 2021; Perego, 2023a; Perego & Callard, 2021; Perego et al., 2020a).

Coined by the author of this chapter in the northern spring of 2020, Long COVID/#LongCovid was one of the patient-made terms and hashtags which COVID survivors created and used in 2020–2021 to draw attention to prolonged COVID symptoms and sequelae, while advocating for treatment and recognition. The term Long COVID, together with other patient-made terms such as Long Haul COVID, moved beyond online advocacy spaces to reach the press, conventional research and policymaking by late northern spring to autumn 2020 (Callard & Perego, 2021; Ladds et al., 2020; Perego et al., 2020a, 2020b; Turner et al., 2023). Patient-made terms and hashtags have remained prominent on social media platforms, such as X/Twitter or Reddit, at the time of writing (early 2025). Some of these terms have also been increasingly, and sometimes explosively, embedded in biomedical publications, policymaking and clinical guidelines (Greenhalgh et al., 2024; Perego, 2023a,

2023b). This novel patient-made terminology, therefore, has dictated recognition of Long COVID as a multi-system disease entity, while building community among allies and survivors.

Another early influential patient-made term which detailed a prolonged course of COVID illness was Long Haul COVID (Perego et al., 2020a). Coined by teacher Amy Watson to name the Facebook support group she created in April 2020 in the USA, it is the source of the term and hashtag long haulers/#longhaulers. 'Long haulers' has been used since the northern spring–summer 2020 to indicate those with long-term symptoms from SARS-CoV-2 infection. It has received widespread recognition on social media, in biomedical literature and in news reporting, including in the work of Pulitzer Prize awardee journalist Ed Yong. The term has also been used on X/Twitter. For example, tweet T58 in the sample by Turner et al. (2023) used long hauler as a hashtag on 25 June 2020 to firmly reassert the reality of non-recovery from COVID: 'This is definitely a thing. A very serious thing. I have friends, including relatively young, formerly quite healthy friends, in the same boat. #LongHauler #COVID19'.

The influential French hashtag #apresJ20 (meaning 'after 20 days') was first used on 12 April 2020 on X/Twitter by clinical psychologist Lapsyrévoltée to address those who were still experiencing symptoms beyond the 20th day from COVID onset.

> *Manque d'info pr les gens qui continuent à avoir des symptômes au delà de J20. Ca serait bien de mettre en commun nos ressentis pr se sentir moins seul.e alors j'ouvre ce sondage/fil pr ceux qui galèrent encore après J20. Commentaires bienvenus*
> *Le RT est doux #COVID19 #apresJ20*
> [There is a] lack of information for people who continue to have symptoms beyond D20 [day 20]. It would be good to share our feelings to feel less alone, so I'm opening this survey/thread for those who are still struggling after D20. Comments welcome. Retweeting is appreciated. [Poll follows in the tweet] (Lapsyrévoltée, 2020; translation from French by E. Perego)

With the #apresJ20 tweet, Lapsyrévoltée (X/Twitter handle @lapsyre-voltee) was piercing together data on experiences of prolonged symptoms, which were largely beyond the medical gaze in France—and elsewhere—at the time. The tweet contained a poll for the audience, with three options for describing symptom clusters: more than 1,200 respondents flagged fatigue/pain (7%) and heart palpitations (4%) among prominent persistent symptoms, with an additional 4% choosing the poll option including all such symptoms together. The tweet openly invited comments and, like many other early tweets on COVID, it was the origin of a long thread where people/Twitter accounts were sharing their experiences with the disease (other examples in Callard & Perego, 2021; Perego & Callard, 2021).

In Lapsyrévoltée's tweet, COVID is also mentioned, specifically as a hashtag, #COVID19. This use of #COVID19 in tweets on persistent symptoms and sequelae is a pattern we can notice in many tweets at the time, including T58 with #longhauler above. The hashtag #COVID19 was also in many tweets I made dating to May–August 2020, which already contained the new term #LongCovid, including the first with the new hashtag (Perego, 2020a); some of which tweets I share in this chapter. #LongCovid itself, therefore, was anchored, and linked explicitly since the beginning, to SARS-CoV-2 infection.

Hashtags such as #apresJ60 ('after 60 days') and #apresJ90 ('after 90 days') emerged weeks after #apresJ20 to draw attention to COVID symptoms and prolonged disease persisting beyond 20 days. These hashtags achieved both local and international circulation. An example is this tweet of mine dating to 13 June 2020. Posted from Italy to address novel policy information coming from Ireland, it featured the three French hashtags together with #LongCovid, and other hashtags in various languages, which were being used by locally situated patient movements in countries such as Finland, Spain, Germany, and Italy:

> Top health official in Ireland warns about long term #COVID19 👇 [pointing hand emoji]. Pattern is consistent w respiratory illness recovery, he says [meaning that other infections can have sequelae, so concern over non-recovery from COVID was justified] #LongCovid

#covid1in20 #apresJ90 #apresJ60 #apresJ20 #covidpersistente #MitCoronaLeben #covidpersistenteItalia #koronaoire [Link to newspaper article in the tweet] (Perego, 2020b)

#ApresJ20/ApresJ20 remains an important term as of 2025. A French patient collective advocating under #apresJ20 contributed to the landmark WHO meeting of 21 August 2020, which recognised the long-term health effects of COVID, including by using the term Long COVID. The association #ApresJ20 Association Covid Long France, created in October 2020 to push for recognition of Long COVID, met with policymakers and remains active at the time of writing (https://www.apresj20.fr/). In 2023, the hashtag #Apres3ans ('after three years') commemorated the creation of #apresJ20 and drew attention to the ongoing fight for Long COVID recognition three years into the pandemic (ApresJ20, 2023).

By mid-2020, patient-made terms and hashtags were also used on X/Twitter to pinpoint the urge to have patient-led knowledge recognised and integrated into pandemic policies. I share as an example a tweet of mine from 4 July 2020, where I commented on a *Nature* article (Callaway et al., 2020) addressing unresolved questions about COVID:

A note on @NatureNews piece 👇 [pointing hand emoji]
♤ A key unresolved question is long term #COVID19 illness/recovery #LongCovid
♤ Patients have hugely contributed to raise awareness of covid dangers. It's not just scholars working hard #apresj20 #covidpersistente #MitCoronaLeben #koronaoire
[Retweet of *Nature* X/Twitter account with link to article in their tweet]. (Perego, 2020c)

In this tweet, the early phrase 'long term COVID illness' (below) is embedded with COVID used as a hashtag and associated with the new term #LongCovid as well as with other hashtags created and/or widely used by the patient community. The tweet, overall, asked prominent scientific journals, such as *Nature*, to address Long COVID and recognise patient contributions to knowledge. This patient-driven work was at risk of being overlooked in favour of conventional medical research (that is, not driven by patients) on acute COVID.

The importance of recognising patient-produced knowledge was therefore strongly felt in at least part of the community already in the early pandemic. Recognition is a prominent topic in some of the earliest papers on Long COVID, all patient-led, published from September/October 2020 (for example, Callard & Perego, 2021; published online on 7 October 2020; Perego et al., 2020a, 2020b). This shows self-awareness about the importance of patient activism and documenting the history of Long COVID, which filtered down in policymaking and scientific publications in the end. On 7 October 2020, for example, *Nature* (2020) published the editorial 'Long COVID: let patients help define long-lasting COVID symptoms'. The editorial included interviews with researchers Nisreen A. Alwan (who launched the campaign #CountLongCovid on 4 September 2020 on X/Twitter) and Felicity Callard, in addition to citing an academic article co-authored by Alwan and Callard with Perego and others (Perego et al., 2020b), significantly titled 'Why we need to keep using the patient made term Long COVID'.

Acknowledgements of patient-produced knowledge has also come from health bodies. For instance, WHO Europe tweeted on 21 February 2021:

> Indeed, we owe a debt to many of these patients, who came together to raise awareness of this condition. As a consequence, we now know much more about the condition we call Long COVID, the name given by patients @martinmckee (WHO Europe, 2021)

The creation of patient-produced hashtags for online advocacy continued into 2021. James Glen, from the support group and charity Long Covid Support @Long_Covid (https://www.longcovid.org/), started #FBLC on X/Twitter on the same 21 February 2021 as a way to further connect the Long COVID community.

> Today I'm starting #FBLC: Follow Back Long Covid – creating a Twitter community to amplify our voices. Stick #FBLC in your bio, follow others who also use #FBLC and support those living with Long Covid. Together

> we can make difference. #LongCovid #CountLongCovid @Long_Covid (Glen, 2021)

In the tweet that introduced the new hashtag, Glen used FBLC together with the other patient-made hashtags #LongCovid and #CountLong-Covid, while tagging @Long_Covid. Once again, this embedded a new advocacy initiative within the collective movement, which had already reached significant milestones, such as WHO recognition, at the time. The FBLC tweet by Glen originated a long thread where patients/accounts with Long COVID shared their support for the initiative, as well as their willingness to tweet #FBLC or add it to their X/Twitter bios or both, thereby fostering community on the platform. Later in 2021, a vast patient-driven campaign spearheaded by @Kelsveil coalesced around the new hashtag #TreatLongCovid, which went viral on X/Twitter on the campaign's awareness day on 24 November 2021 (Perego, 2021a). #TreatLongCovid remains in use today and has been used by high-profile policymakers, such as US Congresswoman Ayanna Pressley for Long Covid Awareness Day on 15 March 2024:

> Long COVID is a growing crisis for our communities and we can't leave our #LongHaulers behind. On #LongCOVID Awareness Day, I'm calling on Congress to take action to #TreatLongCOVID and provide our long-haulers the support and care they deserve. (Pressley, 2024)

Overall, the repeated use of patient-made terms and hashtags in tweets from 2020 to 2021 contributed to building a rich tapestry of inter-connected storytelling, as well as a science-based commentary, which re-wrote how COVID was conceptualised and understood. Some of these terms and hashtags have also been used to push for more effective ways to tackle Long COVID and reached the highest echelons of policymaking. These are themes which I explore further in the second half of this chapter.

Long COVID as a Multi-System Disease Entity

Biomedical and clinical research has increasingly recognised Long COVID as a multi-system condition (Greenhalgh et al., 2024) and this was already evident to the patient community in 2020–2021. Long COVID as a term and a concept embodied the multi-system nature of the disease entity, which reflected growing understanding of COVID itself as not solely a respiratory disease by the northern hemisphere spring 2020 (Wadman et al., 2020).

I share as an example an excerpt, with additional comments, from my email interview with journalist Evan Blake, published in October 2022. There, I summarised aspects of my experience with COVID, which led to my own coinage of Long COVID (Blake, 2022). The multi-system, progressive and fluctuating nature of COVID/Long COVID is evident in my account:

> In early 2020, I was in Lombardy, the first COVID epicentre outside China. As a chronically ill person and a researcher, I was alarmed by the news about the emergence of the novel coronavirus. In January and February, I was following the growing scientific evidence closely.
>
> And then Lombardy was hit very hard. Initially, the situation was like, you know, sensing a storm that you quite feel is coming.
>
> Soon, it became chaotic, tragic. Our healthcare system couldn't cope with SARS-CoV-2. 'Silent' community transmission wasn't detected in time. The world saw the footage of Bergamo.
>
> I was quite ill with acute COVID, but I could not receive any meaningful medical support. I was triaged by phone, to no avail, because healthcare in my area was under duress.
>
> I survived the acute pulmonary phase, but the disease progressed over time, with new symptoms and clinical signs appearing, or returning. Symptoms are too numerous to list. My cognitive impairment was severe, but I was trying to keep up with the emerging scientific data as much as I could. I was on Twitter. I could only read or write little bits at the time.

> I was writing privately to people about this long-term COVID illness. Long Covid is a contraction of similar terms I was using to describe my experience with COVID. This was in March and April 2020. [Long-term COVID illness and similar is a phrase I could still use in tweets with #LongCovid after May 2020, as Perego, 2020b and 2020c above show].
>
> In May 2020, I suffered from a major relapse, with multi-system, cardiovascular, and cardiopulmonary symptoms. My oxygen saturation started to drop again. I was in month three. I had the opportunity to discuss with a healthcare professional the possibility of clotting in my lung, which I had been concerned about. Micro-clotting and vascular damage in the lung and other body parts were being flagged [by then] as key features of severe acute COVID. But they weren't discussed so far into the disease course.
>
> This relapse sealed for me that we were dealing with a prolonged, severe, potentially life-threatening disease, with a strong cardiovascular component.
> There was also discussion, in Italy, about COVID tests that remained positive for weeks. I highlighted this in the #LongCovid hashtag tweet on 20 May 2020[1] (Perego, 2020a) [..]
>
> I simplified the story a lot. I just want to add that I never recovered. Problems like relapsing–remitting hypoxemia, arthritis, coagulopathy, and cardiovascular disease, never left. Some actually became even more prominent, especially in late 2020 and early 2021. I suffered from a severe cardiopulmonary event in early 2021. I have been sharing these data across the networks of advocacy and beyond.
> Cognitive impairment has improved, but I am still very affected, especially with memory loss.
>
> I am too ill to have a normal job for now.

The urge to raise awareness about the multi-system nature of Long COVID, the risk of cardiovascular events, and the potential for viral persistence is already evident in many of my early tweets with #Long-Covid. Some of these tweets weaved together, under the new term Long COVID, the first information about long-term damage affecting multiple organs, which was being increasingly reported from the early epicentres, with particular regard to hospitalised patients at the time. Therefore, I also used Long COVID as a centripetal concept and hashtag to pierce together burgeoning biomedical evidence about COVID and its sequelae, which initially remained scattered across multiple sources, and was being shared anecdotally. These reports, some of which were provided on social and traditional media by healthcare professionals on the frontlines, confirmed the lived experience of survivors going back to March to May 2020, including my own. Some of my early tweets with #LongCovid also made profuse use of other hashtags adopted in the growing patient community, such as #apresJ20, #apresJ90, #covidpersistente, and #1in20. This aimed to attract the attention of other locally situated patient movements, as hashtags make tweets and social media posts easier to search and discover.

On 30 May 2020, for example, I tweeted about an interview by a healthcare provider from Italy, shared on the television channel Rete 4:

> Increasing evidence from [Italy] that #COVID19 can cause long-term, and potentially permanent damage, to the body, with respiratory, cardiac, neurological, kidney and liver problems #1in20 #LongCovid #MildCovid #apresJ90 live @rete4 👇 [pointing hand emoji] [Photo of television screen taken by E. Perego follows][2] (Perego, 2020d)

A few minutes later, still on 30 May 2020, I tweeted about a patient testimony from the same television show:

> #COVID19 G.B., 48, is an [Italian] #coronavirus survivor who has been in ICU for 10 days and covid + for two months. He still suffers chronic cardiovascular and respiratory problems, including a loss of sensation in one leg. Live @rete4 👇 [pointing hand emoji] #LongCovid #apresJ90 [Photo of television screen taken by E. Perego follows. It contains "i postumi del coronavirus" i.e. the after-effects of coronavirus, visible on the screen][3] (Perego, 2020e)

On 12 June 2020, I commented on a newspaper article about a Giulia, a young Italian nurse who suffered from deep vein thrombosis past acute COVID. This reportedly happened around ten days after she became negative to PCR: a negative PCR was, at the time, generally considered evidence of 'recovery':

> Story of Giulia O. (30 ys) a nurse from Italy [Italian flag] that developed thrombosis after #MildCovid. She has been ill for months. #LongCovid #covid1in20 #apresJ90 #apresJ60 #apresJ20 #covidpersistente #MitCoronaLeben #covidpersistenteItalia #covidlungo #koronaoire [Link to article in *Mashable*Italia, 2020] (Perego, 2020f)

Giulia had shared a Facebook post on 29 May 2020, which soon attracted thousands of views and interest from the press. She suffered a severe thrombotic event despite not being hospitalised with acute COVID, which I flagged in the tweet with the hashtag #MildCovid. Her clinical case especially resonated with me at the time, as it showed that delayed thromboembolic events, which I had likely experienced earlier than Giulia's post, could indeed take place after an initial COVID illness. This suggested that my own experience of then-suspected lung clotting in month three from symptom onset was not necessarily an outlier. It is worth mentioning that, while delayed thrombotic sequelae following SARS-CoV-2 infection are now very well-recognised in the literature, it was not so in May 2020.

On 6 July 2020, in responding to concerns about the risks of 'post-viral symptoms' being labelled as 'psychological', I built on stories such as Giulia's and my own to point to a growing understanding of the biological causes of COVID sequelae, which could include a prothrombotic state and attempts at treating it:

> People e.g. in Italy are experiencing, or are under observation/on blood thinners, because of #COVID19 coagulation issues and micro clotting [] #LongCovid #MildCovid #apresJ20 #koronaoire #covidpersistente (Perego, 2020g, with a short thread)

On 1 July 2020, I explicitly tweeted again about Long COVID as a disease entity deriving from COVID, and one in need of treatment and recognition:

> #COVID19 can result in long term illness #LongCovid. Patients need recognition and proper treatment 👇 [pointing hand emoji] #apresJ90 #apresJ60 #apresJ20 #covidpersistente #MitCoronaLeben #covidpersistenteitalia #covid1in20 #koronaoire (Perego, 2020h)

This contrasted with early media and clinical reports on COVID sequelae, which were often described as mere, albeit potentially severe, 'after-effects' of infection: for example, *postumi* (after-effects in Italian, mentioned above). Rather, the concept of Long COVID tackled pathophysiology as a prolonged, multifaceted disease process which extended in time and across the body (Perego & Callard, 2021; Perego et al., 2020a). In commenting upon a newspaper article addressing emerging evidence of sequelae from SARS-CoV-2 infection, for example, I reiterated on 25 July 2020:

> #COVID19 is more than the initial infection caused by #SARSCoV2. The range of symptoms and multi-system damage is potentially huge. The immune system damage can be vast. Lungs can develop permanent fibrosis #LongCovid #apresJ20 #covidpersistente (Perego, 2020i)

The multi-system, prolonged, potentially permanent nature of Long COVID remains a common topic in the dozen thousands of tweets/posts I have shared on X/Twitter since early 2020, in addition to being delineated in my advocacy-research outside the platform. My experience—that of one survivor—blended with the experience of the wider community, which led to the collective building of Long COVID through shared experiences of symptoms, signs, and sequelae. Another example is tweet T322 from the sample in Turner et al. (2023) on 18 July 2020:

> 5 months. I still can't breathe. My heart rate hits 145 easy when I'm laying down multiple times a day If I dare eat anything with calorie intake. I'm on two blood pressure meds and I'm 24. I'm also severely anaemic. My body feels shattered. #LongCovid [Author anonymised in Turner et al., 2023]

If we move to 2021, we can still notice this shared knowledge building embedded in X/Twitter threads. On 27 April 2021, for example, I posted about post-COVID arthritis being diagnosed in Italy, by flagging a tweet from an Italian medical professional sharing their clinical experience (Perego, 2021b). In the thread originating from my tweet, patients/ Twitter accounts from different countries came forward speaking about their own lived experiences and diagnoses of COVID-related arthritis, which, like mine, predated April 2021. In the thread, I shared about both my own experience and patient-driven research, whereby we patient-researchers had been collecting epidemiological and biomedical data on sequelae in Long COVID, often informally through contacts in the patient community: arthritis, in this case, I flagged as 'not rare'. It is worth mentioning that autoimmune and inflammatory rheumatic diseases are now well-documented sequelae of SARS-CoV-2 infection (Karkabayeva et al., 2025).

> I have developed arthritis/ arthritis like features too, with particular regard to my fingers #LongCovid Not rare in the community I am afraid (Perego, 2021c)

In answering another user in the same thread, I tweeted:

> Yes, mine is very visible in the hands, especially in the left one. Joints swallen [sic] and red. More recently arthritis like pain extended to other joints (feet, wrists etc).
>
> It started in May 2020. Medics: buffled! [sic] [referring to surprise over the clinical features of such arthritis, which apparently did not fit the presentation of rheumatoid arthritis, a diagnosis discussed for my case] (Perego, 2021d)

As the scientific (non patient) community zoomed in into specific aspects of Long COVID pathophysiology, the patient community was producing a commentary on these findings by using #LongCovid and pinpointing the multi-system nature of the disease entity. For example, in commenting upon Pérez-Gómez et al. (2021), I tweeted on 22 July 2021:

> Another paper reveals long-term abnormalities in the immune system after SARS-CoV-2 infection. Dendritic cell deficiencies may persist for at least seven months. #LongCovid is a multi-system, often severe condition, with evident biomarkers when in-depth research is carried out [link to account with URL to paper, which mentions the term Long COVID] (Perego, 2021e)

Activists and patient-researchers also advocated by putting together long X/Twitter threads with multiple scientific papers and media coverage. A prominent example is a thread already started by James Glen on 6 June 2020, which shared a link to the Facebook group that was to become Long Covid Support (Glen, 2020a). The thread tagged the group's founder, Claire Hastie, made profuse use of patient-made hashtags such as #covid1in20 and #apresJ20, and started using #LongCovid on 12 June (Glen, 2020b).

Another example is a widely shared thread on paediatric Long COVID I started on 21 September 2021 (Perego, 2021f). I began the thread, which I kept compiling into 2022, by sharing another from @apresJ20, which announced their new webpage on Long COVID in children and a call for action to address paediatric Long COVID (ApresJ20, 2021a). My thread contains hashtags like #LongCovidKids, #LongCovid, #apresJ20, and #CountLongCovid, with @apres20 using #apresJ20, and #LongCovid in turn, while tagging advocates and researchers, including myself, to draw attention to their initiative. The French group also shared a testimony (anonymised screenshot) from an advocate and collaborator whose young son/daughter had evidence of cerebral pathology on a scan 17 months into Long COVID (ApresJ20, 2021b).

In another widely shared thread I started on 12 November 2021, I compiled a list of scientific papers available on Long COVID in adults at the time, which showed damage to multiple organs as well as impacts on the coagulation cascade and the cardiovascular system (Perego, 2021g). In the thread, I used the hashtag #LongCovid even to tag studies where the patient-made term was not adopted, thereby firmly anchoring Long COVID to multi-system pathology, which, by then, was being elucidated in a growing body of peer-reviewed biomedical research on SARS-CoV-2 sequelae. In the first tweet of the thread, I tagged @apresJ20 to foster community and recognition of patient-driven advocacy across geographical borders.

In contributing to the viral #TreatLongCovid patient-driven campaign a few days later, I again underlined the multi-system nature of Long COVID on 24 November 2021:

> I contribute to today's #TreatLongCovid campaign 🔥 [fire emoji] We know SARS-CoV-2 infection can lead to vast long-term symptoms and sequelae | #LongCovid is a multi-system condition(s) that affects multiple organs and body systems. Care and treatment are urgently needed #FBLC (Perego, 2021h)

In the tweet, I used #LongCovid and #FBLC to foster community, while highlighting biomedical and clinical understanding of the disease entity's nature. The tweet comes with a thread of mine addressing both growing biomedical knowledge and the history of Long COVID activism. Tweets in the thread contains #apresJ20 to connect with the French community, as well as the hashtags #MECFS (myalgic encephalitis/chronic fatigue syndrome) and #pwME (people living with ME) to express solidarity to the ME community, which had already been affected by prolonged disease following viral and other infections before the COVID pandemic. These threads I share here are only a few examples of the huge number produced by the patient community across the pandemic, which significantly contributed to rising awareness about Long COVID. Such threads have also highlighted exponentially growing biomedical understanding of COVID: over 400,000 papers are available on the disease at the time of writing, with several thousand on Long COVID alone (LitCovid, 2024).

Discussion and Conclusion

In this chapter, I have provided a summary as well as snapshots of patient advocacy-research on Long COVID. The chapter builds on my own lived experience as patient, activist, and researcher who endured COVID in the early global epicentre of Lombardy. The tweets and quotes provided by myself and others offer direct insights into the massive, painstaking process of knowledge building by the Long COVID community in the early pandemic. Just to give an example, Turner et al. (2023) sampled around 31,000 tweets with #LongCovid and #longhaulers over the period from my first Long COVID 'hashtag tweet' on 20 May 2020 to 21 August 2020, when WHO Director General, Tedros Adhanom Ghebreyesus, publicly recognised Long COVID. This already massive sample does not include tweets on persistent symptoms/sequelae which did not use the hashtags #LongCovid #longhaulers and does not capture advocacy-research taking place in media such as Facebook, Instagram, Slack, the press and private channels, or extending beyond the Turner et al. study period of the northern spring–summer 2020. This evidence alone underscores the magnitude of advocacy-research in Long COVID, the extent of which can be also appreciated by looking at scientific evidence and storytelling produced under other patient-made hashtags and names, such as #apresJ20, #CountLongCovid, #TreatLongCovid, and #FBLC.

This advocacy can be discussed within the framework of what scholars such as Lisa Dietrich have called 'hashtag activism' (Dietrich, 2024a, 2024b). Patient-driven advocacy-research acknowledged and has pushed for the recognition of the multi-system nature of COVID/Long COVID since the dawn of the COVID-related patient movement. This is evident by looking at how advocates tagged themselves on social media, communicated in long threads, and embedded both scientific evidence and personal data within the framework of patient-produced terms and hashtags. These hashtags could be used together in the same tweet to foster solidarity, anchor Long COVID to SARS-CoV-2 infection, and facilitate communication across locally situated patient movements. My own early tweets with #LongCovid in May–July 2020 underscored the multifaceted manifestations and pathophysiology of the disease entity.

A significant portion of Long COVID advocacy-research took place on X/Twitter, while blending with several additional advocacy strategies and research activities, already reaching policymakers and health bodies such as WHO in 2020 and early 2021. In a non-inconsequential number of cases, this advocacy-research was carried out by the very same survivors who were also using X/Twitter, as it was, for example, in my case, or in the case of the French collectives organising under #apresJ20, and members of the US, UK, Finnish, Italian, Spanish, and other nations' patient communities. While this chapter focused on selected advocacy-research dating to 2020–2021, activism and patient-led research on Long COVID continue to this day and deserve further scholarly attention. Recognition of knowledge building in Long COVID is of critical importance for disability activism, I argue, as this ground-breaking patient-driven advocacy-research highlights the power and expertise that lies within patient communities.

Acknowledgements and Disclaimer I thank Deborah Lupton for the kind invitation to contribute to the volume. I thank James Glen for the kind permission to cite his tweets by name. I acknowledge the Long COVID and chronic illness community for support and thought-provoking debate especially on X/Twitter. This chapter was written when I was Long Covid Kids Champion for the Long Covid Kids charity, a volunteer, unpaid role to promote awareness of Long COVID in paediatric patients. All online sources were last accessed in December 2024.

Notes

1. Tweet text is 'The #LongCovid #COVID19 is starting to be addressed on major newspapers in Italy [Italian flag emoji] too: ~ 20% of tested patients remain covid + for at least 40 days 👉 [pointing hand emoji]. Prof from Tor Vergata University of Rome notes: there is a lot we don't know about this virus. [link to newspaper]'.
2. The tweet contains the photograph of a medical professional, presumably the interviewee, in front of a facility, which I took with my phone from television. The Italian flag emoji was used for Italy.
3. The tweet contains the photograph of a person, possibly the interviewee and survivor, which I took with my phone from television. The photo intentionally does not display the face of the person for privacy reasons. I had also decided not to share their full name in the tweet for the same reason, although the information was in the

public domain and shared voluntarily. The emoticon Italian flag is used to refer to the country from which the data came.

References

Al Aly, Z. (2021, 17 October). The WHO is letting down long Covid patients. *The Guardian*. https://www.theguardian.com/commentisfree/2021/oct/17/who-long-covid-patients

Blake, E. (2022, October 10). Long COVID advocate Dr. Elisa Perego speaks about the pandemic and the need for global elimination. *World Socialist*. https://www.wsws.org/en/articles/2022/10/10/elis-o10.html

Callard, F. (2020). Very, very mild: COVID-19 symptoms and illness classification. *Somatosphere*. https://somatosphere.com/2020/mild-covid.html/

Callard, F., & Perego, E. (2021). How and why patients made Long Covid. *Social Science & Medicine, 268*. https://doi.org/10.1016/j.socscimed.2020.113426

Callaway, E., Ledford, H., & Mallapaty, S. (2020). Six months of coronavirus: The mysteries scientists are still racing to solve. *Nature, 583*(7815), 178–179. https://doi.org/10.1038/d41586-020-01989-z

Ciceri, F., Beretta, L., Scandroglio, A. M., Colombo, S., Landoni, G., Ruggeri, A., Peccatori, J., D'Angelo, A., De Cobelli, F., Rovere-Querini, P., Tresoldi, M., Dagna, L., & Zangrillo, A. (2020). Microvascular COVID-19 lung vessels obstructive thromboinflammatory syndrome (MicroCLOTS): An atypical acute respiratory distress syndrome working hypothesis. *Critical Care and Resuscitation, 22*(2), 95–97. https://doi.org/10.51893/2020.2.pov2

Dietrich, L. (2024a). *Illness politics and hashtag activism*. University of Minnesota Press.

Dietrich, L. (2024b). Illness politics and social media mobilisation. *The Lancet, 403*(10446), 2776–2777. https://doi.org/10.1016/S0140-6736(24)01312-6

Greenhalgh, T., Sivan, M., Perlowski, A., & Nikolich, J. Ž. (2024). Long COVID: A clinical update. *The Lancet, 404*(10453), 707–724. https://doi.org/10.1016/S0140-6736(24)01136-X

Karkabayeva, A., Mirakhmedova, K., Khusinova, S., Mamasaidov, A., & Baimukhamedov, C. (2025). COVID-19 is a trigger of autoimmune rheumatic diseases: a hypothesis tested over time. *Rheumatology International 45*(1). https://doi.org/10.1007/s00296-024-05766-3

Ladds, E., Rushforth, A., Wieringa, S., Taylor, S., Rayner, C., Husain, L, & Greenhalgh, T. (2020). Persistent symptoms after COVID-19: qualitative study of 114 "long Covid" patients and draft quality principles for services. *BMC Health Services Research, 20*(1). https://doi.org/10.1186/s12913-020-06001-y

LitCovid. (2024). https://www.ncbi.nlm.nih.gov/research/coronavirus/

Mashable Italia. (2020, 4 June). Io infermiera malata di Covid per 79 giorni, chiedo ai complottisti di ascoltarmi. https://it.mashable.com/coronavirus/3446/sono-uninfermiera-malata-di-covid-ascoltatemi-complottisti?s=03

Nature. (2020). Editorial: Long COVID: Let patients help define long-lasting COVID symptoms. *Nature, 586*(7828), 170. https://doi.org/10.1038/d41586-020-02796-2

Ng, Q. X., Wee, L. E., Lim, Y. L., Ong, R. H. S., Ong, C., Venkatachalam, I., & Liew, T. M. (2024). Piecing together the narrative of #longcovid: An unsupervised deep learning of 1,354,889 X (formerly Twitter) posts from 2020 to 2023. *Frontiers Public Health, 12*,. https://doi.org/10.3389/fpubh.2024.1491087

Perego, E. (2023a). Long COVID perspectives: history, paradigm shifts, global challenges. *SocArXiv*. https://doi.org/10.31235/osf.io/u3bfy

Perego, E. (2023b). Observations on the US working definition for Long COVID as of May 2023. *SocArXiv*. https://doi.org/10.31235/osf.io/hfa8e

Perego, E., & Callard, F. (2021). Patient-made Long Covid changed COVID-19 (and the production of science, too). *SocArXiv*. https://doi.org/10.31235/osf.io/n8yp6

Perego, E., Callard, F., Stras, L., Melville-Jóhannesson, B., Pope, R., & Alwan, NA. (2020a). Why the patient made term 'long COVID' is needed. *Welcome Open Research 5*, 224. https://doi.org/10.12688/wellcomeopenres.16307.1

Perego, E., Callard, F., Stras, L., Melville-Jóhannesson, B., Pope, R., & Alwan, NA. (2020b). Why we need to keep using the patient made term "Long COVID". *British Medical Journal.* https://blogs.bmj.com/bmj/2020/10/01/why-we-need-to-keep-using-the-patient-made-term-long-covid/

Perez-Gomez, A., Vitalle, J., Gasca-Capote, M., Gutierrez-Valencia, A., Trujillo-Rodriguez, M., Serna-Gallego, A., Muñoz-Muela, E., Jimenez-Leon, M., Rafii-El-Idrissi Benhnia, M., Rivas-Jeremias, I., Sotomayor, C., Roca-Oporto, C., Espinosa, N., Infante-Dominguez, C., Crespo-Rivas, J.,

Fernández-Villar, A., Pérez-González, A., Lopez-Cortes, L., Poveda, E., & Ruiz-Mateos, E. (2021). Dendritic cell deficiencies persist seven months after SARS-Cov-2 infection. *Cellular & Molecular Immunology, 18*, 2138–2139. https://doi.org/10.1101/2021.03.18.436001

Turner, M., Beckwith, H., Spratt, T., Vallejos, E. P., & Coughlan, B. (2023). The #longcovid revolution: A reflexive thematic analysis. *Social Science & Medicine, 333*,. https://doi.org/10.1016/j.socscimed.2023.116130

Wadman, M., Couzin-Frankel, J., Kaiser, J., & Matacic, C. (2020). A rampage through the body. *Science, 368*(6489), 356–360. https://doi.org/10.1126/science.368.6489.356

Appendix: Tweets Referred to in the Chapter

ApresJ20 [@apresj20]. (2021a, September 21). *NEW Our association @apresj20 has just published a page on our website specifically dedicated to paediatric #longcovid! Why? Because there is an EMERGENCY in [France] on the Recognition & Appropriate Care Management of Paediatric #Long-Covid! 9/ [Tweet]. Twitter/X.* https://x.com/apresj20/status/1439837063197728769?t=kcMRpPKIGulILSrT92QMsg&s=19

ApresJ20 [@apresj20]. (2021b, September 21). Ns tenons tt particulièrement à remercier @lilystbarth pour son aide sur la construction de ce contenu sur notre site et pour son implication sans relâche - chaque jour - pour soutenir et aider les familles concernées par le #covidlong pédiatrique! urlr.me/37GcD 7/ [Tweet]. Twitter/X. https://x.com/apresj20/status/1439837056654524420?t=npC-SwLzG-InCIr3DLmZ9w&s=19

ApresJ20 [@apresj20]. (2023, April 12). *Nous vous invitons aujourd'hui à poster vos témoignages sous la forme: « Prénom, #CovidLong depuis X jours, vos symptômes, vos difficultés et/ou tout ce que vous souhaitez partager à ce sujet ! » accompagnés des hashtags #ApresJ20 & #Apres3ans. 10/10* [Tweet; image included]. Twitter/X. https://x.com/apresj20/status/1646095913134243840?t=8V04KGo9yhnKWi2f-79VUQ&s=19

Glen, J. [@james_glen]. (2020a, June 6). *In order to help raise awareness of the COVID long-termers - mild-to-moderate cases that have people struggling for months - this is a curated list of English-language press coverage of the #covid1in20 #covid1in10 experience. Join the Facebook group* [Tweet; facebook.com/groups/6253494…]. Twitter/X. https://x.com/james_glen/status/1269361160198983681?t=HauOmVgehYddOe3Sgoc8MQ&s=19

Glen, J. [@james__glen]. (2020b, June 12). "*These people have been sick with coronavirus for more than 60 days. Doctors aren't sure why.*" *Thank you for writing this @arianaeunjung @LennyMBernstein #covid1in10 #covid1in20 #longcovid* [Tweet; https://www.washingtonpost.com/health/2020/06/11/coronavirus-chronic/]. Twitter/X. https://x.com/james__glen/status/1271363694623182848?t=W84v8DA546JZEzXuojY9Mg&s=19

Glen, J. [@james__glen]. (2021, February 21). *Tweet in chapter* [Tweet]. Twitter/X. https://x.com/james__glen/status/1364906517158371328?t=sZYTpj3EFFmfHkvll-rO0g&s=19

Lapsyrévoltée [@lapsyrevoltee]. (2020, April 12). *Tweet in chapter* [Tweet]. Twitter/X.

https://x.com/lapsyrevoltee/status/1249339563232899073?t=nSPtoDVjmTSH5UI0oLASbQ&s=19

Perego, E. [@elisaperego78]. (2020a, May 20). *Tweet in chapter* [Tweet; https://t.co/c1cHRHi86h]. X/Twitter.

https://x.com/elisaperego78/status/1263172084055838721?t=nnvYn7SNgC25sEGM9nDm5Q&s=19

Perego, E. [@elisaperego78]. (2020b, June 13). *Tweet in chapter* [Tweet; https://t.co/TDjfALejSN]. X/Twitter. https://x.com/elisaperego78/status/1271850583360704512?t=_QhqV101NUoSotHvJQjXlw&s=19

Perego, E. [@elisaperego78]. (2020c, July 4). *Tweet in chapter* [Tweet]. X/Twitter.

https://x.com/elisaperego78/status/1279495275296456705?t=uDNL_M-sggeUjIrN0E20Sw&s=19

Perego, E. [@elisaperego78]. (2020d, May 30). *Tweet in chapter* [Tweet]. X/Twitter.

https://x.com/elisaperego78/status/1266498654355050502?t=ERdyUowC_IW6LHxUGAx8HA&s=19

Perego, E. [@elisaperego78]. (2020e, May 30). *Tweet in chapter* [Tweet]. X/Twitter. https://x.com/elisaperego78/status/1266502111556186112?t=U_-c8Qr7MmcznoraTlXezg&s=19

Perego, E. [@elisaperego78]. (2020f, June 12). *Tweet in chapter* [Tweet; https://t.co/q8GdV2BAVO]. X/Twitter.

https://x.com/elisaperego78/status/1271492731412586501?t=h40-ycUsS2rhcDRo07VTuw&s=19

Perego, E. [@elisaperego78]. (2020g, July 6). *People e.g. in Italy are experiencing, or are under observation/ on blood thinners, because of #COVID19 coagulation issues and micro clotting. Let's hope the UK is careful with the psychology stuff. It can cost lives. #LongCovid #MildCovid #apresJ20 #koronaoire #covidpersistente* [Tweet]. X/Twitter. https://x.com/elisaperego78/status/1280205299643756545?t=_H6GjRsrcBTzZEnFB4hSag&s=19

Perego, E. [@elisaperego78]. (2020h, July 1). *Tweet in chapter* [Tweet]. X/Twitter. https://x.com/elisaperego78/status/1278381312005545986?t=zrhn2xSVxqI-TYvg2oSxww&s=19

Perego, E. [@elisaperego78]. (2020i, July 25). *Tweet in chapter* [Tweet; https://t.co/qGvhN6nuns]. X/Twitter. https://x.com/elisaperego78/status/1287065933643685888?t=NWE6TC_SSRBuh-4RRx6GDA&s=19

Perego, E. [@elisaperego78]. (2021a, November 24). *#TreatLongCovid is trending in the UK Thanks so much to @Kelsveil for organising and thinking about today's campaign. Another milestone for #LongCovid advocacy and patient led community #FBLC [Tweet]. X/Twitter.* https://x.com/elisaperego78/status/1463455008498896901?t=BgKayGPA05YWio5JWR9egQ&s=1

Perego, E. [@elisaperego78]. (2021b, April 27). *Italy is reporting new cases of post covid arthritis. The long term effects of #COVID19 are numerous [] #LongCovid #LongCovidItalia #apresJ20 @apuakoronaan @LongCovidKids @longcoviditalia @MartaEsperti @apresj20 @CPersistente @longcovidsos @long_covid* [Tweet]. X/Twitter. https://x.com/elisaperego78/status/1387108977637429251?t=MAa2ZP1gLD9IGLYw-S0cEw&s=19

Perego, E. [@elisaperego78]. (2021c, April 27). *Tweet in chapter* [Tweet]. X/Twitter. https://x.com/elisaperego78/status/1387113492805832704?t=uroGVfhWu5gftIV0_-tWhg&s=19

Perego, E. [@elisaperego78]. (2021d, April 27). *Tweet in chapter* [Tweet]. X/Twitter. https://x.com/elisaperego78/status/1387115291872743428?t=HFIt_NTTeSXojUyev3t7IA&s=19

Perego, E. [@elisaperego78]. (2021e, July 22). *Tweet in chapter* [Tweet]. X/Twitter. https://x.com/elisaperego78/status/1418216108134305796?t=FvRnbG-jHdexe8k5qexRJQ&s=19

Perego, E. [@elisaperego78]. (2021f, September 21). *Information on #LongCovid in children is available on @apresj20 website. The emerging scientific evidence shows that a non insignificant percentage of children develops long-term symptoms and sequelae following SARS-CoV-2 infection #LongCovidKids*

I share some papers 🔽🧵 X/Twitter. https://x.com/elisaperego78/status/1439966792760365064?t=dQt093c8S1mu8dVJYu9XMw&s=19

Perego, E. [@elisaperego78]. (2021g, November 12). *It's now proven by a very significant number of publications: sadly, SARS-CoV-2 infection causes prolonged symptoms and damage in multiple organs and body systems [thread]. My gratitude to @apresj20 for their constant effort to promote top-notch science | advocacy on #LongCovid* [Tweet]. X/Twitter. https://x.com/elisaperego78/status/1459215406439272449?t=Agr2eMDczdioztvcYshH9w&s=19

Perego, E. [@elisaperego78]. (2021h, November 24). *Tweet in chapter* [Tweet]. X/Twitter. https://x.com/elisaperego78/status/1463436567926689795?t=C1mrrX-GY519j6kqmZQl6Q&s=19

Pressley, A. [@RepPressley]. (2024, March 15). *Tweet in chapter* [Tweet; photo in tweet]. X/Twitter. https://x.com/RepPressley/status/1768623183526039837?t=OjK4FrNpQrZBRO5BZOkTeQ&s=19

WHO Europe. [@WHO_Europe]. (2021, February 21). *Tweet in chapter* [Tweet]. X/Twitter. 2021 https://x.com/WHO_Europe/status/1364886660098510848?t=HsYaHNI-LMK9ESiRD_qfpg&s=19

3

Long COVID Times: An X/Twitter-Informed Rhythmanalysis of Pacing

Sam Martin and Emma Uprichard

Introduction

Long COVID is a growing global health crisis (Davis et al., 2021). While much research has focused on the causes, symptoms, and treatments of Long COVID, this chapter uniquely explores the phenomenological experiences of time and temporality among those living with the condition. We employ Lefebvre's (2013) rhythmanalysis as a theoretical and methodological lens to expose the complex temporal experiences of Long COVID. Rhythmanalysis posits that the multiple rhythms of everyday

S. Martin (✉)
Rapid Research Evaluation and Appraisal Lab (RREAL), Department of Targeted Intervention, University College London (UCL), London, UK
e-mail: sam.martin@paediatrics.ox.ac.uk

Oxford Vaccine Group, University of Oxford, Oxford, UK

E. Uprichard
Centre for Interdisciplinary Methodologies, University of Warwick, Coventry, UK
e-mail: E.Uprichard@warwick.ac.uk

D. Lupton (ed.), *Long COVID and Society*,
https://doi.org/10.1007/978-981-96-9168-5_3

life provide insight into society and its divisions by examining how time is spent and how it shapes experiences (Lyon, 2020). In the context of Long COVID, this approach illuminates the disruption and reshaping of daily rhythms caused by the onset and fluctuation of symptoms. Our study extends the work on chronic illness, particularly Michael Bury's (1982) concept of 'biographical disruption', by arguing that the disruption experienced by those with Long COVID is not a singular event but a complex, multi-dimensional, and ongoing process. The unpredictable and ever-changing nature of Long COVID symptoms, which can be exacerbated through multiple infections (Boufidou et al., 2023; Davis et al., 2023), creates an ongoing 'disrupting disruption' that ripples through all aspects of life, requiring continuous adaptation.

While previous research has explored the temporality of illness experiences (Hannum & Rubinstein, 2016; Jowsey, 2016; Ricoeur, 1981, 1984), we argue that the temporal disruption of Long COVID is uniquely layered and complex. This chapter analyses social media data from X (formerly Twitter) to uncover the lived experiences of those with Long COVID, focusing on the themes of biographical disruption, collective experiences, self-tracking practices, and the challenges of pacing and post-exertional malaise (PEM). By drawing on the example of living with Long COVID and incorporating insights from the self-tracking approach, we propose the term 'complex multi-dimensional polyrhythms' to synthesise and extend the understanding of the temporal experience of being chronically ill. Through this lens, we reveal the 'long' aspect of Long COVID and argue for greater attention to the politics of time in shaping social divisions for those living with chronic illnesses.

Whereas research on chronic illness has explored the temporality of being and becoming unwell over time, we argue that temporal disruption is layered, complex, and evolves dynamically. Self-tracking offers a unique lens to examine this disruption, highlighting the intricate interplay between objective data and subjective experience. Studies of self-tracking practices by people with Long COVID have found that the use of various tracking wearables to monitor symptoms has come to play a significant role in understanding the temporal disruption caused by the lived experience of Long COVID symptoms (Enichen et al., 2024). As individuals grapple with the complex and ever-changing nature of their condition, many have turned to self-tracking tools to better understand and manage their symptoms (Lewis, 2022). Because medical understanding of Long COVID is still evolving, patients have filled the gap by diligently recording their symptoms, triggers, and recovery patterns. This ranges from using wearable devices (fitness trackers, smartwatches, pulse oximeters) to manual symptom diaries and fatigue logs.

Using self-tracking technologies can sometimes exacerbate the sense of temporal disruption experienced by those with Long COVID. The constant monitoring and measuring of symptoms can heighten awareness of the body's unpredictable rhythms, leading to increased anxiety and frustration (Pietrzak-Franger, 2023). This is particularly true when the data collected do not align with the individual's subjective experience of their symptoms. Despite these limitations, the self-tracking approach can still provide a valuable tool for those living with Long COVID to communicate their experiences to healthcare providers and researchers. By tracking symptoms over time, individuals can help to identify patterns and triggers that may not be immediately apparent, contributing to a more comprehensive understanding of the condition (Tempini, 2023).

X (formerly Twitter) has been widely used by individuals with chronic illnesses to share experiences and find support (Martin et al., 2020). During the initial and latter stages of the pandemic (April 2020-December 2022), X served as a valuable resource for public health agencies, governments, healthcare workers, academics, and lay people to share information and experiences related to the pandemic (Aldosery et al., 2024; Boon-Itt & Skunkan, 2020; Rosenberg et al., 2020; Snow et al., 2024; Xue et al., 2020). X data has also been used to better understand health-related topics over time (de Carvalho et al., 2022). We employed X data to explore the phenomenological experience of the 'long' aspect of Long COVID over time. Following Lefebvre's (2013) rhythmanalysis approach, we examined concepts with an embodied temporal dimension, such as symptoms experienced and shared over days, weeks, and years. We analysed these concepts quantitatively and qualitatively using discourse analysis to understand how they are communicated and how their fluctuating temporality is integral to the experience of living with Long COVID.

We used rapid appraisal analysis (Green & Thorogood, 2018) to collect and analyse data within a limited timeframe, which was well-suited to the complexities of the COVID-19 pandemic (Vindrola-Padros & Johnson, 2020) and the emerging experiences of Long COVID. We employed an advanced Boolean search (see Appendix 1) to collect a 40% sample of tweets from UK users who identified as having Long COVID between 1 April 2020, and 1 May 2022, resulting in 43,916 posts. We then extracted tweets that specifically discussed symptoms in relation to time, using a sub-Boolean search isolating keywords related to symptoms and time (Appendix 1). This resulted in 27,786 tweets (63% of the original sample). We prioritised tweets with engagement (quoted, retweeted, liked, or part of a high-visibility X thread), reducing the final analysed sample to 2253 tweets. Formal ethical clearance was obtained from the University of Warwick. To preserve user anonymity and confidentiality, we summarise themes and paraphrase tweets instead of directly quoting them, ensuring that users remain non-identifiable in internet and social media searches in accordance with X's research regulations implemented in 2023.

Polyrhythmic Biographical Disruption

Michael Bury's (1982) theory of biographical disruption posits that chronic illness significantly disturbs one's life narrative and underlying social structures, requiring a re-evaluation of identity, daily routines, plans, and social relationships. Bury explains:

> My contention is that illness, and especially chronic illness, is precisely that kind of experience where the structures of everyday life and the forms of knowledge which underpin them are disrupted. Chronic illness involves recognition of the worlds of pain and suffering, possibly even of death, which are normally seen as distant possibilities or the plight of others […] Further, the expectations and plans that individuals hold for the future have to be re-examined. Thus, I want to maintain that the development of a chronic illness like rheumatoid arthritis is most usefully

> regarded as a 'critical situation', a form of biographical disruption. (Bury, 1982, p. 169)

While we agree with Bury's thesis, we argue that his work overlooks the temporal experience of 'becoming' chronically ill. That is to say, for those living with Long COVID, the disruption is experienced at a deep phenomenological level that is also temporal. Temporality is even inscribed in the names given to the condition—'Long COVID', 'long haulers'. Official diagnosis is set after 12-weeks of the acute phase of a COVID infection, but for many, this marker is nonsense, as symptoms can last for much longer. Furthermore, like many post-viral conditions, the biographical disruption is rarely a simple rupture marking a sudden change in direction or velocity of trajectory; instead, it is a complex, multi-dimensional disruption affecting multiple areas of life. Hence, the term 'biographical disruption-ing', used as a gerund, which is a noun functioning as a verb-like state, is perhaps more apt to emphasise the ongoing, ever-changing nature of the disruption-ing that ripples through the biography and all aspects of life, as the narratives of self are continually re-reconstructed to make sense of the new state of being thereafter.

The onset of Long COVID and its unpredictable, fluctuating and disrupting symptoms force a reshaping of everyday routines. Work, leisure, family time, and even basic tasks can be interrupted, creating a sense of disorder and unpredictability (Leggat et al., 2024). Managing symptoms often requires establishing new rhythms, such as pacing activities, incorporating rest periods, and reorganising the day (Merikanto et al., 2022). We would add that these management strategies need to be done on the day and even throughout the day, every day, to more or less extent, depending on how the trajectory of a person's Long COVID journey. These adaptive rhythms highlight the tension between the body's internal rhythms and the external social rhythms imposed by work, family commitments, and societal expectations.

In turn, the experience of Long COVID often involves a profound sense of losing one's previous sense of self, as if parts of the adult self have become fractured. This loss is not a simple, linear process but rather a complex, multi-dimensional disruption affecting multiple aspects of an individual's life. The complex multi-dimensional polyrhythms (CMDP) of Long COVID contribute to this sense of biographical disruption-ing, creating a dizzying and ever-shifting landscape that can be difficult to navigate. The loss of self-experienced by those with Long COVID is not merely a 'bump in the road', but a fundamental disruption to the very fabric of their being. It requires individuals to reconstruct their sense of self and find new ways to navigate the world in the face of constantly fluctuating symptoms and unpredictable rhythms. This process of adaptation and resilience-building may, in a way, be likened to the Japanese art of Kintsugi, which embraces the beauty of broken objects by mending them with gold. Similarly, individuals with Long COVID must learn to find new ways to thrive and create meaning in the face of adversity.

PEM: When Fatigue Goes On and On and On and On …

Post-exertional malaise (PEM) is a hallmark symptom of Long COVID, characterised by a worsening of symptoms following physical or mental exertion. PEM is more than just tiredness; it is an exhaustion that persists even after rest. As Chu et al. (2018) explain, PEM can involve a range of symptoms beyond fatigue, such as flu-like feelings, pain, cognitive problems, and decreased functional capacity. How PEM is defined varies, but as Chu et al. sum up,

> Whatever the term, each definition identifies both cognitive and physical exertion as impetuses of PEM, provides a list of specific symptoms beyond post-exertional fatigue (e.g. flu-like feelings, pain, sore throat, cognitive problems, decreased functional capacity), indicates that PEM could vary depending on the individual, and remarks on the sometimes delayed and prolonged nature of PEM. (Chu et al., 2018, p. 3)

The temporality of PEM differs from that of normal tiredness. As Morris (2019) notes, fatigue accumulates over time in a manner distinct from the usual daily buildup of tiredness, and it dissipates according to its own timeline, which varies from case to case. The exhaustion of PEM can be debilitating, often accompanied by a flare-up of old and new symptoms, exacerbating the recovery period. Managing PEM requires careful activity pacing and a keen awareness of one's energy levels. However, this is complicated by the ever-changing nature of Long COVID symptoms and the demands of daily life. Long haulers must learn to navigate this complex landscape, adapting to their new reality while still holding onto aspects of their pre-illness self. Furthermore, many people with Long COVID have been well or at least not as unwell. Therefore, most come to their new way of being from an ableist space where being as fast or slow to recover or do something with Long COVID is compared with how things used to be—who they used to be. The PEM relapse or crash is usually contrasted to some other former state of being, moving from a state of better unwellness to worse unwellness as if forcing the mind to surrender and acknowledge that, 'Oh, I'm still ill'. The unwellness is still there despite the mind suggesting otherwise. Many report that, at times, it is easy to 'forget' who you are, as the newness of self takes its own time to set in. Indeed, long haulers frequently comment on how difficult it is to know what is even possible. In moments of better well-being, it is easy to 'slip back' into trying to be the person that was once there, only to re-learn that a new space of possibilities is now in place. The body is merciless in its teachings and will say, 'This is how it is. Adapt to the present or get more unwell'.

This complex process of adaptation is further complicated by the possibility of COVID reinfection, which can create what we term 'nested disruptions' within the already disrupted biographical narrative. Our data reveals that many Long COVID sufferers experience significant setbacks following reinfection, which can either intensify existing symptoms or introduce entirely new ones. As one participant described: 'Just when I thought I was making progress with my Long COVID symptoms, I caught COVID again and it's like starting from zero, but worse. All my old symptoms are back plus new ones. It's like #LongCovid-Me 2.0.' These reinfections force individuals to repeatedly recalibrate their understanding of their condition and reset their expectations for recovery. The polyrhythmic nature of Long COVID is thus not only characterised by daily or weekly fluctuations in symptoms but also by these larger disruptions caused by subsequent infections. Each reinfection can trigger new inflammatory responses and immune dysregulation (Boufidou et al., 2023; Davis et al., 2023), creating additional layers of temporal complexity that must be incorporated into the evolving biographical narrative.

Pacing: A Delicate Balancing Act

Pacing is a crucial strategy for managing Long COVID symptoms, particularly PEM. Over time, for much of the time, to be able to cope with the experience of Long COVID, long haulers eventually learn to live with the need for constant pacing. The UK's NHS describes pacing in terms of the 3 Ps: Planning (daily, weekly, monthly, etc.); Pacing (e.g. taking your time, taking breaks, not overdoing things when feeling better); and Prioritising (e.g. deciding which tasks are most important). Pacing is part of many post-viral treatment plans and living with chronic illness in general.

Pacing sounds so simple to do. The concept of pacing is familiar, as it is part of the human experience: We all need to sleep, rest, recharge. We all get tired, have limited energy at some point, and also go in and out of periods of wellness. Energy levels fluctuate and need to be managed every day, and they vary vastly depending on all kinds of individual attributes as well as environmental ones and of course, life events too. As Kauffman puts it (2000), being alive is work, and work needs energy. But it would be a mistake to think that pacing with Long COVID is easy or straightforward to do, simply because we are familiar with the term. Indeed, this is perhaps what is difficult about it: What was thought to be known about oneself needs to be relearned, including the kinds of activities that are now im/possible to do, or how and when to do them. As Frank (1995: 1) states, 'ill people have to learn to think differently'.

> Let's talk about #pacing. When I got sick with #longCOVID, I thought pacing meant just slowing down. How wrong I was! True pacing is about breaking your day into manageable chunks and actively scheduling

rest periods. It's not just about doing things more slowly. #Long-COVIDRecovery. (Anonymised and paraphrased long hauler, X/Twitter, 2022)

Pacing in Long COVID is a complex and often messy process that takes time to learn and adapt to. It is not only about going more slowly, nor is it a simple routine or habit that can be easily repeated. Initially, it might seem like a straightforward matter of identifying triggers and figuring out one's limits, but long haulers soon discover that pacing is far more dynamic. The quality and experience of pacing can change daily, weekly, or monthly, depending on fluctuations in health. It requires a level of precision that can feel almost military-like, as the consequences of getting it wrong can be severe, such as relapsing or hindering recovery. However, achieving this precision is challenging, as planning itself is an evolving concept.

Linear-controlled and predictable planning is impossible. Planning requires micro-planning and is a balancing act. It is as if the system or algorithm required to work out what to plan and prioritise keeps needing to be updated every hour, every day, every day, every week, and reshuffling of tasks and priorities needs to happen both in real time. This is partly because symptoms are changeable over time and according to whatever is happening or has recently happened. If something happens in the moment, it is necessary to adapt and update the energy bank. An unexpected symptom, phone call, or email can mean needing to replan the whole day.

Spoonies: Measuring Energy and Time

The concept of 'spoonies' has become increasingly relevant for those living with Long COVID, as they navigate the challenges of managing limited energy reserves while simultaneously grappling with the profound biographical disruption caused by the onset of chronic illness (Bury, 1982). The spoon theory, coined by Christine Miserandino in (2003), uses spoons as a metaphor for the limited amount of physical and mental energy available for daily activities. Activities or tasks are said consume a certain number of spoons. 'Spoonies' refers to people who have adopted the spoons metaphor to describe their energy levels. This approach has been adapted by those with chronic illnesses, including Long COVID, to communicate the need for careful pacing and energy management, as well as to convey the ongoing, multi-dimensional nature of the disruption to their lives and sense of self.

Our analysis of X (formerly Twitter) data reveals the sociocultural aspects of Long COVID, including the sense of stigma, frustration, and isolation often associated with chronic illnesses. These affective components are closely tied to the temporal experience of the disease, highlighting the concept of 'emotional temporality' as a crucial aspect of the Long COVID experience. As one long hauler shared on X:

> A big thing with #LongCOVID is the frustration that comes with relapses after prolonged better health periods. Obviously it's justified as relapses tend to disrupt life in big ways, but important not to self-blame under the illusion that relapse triggers are fully controllable. (Anonymised and paraphrased long hauler, X/Twitter, 2022)

This quote illustrates how the unpredictable nature of Long COVID symptoms contributes to the ongoing biographical disruption experienced by spoonies, as relapses continually disrupt their attempts to establish a 'new normal'.

Discussions about pacing and PEM were prevalent among Long COVID spoonies. While official guidelines, such as the NHS Trust Long COVID rehabilitation booklet for patients (2024) or the WHO (2021) 'Support for rehabilitation' leaflet provide advice on managing energy exertion, many long haulers found that recovery from PEM was a complex, non-linear process that required continual learning, adaptation, and acceptance of the chronic nature of their condition. As one individual shared:

> I am doing less, and the less I do, it seems the less I am able to do. I did not think rest and pacing was supposed to work like this. I feel just as ill as when I was doing more. Make it make sense #LongCOVID #POTS #MECFS. (Anonymised and paraphrased long hauler, X/Twitter, 2022)

This quote highlights the frustration and confusion that can arise as Long COVID spoonies attempt to navigate the complex temporality of their symptoms and adapt to the limitations imposed by their condition. The intersection of biographical disruption and the spoonie identity is further evident in the co-related hashtags used by Long COVID sufferers on X. Hashtags such as #chronicillness, #mecfs, #pwme, #pots, #fibromyalgia, and #myalgicencephalomyelitis were frequently used alongside #longCOVID and #spoonie, highlighting the similarities between Long COVID and pre-existing chronic conditions. The shared language and experiences of the spoonie community provide a sense of solidarity and support as individuals adapt to the profound disruptions caused by Long COVID.

Sentiment analysis of keywords used by Long COVID spoonies revealed a mix of positive and negative experiences. Positive sentiments were associated with the sense of community and support found online, and practical advice for managing symptoms. Negative sentiments arose in discussions about the perceived lack of understanding from others regarding the fluctuating nature of Long COVID symptoms, as well as frustration with the slow pace of biomedical research and the need for formal recognition of Long COVID as a multi-system disease.

Overall, the experiences shared by Long COVID spoonies on X provide valuable insights into the complex, multifaceted nature of the condition, encompassing physical, emotional, and social challenges. The application of the spoon theory and the emphasis on pacing and fatigue management highlight the centrality of temporal disruption in the lived experience of Long COVID, as individuals navigate the ongoing impacts of the disease on their daily lives and sense of self. By adopting the spoonie identity, Long COVID sufferers are actively engaging in the process of reconstructing their biographical narratives and finding meaning in the face of profound disruption.

Self-Tracking and Long COVID

Since the pandemic, the self-tracking movement (Lupton, 2016, 2019a) has gained significant traction among individuals living with Long COVID as they seek to better understand, manage, and communicate their symptoms. Analysis of our data and the wider literature found that Long COVID sufferers have turned to self-tracking tools, such as wearable devices, smartphone apps, and symptom logs, to quantify their experiences and navigate the temporal disruptions caused by the condition (Alavi et al., 2022; Homewood, 2023; Khondakar and Kaushik, 2023; Mitratza et al., 2022).

One common metric used by Long COVID spoonies is heart rate variability (HRV), which measures the variation in time between each heartbeat. HRV has been shown to be a useful indicator of autonomic nervous system function and can help individuals track their body's response to various stressors, including physical exertion and emotional stress (Corrado et al., 2022). By monitoring their HRV, Long COVID sufferers can gain insights into their body's recovery process and make informed decisions about pacing their activities to avoid PEM. As one Long COVID spoonie shared on Twitter:

> Using my smartwatch to track HRV has been a game-changer for managing my #LongCOVID symptoms. If I do it in the morning, I can identify when I need to rest and pace myself to avoid crashes #spoonie #invisibleillness #longhauler. (Anonymised and paraphrased long hauler, X/Twitter, 2022)

Sleep tracking is another popular tool among Long COVID spoonies, as sleep disturbances are a common symptom of the condition (Khosla et al., 2023). Wearable devices, such as smartwatches and fitness trackers, can provide detailed information about an individual's sleep patterns, including the duration and quality of sleep, as well as any disruptions throughout the night. This information can help Long COVID sufferers identify patterns in their sleep and adjust their sleep hygiene to improve their overall well-being. One individual tweeted:

> My fitness tracker has been invaluable for monitoring my fully disrupted sleep patterns since getting #LongCOVID. Symptoms can = sleep quality. And if I'm lucky, making changes can help my sleep/energy the next day. #spoonie #sleeptracking. (Anonymised and paraphrased long hauler, X/Twitter, 2022)

Symptom logs, either in the form of physical journals or digital apps, are also widely used by Long COVID spoonies to track the frequency, intensity, and duration of their symptoms (Hirten et al., 2021; Radin et al., 2024). By regularly recording their symptoms, individuals can identify potential triggers and patterns in their condition, which can inform their pacing strategies and help them communicate their experiences to healthcare providers. A Long COVID spoonie shared their experience on Twitter:

> Keeping a daily symptom log has been crucial for managing my #LongCOVID. It helps me identify patterns and triggers, and valuable data to share with my doctors (well, when they listen to me...) #LongCOVID #spoonie #invisibleillness #longhauler #chronicillness. (Anonymised and paraphrased long hauler, X/Twitter, 2022)

However, while these self-tracking tools can provide valuable insights, they can also contribute to the polyrhythmic biographical disruption experienced by Long COVID spoonies. The constant monitoring and tracking of symptoms can serve as a persistent reminder of the individual's altered state of being and can exacerbate feelings of frustration and loss of control. As one individual expressed put it:

> As much as tracking my symptoms helps me manage my #LongCOVID, it can also be a constant reminder of how much my life has changed. It's a freakin' double-edged sword. #LongCOVID #spoonie #alteredlife #longhauler. (Anonymised and paraphrased long hauler, X/Twitter, 2022)

The 'double-edged sword' of tracking Long COVID symptoms digitally is one that long haulers also need to adapt to. After all, the data generated by these tools may not always align with the individual's subjective experience, leading to a sense of disconnect between the tracked self and the lived reality of Long COVID. This can further compound the biographical disruption as individuals struggle to reconcile their pre-illness identity with their current condition (Lupton, 2016, 2019b). A Long COVID spoonie shared their thoughts on this disconnect:

> Sometimes the data from my #apps doesn't match how I feel. It can be frustrating when the numbers don't reflect the reality of living with #LongCOVID #spoonie #alteredlife #longhauler. (Anonymised and paraphrased Long hauler, X/Twitter, 2022)

Despite these challenges, self-tracking practices remain an important aspect of the Long COVID experience, as they provide a means for individuals to gain a sense of agency and control over their condition. By using these tools in conjunction with other self-management strategies, such as pacing and energy conservation, Long COVID spoonies can work towards finding a new equilibrium within the complex multi-dimensional polyrhythms of their lives.

Discussion

This study has employed a rhythmanalysis approach to shed light on the complex temporal disruptions experienced by individuals with Long COVID. By analysing X/Twitter data through the lens of Lefebvre's rhythmanalysis and extending Bury's concept of biographical disruption, we have developed the concept of complex multi-dimensional polyrhythms to better understand the lived experience of Long COVID. The biographical disruption caused by Long COVID is layered, complex, and evolves dynamically. It is not a singular event, but rather an ongoing process that requires continuous adaptation and re-evaluation of a person's identity, routines, and future plans. By understanding the complex multi-dimensional polyrhythms of Long COVID, we can better appreciate the profound impact it has on individuals' lives and the challenges they face in navigating this ever-changing landscape. This understanding is crucial for developing effective support systems and interventions that acknowledge the temporal dimensions of living with Long COVID and other chronic illnesses.

Self-tracking practices and the use of social media have long been recognised as part of the self-management of chronic illness. We see that work 'come to life' here in the context of Long COVID. Digital self-tracking has emerged as a critical area of study within medical sociology, with scholars such as Lupton (2016, 2019a, 2019b) examining how the quantification of health data transforms illness experiences and embodiment. While previous research has explored how individuals with chronic conditions use digital technologies to monitor and manage their symptoms (Fotopoulou & O'Riordan, 2017; Pols, 2014), our analysis of Long COVID experiences offers new insights into the temporal dimensions of self-tracking in the context of a novel post-viral condition. The self-tracking practices described by Long COVID sufferers in our data align with what Lupton (2016) terms 'communal self-tracking', where individuals share their data and experiences within online communities to generate collective knowledge. Our findings expand on this and suggest that for Long COVID patients, self-tracking serves a unique purpose beyond symptom management: It provides evidential validation for a condition that has faced medical scepticism and institutional barriers to recognition. This extends Dumit's (2006) concept of 'illnesses you have to fight to get', where patients must produce evidence to medical practitioners to legitimise contested conditions.

Additionally, our analysis reveals an important tension in self-tracking practices for Long COVID that previous sociological work has not fully addressed. While tracking tools offer a means to quantify and communicate symptoms, they simultaneously heighten awareness of the body's unpredictable rhythms, potentially intensifying the temporal disruption that characterises the condition. This paradox challenges the often optimistic framing of self-tracking technologies in chronic illness management (Sharon, 2017) and highlights the need for a more nuanced understanding of how these practices intersect with biographical disruption.

The concept of complex multi-dimensional polyrhythms can provide a valuable framework for understanding the dynamic interplay between biological, social, and emotional rhythms in the lived experience of chronic illness. The findings have key implications for healthcare practices, public health policies, and social support systems for individuals living with Long COVID and other chronic illnesses. By employing a rhythmanalysis approach and incorporating insights from the literature on self-tracking, we have demonstrated the complex, multi-dimensional nature of the temporal disruptions experienced by Long COVID sufferers.

Healthcare professionals may benefit from understanding the concept of complex multi-dimensional polyrhythms when treating patients with Long COVID. Recognising the dynamic interplay between biological, social, emotional, and temporal rhythms can help providers develop more holistic and personalised treatment plans that account for the unique challenges faced by each individual. This may involve collaborating with patients to develop strategies for pacing, energy management, and symptom tracking, as well as providing emotional support and validation of their experiences. Public health policies would also benefit from taking into account the long-term, multifaceted impact of Long COVID on individuals and society as a whole. This may involve allocating resources for research into the underlying mechanisms of Long COVID, as well as developing targeted support programmes for those affected by the condition. Such programmes could include financial assistance, job accommodations, and access to specialised healthcare services. By universally recognising Long COVID as a chronic condition that requires ongoing support, especially as reinfection can flare up or worsen symptoms (Davis et al., 2023), policymakers can help mitigate current and future social and economic consequences of the pandemic.

The polyrhythmic nature of Long COVID is further complicated by the impacts of reinfection. Emerging research suggests that subsequent SARS-CoV-2 infections can trigger new inflammatory cascades and immune dysregulation that exacerbate existing symptoms or introduce new ones (Boufidou et al., 2023; Davis et al., 2023). This creates what might be described as 'nested disruptions'—biographical disruptions within disruptions—that force individuals to repeatedly recalibrate their understanding of their condition and its trajectory. The cumulative physiological effects of multiple infections include potential impacts on organ systems already compromised by Long COVID, creating compounding biological rhythms that further complicate recovery. These findings have significant implications for healthcare planning and policy. The recognition that Long COVID symptoms can be exacerbated by reinfection necessitates preventative strategies that go beyond acute management, including ongoing protection measures for vulnerable populations and reintegration programmes that acknowledge the non-linear recovery patterns documented in our analysis. More broadly, our concept of complex multi-dimensional polyrhythms offers a framework for understanding other post-viral conditions and chronic illnesses characterised by fluctuating symptoms and temporal unpredictability.

The importance of online communities, such as the spoonie community on X and other social media platforms (for example, Instagram, Reddit, and Facebook), highlights the need for platforms that allow individuals to connect with others who share similar experiences. These communities can provide emotional support, practical advice, and a sense of belonging for those navigating the challenges of chronic illness. Healthcare providers and policymakers should work to facilitate the growth and accessibility of such communities, as they play a crucial role in supporting the well-being of those with Long COVID. The experiences of Long COVID spoonies on X highlight the importance of community and connection in the face of chronic illness. The shared language, experiences, and support found within the spoonie community provide a sense of solidarity and validation for those navigating the challenges of Long COVID. As we move forward, it is crucial to foster and support these communities, both online and in-person, as a vital resource for those living with chronic illness.

By understanding the complex multi-dimensional polyrhythms of Long COVID and working together to support those affected, we can help ensure that individuals with this condition are able to find meaning, purpose, and joy in their lives, despite the challenges they face. The story of Long COVID is one of resilience, adaptation, and the power of the human spirit in the face of adversity, and it will require ongoing attention, research, and advocacy in the years to come. However, it is important to acknowledge the limitations of this study. The reliance on social media data from X may not capture the full range of experiences of individuals with Long COVID, particularly those who do not use the platform or engage with the specific hashtags analysed. Additionally, the study's focus on the UK context may limit the generalisability of the findings to other cultural and healthcare settings. Future research should aim to include a more diverse sample of Long COVID sufferers and explore the impact of cultural factors on the experience of living with the condition.

Another area for future research is the long-term impact of Long COVID on individuals and society. As the pandemic continues to evolve and more people experience the long-term effects of the SARS-CoV-2 virus, it will be crucial to track the trajectory of Long COVID over time and identify factors that contribute to recovery or ongoing disability. This may involve longitudinal studies that follow individuals with Long COVID over an extended period, looking at the impacts of further infections, as well as research that examines the broader social and economic implications of the condition.

Funding The authors disclose receipt of the following financial support for the research, authorship, and/or publication of this chapter: This work was supported by the Economic and Social Research Council (grant numbers ES/N012550/1 and ES/S000402/1).

Appendix 1

Boolean Search Terms

("Long COVID" OR "Post-COVID*" OR "PASC" OR "longhauler*" OR "spoonie") AND (symptom* OR "chronic* condition*" OR fatigue OR "shortness of breath" OR cough* OR "chest pain" OR "joint pain" OR palpitations OR fever OR "loss of taste" OR "loss of smell" OR anosmia OR "disrupt*" OR "brain fog" OR headache* OR dizziness OR depression OR anxiety OR insomnia* OR "tired*" OR "wiped*t" OR "worn out" OR breathless* OR "can't breathe" OR "weird taste" OR "weird smell" OR "shortness of breath" OR "#SOB" OR tingl* OR "forgetful*" OR "sleep*" OR "low mood" OR "worried all the time"

OR "worry*" OR "heart flutter*" OR "irregular heartbeat" OR "tumm*" OR "stomach ache*" OR "gastro*" OR "gut*" OR nausea* OR vomiting OR "sore*" OR "muscle*" OR "aching joints" OR "faint" OR "tingl*" OR numb* OR "hair loss" OR "alopeci*" OR "taste*" OR rash* OR "COVID toe*" OR "tachycardi*" OR "weak" OR "blurred vision" OR "hard to move" OR "brainfog" OR "cognitive*" OR "stomach cramp*" OR "gut issue*" OR "weight loss" OR "time*" OR "day*" OR "week*" OR "month*" OR "year*" OR "aniv*").

References

Alavi, A., Aditya, T., Alavi, A. A., Bogu, G. K., Brooks, A. W., Bhasin, R., Celli, A., Celis, D., Cha, K., Honkala, A., Higgs, E., Knowles, P., Metwally, A. A., Mishra, T., Panchamukhi, S., Rangan, E. S., Rolnik, B., Wang, M., Wang, Q., … & Snyder, M. P. (2022). Real-time alerting system for COVID-19 and other stress events using wearable data. *Nature Medicine, 28*(1), 175–184. https://doi.org/10.1038/s41591-021-01593-2

Aldosery, A., Carruthers, R., Kay, K., Cave, C., Reynolds, P., & Kostkova, P. (2024). Enhancing public health response: A framework for topics and sentiment analysis of COVID-19 in the UK using Twitter and the embedded topic model. *Frontiers in Public Health, 12.* https://doi.org/10.3389/fpubh.2024.1105383

Boon-Itt, S., & Skunkan, Y. (2020). Public perception of the COVID-19 pandemic on Twitter: Sentiment analysis and topic modeling study. *JMIR Public Health and Surveillance, 6*(4). https://doi.org/10.2196/21978

Boufidou, F., Medić, S., Lampropoulou, V., Siafakas, N., Tsakris, A., & Anastassopoulou, C. (2023). SARS-CoV-2 reinfections and Long COVID in the post-omicron phase of the pandemic. *International Journal of Molecular Sciences, 24*(16). https://doi.org/10.3390/ijms241612962

Bury, M. (1982). Chronic illness as biographical disruption. *Sociology of Health & Illness, 4*(2), 167–182. https://doi.org/10.1111/1467-9566.ep11339939

Bury, M. (1991). The sociology of chronic illness: A review of research and prospects. *Sociology of Health & Illness, 13*(4), 451–468. https://doi.org/10.1111/j.1467-9566.1991.tb00522.x

Chu, L., Valencia, I. J., Garvert, D. W., & Montoya, J. G. (2018). Deconstructing post-exertional malaise in myalgic encephalomyelitis/chronic fatigue syndrome: A patient-centered, cross-sectional survey. *PloS One, 13*(6). https://doi.org/10.1371/journal.pone.0197811

Corrado, J., Halpin, S., Preston, N., Whiteside, D., Tarrant, R., Davison, J., Simms, A. D., O'Connor, R. J., Casson, A., & Sivan, M. (2022). Heart rate variability biofeedback for long COVID symptoms (HEARTLOC): Protocol for a feasibility study. *BMJ Open, 12*(11). https://doi.org/10.1136/bmjopen-2022-066044

Davis, H. E., Assaf, G. S., McCorkell, L., Wei, H., & Low, R., & Re'em, Y. (2021). Characterizing long COVID in an international cohort: 7 months of symptoms and their impact. *eClinicalMedicine, 38*. https://doi.org/10.1016/j.eclinm.2021.101019

Davis, H. E., McCorkell, L., Vogel, J. M., & Topol, E. J. (2023). Long COVID: Major findings, mechanisms and recommendations. *Nature Reviews Microbiology, 21*(3), 133–146. https://doi.org/10.1038/s41579-022-00846-2

de Carvalho, V. D. H., Nepomuceno, T. C. C., Poleto, T., & Costa, A. P. C. S. (2022). The COVID-19 infodemic on "X" (formerly Twitter): A space and time topic analysis of the Brazilian immunization program and public trust. *Tropical Medicine and Infectious Disease, 7*(12), 425. https://doi.org/10.3390/tropicalmed7120425

Dumit, J. (2006). Illnesses you have to fight to get: Facts as forces in uncertain, emergent illnesses. *Social Science & Medicine, 62*(3), 577–590. https://doi.org/10.1016/j.socscimed.2005.06.018

Enichen, E. J., Heydari, K., Wang, S., Nickel, G. C., & Kvedar, J. C. (2024). The utility of personal wearable data in long COVID and personalized patient care. *NPJ Digital Medicine, 7*(1), 326. https://doi.org/10.1038/s41746-024-01341-z

Fotopoulou, A., & O'Riordan, K. (2017). Training to self-care: Fitness tracking, biopedagogy and the healthy consumer. In D. Lupton (Ed.), *Self-tracking, health and medicine* (pp. 54–68). Routledge. https://doi.org/10.4324/9781315108285

Frank, A. W. (1995). *The wounded storyteller: Body, illness & ethics*. University of Chicago Press.

Green, J., & Thorogood, N. (2018). *Qualitative methods for health research*. SAGE Publications.

Hannum, S. M., & Rubinstein, R. L. (2016). The meaningfulness of time: Narratives of cancer among chronically ill older adults. *Journal of Aging Studies, 36*, 17–25. https://doi.org/10.1016/j.jaging.2015.12.006

Hirten, R. P., Danieletto, M., Tomasev, N., Steinhubl, S. R., Wenzhe, S., Han, Y., Golden, E., Sadasivam, N., Makhnevich, A., Tinsley, A., Glicksberg, B. S., Levin, M. A., Charney, A. W., & Keefer, L. (2021). Use of physiological data from a wearable device to identify SARS-CoV-2 infection and symptoms and predict COVID-19 diagnosis: Observational study. *Journal of Medical Internet Research, 23*(2). https://doi.org/10.2196/26107

Homewood, S. (2023). Self-tracking to do less: An autoethnography of long COVID that informs the design of pacing technologies. *Proceedings of the 2023 CHI Conference on Human Factors in Computing Systems*, 1–14. https://doi.org/10.1145/3544548.3581505

Jowsey, T. (2016). Time and chronic illness: A narrative review. *Quality of Life Research, 25*(5), 1093–1102. https://doi.org/10.1007/s11136-015-1169-2

Khondakar, K. R., & Kaushik, A. (2023). Role of wearable sensing technology to manage long COVID. *Biosensors, 13*(1), Article 62. https://doi.org/10.3390/bios13010062

Khosla, S., Cheung, J., & Gurubhagavatula, I. (2023). Sleep assessment in long COVID clinics: A necessary tool for effective management. *Neurology Clinical Practice, 13*(1). https://doi.org/10.1212/cpj.0000000000200079

Leggat, F. J., Heaton-Shrestha, C., Fish, J., Siriwardena, A. N., Domeney, A., Rowe, C., Patel, I., Parsons, J., Blair, J., & Jones, J. (2024). An exploration of the experiences and self-generated strategies used when navigating everyday life with long COVID. *BMC Public Health, 24*(1), 789. https://doi.org/10.1186/s12889-024-18267-6

Lefebvre, H. (2013). *Rhythmanalysis: Space, time and everyday life*. Bloomsbury Publishing.

Lewis, D. (2022). Barriers to citizen science and dissemination of knowledge in healthcare. *Citizen Science: Theory and Practice, 7*(1), 40. https://doi.org/10.5334/cstp.511

Lupton, D. (2016). *The quantified self: A sociology of self-tracking*. Polity Press.

Lupton, D. (2019a). 'It's made me a lot more aware': A new materialist analysis of health self-tracking. *Media International Australia, 171*(1), 66–79. https://doi.org/10.1177/1329878X19844042

Lupton, D. (2019b). *Data selves: More-than-human perspectives*. Polity Press.

Lyon, D. (2020). Sensing rhythm. In H. Holmes & S. M. Hall (Eds.), *Mundane methods* (pp. 121–136). Manchester University Press.

Martin, S., Kilich, E., Dada, S., Kummervold, P. E., Denny, C., Paterson, P., & Larson, H. J. (2020). "Vaccines for pregnant women…?! Absurd": Mapping maternal vaccination discourse and stance on social media over six months. *Vaccine, 38*(42), 6627–6637. https://doi.org/10.1016/j.vaccine.2020.07.036

Merikanto, I. et al. (2023). 'Sleep symptoms are essential features of long-COVID—Comparing healthy controls with COVID-19 cases of different severity in the International COVID Sleep Study (ICOSS-II)'. *Journal of Sleep Research, 32*(1), e13754.

Miserandino, C. (2003). The spoon theory. *But You Don't Look Sick.* https://butyoudontlooksick.com/articles/written-by-christine/the-spoon-theory/

Mitratza, M., Goodale, B. M., Shagadatova, A., Kovacevic, V., van de Wijgert, J., Brakenhoff, T. B., Dobson, R., Franks, B., Veen, D., Folarin, A. A., Stolk, P., Grobbee, D. E., Cronin, M., & Downward, G. S. (2022). The performance of wearable sensors in the detection of SARS-CoV-2 infection: A systematic review. *Lancet Digital Health, 4*(5). https://doi.org/10.1016/S2589-7500(22)00019-X

Morris, K. (2019). Toward a phenomenology of fatigue. In E. Dahl, C. Falke, & T. E. Eriksen (Eds.), *Phenomenology of the broken body* (pp. 137–154). Routledge.

NHS. (2024). *Long COVID rehabilitation booklet: Information for patients.* The leeds community healthcare, NHS trust (ref: 2489). *Medical illustration services,* MID code: 2040905_014/BP. https://flipbooks.leedsth.nhs.uk/LN005039.pdf

Pietrzak-Franger, M. (2023). Postdigital health practices: New directions in medical humanities. *Medical Humanities, 49*(4), 503–510. https://doi.org/10.1136/medhum-2023-012611

Pols, J. (2014). Knowing patients: Turning patient knowledge into science. *Science, Technology, & Human Values, 39*(1), 73–97. https://doi.org/10.1177/0162243913504306

Radin, J. M., Vogel, J. M., Delgado, F., Dunn, J., & Topol, E. J. (2024). Long-term changes in wearable sensor data in people with and without Long COVID. *NPJ Digital Medicine, 7*, 246. https://doi.org/10.1038/s41746-024-01238-x

Ricoeur, P. (1981). Narrative time. In W. J. T. Mitchell (Ed.), *On narrative.* University of Chicago Press.

Ricoeur, P. (1984). *Time and narrative (Vol I).* University of Chicago Press.

Tempini, N. (2023). The ethics of data self-reporting: important issues and best practices. *F1000Research, 12*(485), 485. https://doi.org/10.12688/f1000research.128911.1

Rosenberg, H., Syed, S., & Rezaie, S. (2020). The Twitter pandemic: The critical role of Twitter in the dissemination of medical information and misinformation during the COVID-19 pandemic. *Canadian Journal of Emergency Medicine, 22*(4), 418–421. https://doi.org/10.1017/cem.2020.361

Sharon, T. (2017). Self-tracking for health and the quantified self: Re-articulating autonomy, solidarity, and authenticity in an age of personalized healthcare. *Philosophy & Technology, 30*(1), 93–121. https://doi.org/10.1007/s13347-016-0215-5

Snow, E., Weir, N., & Mueller, T. (2024). What does Twitter say about COVID-19 vaccines? *Research in Social and Administrative Pharmacy, 20*(2), 229. https://doi.org/10.1016/j.sapharm.2023.09.061

Vindrola-Padros, C. & Johnson, G. A. (2020). Rapid techniques in qualitative research: A critical review of the literature. *Qualitative Health Research, 30*(10), 1596–1604.

World Health Organization, Regional Office for Europe. (2021). *Support for rehabilitation: Self-management after COVID-19-related illness* (2nd ed.). World Health Organization, Regional Office for Europe. https://iris.who.int/handle/10665/344472

Xue, J., Chen, J., Hu, R., Chen, C., Zheng, C., Su, Y., & Zhu, T. (2020). Twitter discussions and emotions about the COVID-19 pandemic: Machine learning approach. *Journal of Medical Internet Research, 22*(11), Article e20550. https://doi.org/10.2196/20550

Part III

Medical Responses

4

'Just Because You Didn't Detect It, Doesn't Mean It's Not There': Long COVID, ME/CFS and the Social Dynamics of Biomedical Knowledge Production

Kathy S. Anderson

Introduction

Shortly after the start of the COVID-19 pandemic, accounts of a new post-viral condition began to surface. The illness, which came to be known as Long COVID, has prompted debates about the similarities between Long COVID and other post-infective illnesses, namely myalgic encephalomyelitis/chronic fatigue syndrome (ME/CFS).[1] In particular, debates about the nature, treatments and management of these conditions, as well as their biological or psychological/psychosomatic origins, have intensified in recent years. Whereas prevailing biomedical models treat both these contested chronic illnesses as originating primarily in the psychological or psychosomatic domain, this is challenged by people with lived experience, who often argue their conditions are primarily biological.

K. S. Anderson (✉)
Sydney Centre for Healthy Societies, University of Sydney, Sydney, NSW, Australia
e-mail: kfac4518@uni.sydney.edu.au

D. Lupton (ed.), *Long COVID and Society*,
https://doi.org/10.1007/978-981-96-9168-5_4

There are many documented similarities between Long COVID and ME/CFS, both in terms of symptomology and social difficulties, such as disablist attitudes towards those living with the conditions (Hunt et al., 2022; Spence et al., 2023). One notable difference is that many medical practitioners and other healthcare professionals have been diagnosed and are living with Long COVID. Some of these professionals have joined Long COVID communities and advocacy movements, complicating the 'expert/lay' person divide, and bolstering the claims made by those with lived experience. Collectively, these lay and expert advocates have challenged the prevailing biomedical view of post-infective illnesses (for example, Hunt et al., 2022).

There is a need to incorporate embodied perspectives in considerations of emerging and contested illnesses. Failing to do so has ongoing material consequences in the day-to-day lives of those with such conditions. While there have been several studies examining how knowledges around contested chronic illnesses are socially produced (for example, Aronowitz, 1998; Barker, 2005; Dumes, 2020), there has been a dearth of empirically based, comparative studies in an Australian context examining the development of biomedical knowledges for contested chronic illnesses and the connections between illness classifications and lived experiences.

The purpose of this chapter is to examine how biomedical knowledges of contested chronic illnesses have been socially produced in Australia in relation to both Long COVID and ME/CFS. I build on prior research into the knowledge production of contested chronic illnesses, in particular studies of ME/CFS and Long COVID, by using a sociology of knowledge and sociology of contested chronic illness theoretical framework. This chapter aims to extend how these biomedical knowledges are socially produced and how they become 'scientific facts': that is, embedded in institutional structures, including in the medical curricula and as applied knowledges in the clinical setting. The analysis uses the concepts of 'thought styles' and 'thought collectives', developed by the prominent scholar of the sociology of knowledge, Ludwik Fleck (1979), as an analytical tool to examine what counts as knowledge, and in particular, to identify how the development of biomedical knowledges of ME/

CFS and Long COVID are contingent upon social as well as biological factors.

In what follows, the development of clinical guidelines and biomedical classifications for ME/CFS and Long COVID is examined, providing a unique lens for discovering the various non-scientific factors influencing decisions made and actions taken with regard to the development and reproduction of biomedical knowledges. Drawing on interviews with 20 clinicians, researchers and advocates in ME/CFS and Long COVID knowledge production, the shifting influence of lived experience as a credible form of expertise in shaping biomedical knowledges is demonstrated.

Biomedical Knowledge Construction: A Neutral Endeavour?

For Fleck (1979), knowledge is never created as an individual endeavour. Rather it results from socialisation into and work in relation to a specific knowledge cohort or group and is therefore socially constructed. Further, Fleck claims there are no scientific 'facts' to be discovered 'objectively' in nature. Rather, the 'facts' are a process of socialisation into our discipline or group. Fleck used the concepts of thought style and thought collective to explain why researchers in different disciplines can have conflicting perspectives on the phenomena they are researching. A thought collective is a community of professionals/scientists who produce knowledge based on the agreed upon principles of knowledge of a particular group, known as their thought style (White, 2017).

Chronic illnesses have long been a major focus of research in the sociology of health and illness. Contested chronic illnesses have been defined in different ways, including where environmental causation is disputed as a cause of the illness and which is only partly explained in biomedical terms; in the case of those conditions currently lacking 'objective' measurements or biomarkers, with the aetiology yet to be determined and where the condition is biomedically framed as primarily psychological (see Brown et al., 2004; Spandler & Allen, 2018; Ware, 1992).

ME/CFS is widely considered a contested illness (Millen et al., 1998; Ware, 1992;). It is defined as a complex, disabling and debilitating long-term chronic illness, with a variety of bodily symptoms and its core feature known as post-exertional malaise (PEM) (Spandler & Allen, 2018). The emerging literature on Long COVID also defines it as a contested chronic illness (Spence et al., 2023; Wild et al., 2024). In both cases, those living with these conditions have challenged the medical profession's characterisation of and lack of attention to their illnesses. People living with Long COVID, similar to the experiences of those with ME/CFS, are increasingly subject to dismissiveness from medical professionals, family, friends and the broader public, where it is implied that their illness is not 'real' but rather is psychosomatic (Au et al., 2022; Wild et al., 2024).

Challenges to the biomedical framing of ME/CFS have a long history. The illness was provided with a new definition and the name 'chronic fatigue syndrome' in 1988 by the USA Centers for Disease Control (CDC) in response to the many ME/CFS cluster outbreaks around the world in the 1980s (Ankeny & Mackenzie, 2016; Carruthers et al., 2003). This new definition and name led to many contestations from those with lived experience who argued, in particular, that this case definition and the term chronic fatigue syndrome did not adequately capture the seriousness of their condition. The predominant biomedical framing of their illness was incongruous with their lived experience, which was characterised by far more than ongoing tiredness. People with ME/CFS claim that the focus on only one symptom, 'fatigue', trivialised the level of debilitation and the other severe symptomology they experienced, and essentially refuted the physical nature of their condition. This trivialising of their condition and the resultant stigma may be partially attributable to ME/CFS being labelled as 'psychosomatic' and those living with the condition as 'malingerers' (Ankeny & Mackenzie, 2016; Jason & Richman, 2007; Ware, 1992). It has led patients to mobilise collectively through self-help groups to provide support and knowledge of the condition lacking in the biomedical domain, raise awareness and reject the 'psychologising' of their condition and call for more biomedical research (Ankeny & Mackenzie, 2016; Aronowitz, 1998; Millen et al., 1998).

These historical challenges by people with ME/CFS occurred simultaneously alongside two significant cultural shifts. The first, which began in the early 1990s, was the move towards the model of evidence-based medicine (EBM). EBM in essence entails the standardisation of medical care through measures such as clinical practice guidelines, with scientific evidence underpinning decisions made by doctors on behalf of patients. The EBM approach valorises scientific or 'objective' evidence over expert opinion or subjective or embodied forms of evidence, with randomised control trials viewed as the pinnacle in the hierarchy of evidence underpinning clinical practice guidelines (Timmermans & Angell, 2012).

Social scientists have criticised the seemingly 'benign' concept of EBM and have raised questions about what counts as 'evidence' and, as such, whose ideas are included or excluded. They have asked whether standardisation is the best way to achieve best practice in medical care and if randomised control trials should be privileged in every context (Broom & Adams, 2012; Timmermans & Angell, 2012). For those living with contested chronic illnesses, the type of evidence chosen and who makes these choices are vital when creating knowledges around these conditions, as they are formal mechanisms for recognising suffering (Dumes, 2020). In addition, EBM has been portrayed as exempt from external influence or human bias, with politics eliminated from decisions that are 'scientifically' driven. In practice, however, the purported objectivity of EBM has not reflected the 'reality of knowledge work' (Broom & Adams, 2012, p. 5). Ankeny and Mackenzie (2016) concur, suggesting that subjective factors influence the development and use of clinical practice guidelines, as these are more readily accepted if they are developed by trusted peers in the medical profession.

The second shift entailed the emergence of illness-specific patient advocates and 'disease-based' patient advocacy groups which challenged the power dynamics in the patient/doctor relationship and the dominance of medicine more broadly. These groups were emboldened by the growth of the healthcare consumer movement and democratisation of knowledge since the late twentieth century, particularly through the emergence of the internet, providing enhanced opportunities for patients to readily access biomedical knowledge and mobilise collectively via websites, discussion forums, blogs and social media (Brown et al., 2004; Callard & Perego, 2021; Epstein, 2008). The challenges led to a shift in medical dominance and power, with patients highlighting their autonomy, rights and the importance of embodied knowledges in biomedical knowledge production, particularly in clinical practice guidelines (Ankeny & Mackenzie, 2016; Callard & Perego, 2021; Medina-Aedo et al., 2024).

Methods

I conducted qualitative interviews with 20 experts based in Australia (four clinicians, ten clinician/researchers, three advocates and three researchers), three of whom identified as living with Long COVID. The study was conducted as part of a broader programme of research into the knowledge politics and lived experiences of Long COVID and ME/CFS in Australia. Ethics approval was obtained from the University of Sydney Human Research Ethics Committee [HREC 2022/585]. Purposive non-probability sampling was used to recruit participants. Interviews were conducted via video call, telephone or in person between March and December 2023. To ensure anonymity, all interviewees are referred to using the pronoun 'they' and any identifying information has been omitted. The analysis was guided by the principles of reflexive thematic analysis (Braun & Clarke, 2022), beginning with familiarisation of the data during the initial transcription of the interviews, followed by systematic coding, then identifying clusters of codes with similar or inter-related meanings to produce potential themes. The development from initial to final themes was an iterative process reflecting on and analysing the potential themes and subsequent findings to further develop the overall conceptual development and rigour of the analysis.

Findings

Two themes were developed, encompassing the multifaceted factors influencing biomedical knowledge production in contested chronic illnesses and the biases within the medical profession that are legacies of 'psychological' thought styles.

Epistemic Hierarchies: Clinical Guidelines, Diagnostic Categories and the Development of 'Scientific Facts'

Many of the participants claimed that politics, and associated economic factors, play a role in decisions made about knowledge production in ME/CFS and Long COVID, including the privileging of certain illnesses over others. It was noted that the involvement of politicians influencing the direction of medical knowledge was evident in responses around the impetus for the development of the Australian ME/CFS clinical practice guidelines (Toulkidis, 2002). For example:

> [W]hilst I don't want to make too much point of it, whilst we might have, we would have got round to doing something like [developing clinical guidelines], there is no question it got a boost because of the federal Health Minister's interest in it. (clinician/researcher, participant 1)

Another clinician's response echoes the above sentiments about the impetus for developing the ME/CFS guidelines being driven partly by political concerns, stating:

> [t]he Health Insurance Commission who pays for the tests under Medicare said we will give you some money to provide guidelines on appropriate testing for chronic fatigue syndrome just like we did for HIV. (clinician/researcher, participant 2)

However, when questioned further, this interviewee suggested that the impetus for the clinician/researchers to be involved in the development of the guidelines was due to the receipt of government funding, which was viewed as necessary to find a solution to the increase in the number of ME/CFS patients attending clinics and hospitals:

> [T]hey just gave us the money to do it, and an offer of money stimulated an agreed desire to put together guidelines, which would put everything into the right kind of perspective. [We] were really keen to do this because there was so much misinformation going around and everything – and so much, you know. It is kind of hard to think back to how much drama there was. But at the hospital for example, I think I was considered to be a little bit, you know, odd, because I was seeing these patients but I didn't make any secret about it. And like rheumatology people, all of whom thought [ME/CFS] was all, you know, psychological. (clinician/researcher, participant 2)

However, in contrast to the previous responses from clinicians, an advocate claimed that the impetus for the ME/CFS guidelines was mainly due to lobbying from patient advocacy groups, stating: 'Oh absolutely, it was the patient support groups that did it' (advocate, participant 12). This response indicates the prevalence of the contestations occurring at the macro level of biomedical knowledge production.

Other indications of the way in which contested chronic illnesses are shaped by community or public support are conveyed by numerous participants. These perspectives are succinctly encapsulated by a clinician who also lives with Long COVID. In responding to a question about how Long COVID is being categorised or defined in real time, this interviewee highlighted how the broader sociopolitical landscape infiltrates the medical profession:

> [I]t's happening with a lot of political overlay and hyper-scrutiny that you don't see anywhere else in the medical field [...] with Long COVID there is all this political overlay of, 'Oh no, it's just like the flu'. There is like all of these very polarised political camps within the medical profession, that even in the science it is manifesting so that, you know, the hyper-criticism of information is becoming really counter-productive. All of these controversies are actually politically motivated, although people don't know that. Like, the clinician or the scientist think that they are not influenced, but we are human, so of course you are influenced, you are

> influenced by, saying 'Ah I'm not sure this thing is real' [emphasis added]. You know, how can you not be, it's foolish to think that you wouldn't be. (clinician/researcher, participant 8)

The responses from many of the participants demonstrate that some actors in powerful positions consider these illnesses to be 'socially unimportant disease[s]' (Fleck, 1979, p. 77), or 'low prestige' diseases (Grue, 2016). Another example can be given that illustrates this point, comparing HIV/AIDS with ME/CFS:

> So, you develop a hardness, but you also never lose that soft core, but it gets to you at times. And you see people who shouldn't be, particularly in the HIV pandemic, young men that, mostly men, and so you saw people with horrible illnesses battling on, doing everything they can to get on top of their lives. And then you see somebody who you think, ah, look, you know, just get a kick in the bum and maybe you would be up and doing it. And so, I think that it was inevitable that there would be an element of that [in relation to ME/CFS]. Not that people were even thinking that they were malingering but thinking that they could just try harder. So, I'm not trying to justify that, but I'm trying to explain it, rather than justify it. (clinician/researcher, participant 1)

The claim that ME/CFS and Long COVID may be considered as 'socially unimportant diseases' is bolstered by the many testimonies by those explicating the burdens they face not only from the debilitating symptoms, but also the lack of social recognition for their conditions (for example, Mullard et al., 2024; Spandler & Allen, 2018). The lack of interest indicates that ME/CFS and Long COVID have not reached the status of a 'social event' (Fleck, 1979, p. 76): that is, illnesses which have garnered sufficient community interest to attract funding and build the capacity for ongoing research.

One participant highlights the 'raw' politics involved in determining which illnesses become a social event. Their comment also provides a social overlap between ME/CFS and Long COVID, and is indicative of how the prevailing historical attitudes or thought style towards ME/CFS (that it is primarily psychological) may lead to a reduction in support for those living with Long COVID:

> COVID runs the risk of being a bit like the Gulf War syndrome, becoming very political. You know, if a couple of politicians get Long COVID it will be adequately funded [laughs] or if their children do, but if they don't then no-one will fund it at all. And if people [state] very loudly and publicly, 'oh it's just another name for chronic fatigue', then [...] that's likely to lead to a diminution of support for funding. (clinician/researcher, participant 3)

Similarly, another participant directly expresses the politics of knowledge production with suggestions that the low disease prestige of Long COVID as a chronic illness, as well as the amount of funds required to help those disabled by chronic illness, is a significant factor in suitable funds not being allocated for research in Australia:

> [T]hey're not interested at all. I mean, if 37 million [Australian] dollars, that's 23 million US dollars, well the Biden Administration has spent a billion [on Long COVID research]. Now we don't have anywhere near that level of interest or philanthropy. So, we have nothing. We have a growing cohort of people [with Long COVID], and with every wave, 10 percent of whatever's under that wave are going to be Long COVID. So, it just keeps mounting. And, so at some point the burden of cost of both Long COVID itself, those who cannot work plus [...] I mean, those are all chronic diseases, they are the greatest burden of health care costs that we endure. And so the lack of recognition that this is causing a profound social shift towards chronic illness that is already poorly organised and poorly funded, you know, speaks volumes about what politicians think. (clinician/researcher, participant 20)

Some of the comments participants offered around the development of the ME/CFS guidelines suggest the importance of patient inclusion in the process of knowledge production from an early stage. It also indicates the medical profession's resistance to relinquishing some epistemic ground to those for whom they care:

> I learnt this, and I think the profession learnt it from the AIDS epidemic and I applied to CFS, you don't write guidelines about people without including those people. I don't think we had a bolt of lightning that

> made us into better people. We were forced into it by a fantastically effective community organisations that formed around HIV/AIDS, because it was affecting young, often highly educated, articulate men who formed fantastic organisations. So I'd learnt the lesson well. I think by the time we got to that, the whole profession had understood that you just simply don't, you will have a poorer outcome in an educational sense if you don't include people about their disorder. (clinician/researcher, participant 1)

All the advocate participants emphasised the importance of the incorporation of meaningful patient experience in the development of biomedical knowledges. This aligns with the increasing importance placed on patient experiences in the production of clinical practice guidelines (see Medina-Aedo et al., 2024). For example, one advocate states that:

> Doctors are not the font of all knowledge. The lived experience of CFS patients and their carers is a relevant consideration in the formulation of appropriate policy responses and treatments. (advocate, participant 12)

Similarly, another advocate highlights how the patient, as the end-user of healthcare, needs to be central in the production of biomedical knowledge:

> Oh, absolutely vital [...] you are not getting consumers there to evaluate whether this was a good trial, or that was a good trial, or, whether X drug needs to have more molecule B in it. You are getting consumers there because all clinical decisions have to remember that it's bodies, that it's people's bodies at the end of the rope, it's people's kids, it's people's spouses, it's their mother, it's their father. And if you don't have a consumer involved at all then, you know, you are really just circling around your own drain, and you see this all the time. I mean, that's why a lot of our health system goes nowhere, because it's not done with the person who's going to use the service at the end of the day in the room. (advocate, participant 11)

However, in spite of the increasing rhetoric and policies championing patient inclusion in knowledge production, the following comments from a clinician/researcher discussing Long COVID vividly demonstrate the thinly veiled mistrust of the patient voice:

> [S]o, in formulation of the new case definition, we will definitely have to have consumer input, and in formulation of the clinical practice guidelines. To be honest, from my experience from the chronic fatigue syndrome world, is that it is a double-edged sword. Because quite a lot of, there's just a bunch of researchers that I know of who have said that vocal, social media, radical, anti, anti-academic, anti-evidence based, anti-psychiatry, anti-exercise, anti-CBT [cognitive behaviour therapy], that voice, that just scares credible academic researchers off. And so, this consumer voice needs to be carefully curated is what I would say – otherwise the consumers shoot themselves in the foot, which is what they have done effectively in chronic fatigue syndrome. (clinician/researcher, participant 7)

The characterisation of some patients as 'militant' or 'radical' can be used as a rhetorical tool to shut down genuine discussions between patients, researchers and clinicians, creating a form of epistemic injustice towards the already marginalised ME/CFS community (Blease & Geraghty, 2018). While it has been demonstrated in this chapter that the sociopolitical landscape is shifting towards recognising the value of lived experience knowledges, there is evidence of an ongoing mistrust of 'subjective' knowledges remaining. This is powerfully demonstrated by a clinician/researcher who lives with Long COVID, documenting a reduction in status since inhabiting the 'sick role':

> I actually made contact with one of the leads of that [Long COVID] clinic. And I said, 'Look, have you ever thought about co-designing with patients, and if you are interested, I am happy to assist.' I heard nothing – I was treated as a non-expert; I was treated as a patient or a sufferer. I actually went into the hospital, and I said, 'Look you got to be careful in how you articulate this, because some of this data is not accurate, it's not validated'. And I was met with, 'You are not the expert – back off'. So I immediately realised that my standing as a physician, my standing as a researcher, in my own right, and including in COVID, that having Long COVID demoted me immediately [laughs]. (clinician/researcher, participant 8)

The Legacy of Historical Thought Styles

The continuing ontological debates about the nature of ME/CFS and Long COVID were a prominent theme discussed, either implicitly or explicitly, by the interviewees. This includes comments from clinicians who had awareness of and/or experience with ME/CFS patients from the 1970s onwards. Their comments provide evidence for the origins of the 'psychological' thought style via the historical views held within the medical profession. One clinician/researcher made direct reference to the controversial research by British psychiatrists Colin P. McEvedy and his colleague, A. W. Beard, who published a study in 1970 that claimed ME/CFS was a form of 'mass hysteria' (McEvedy & Beard, 1970a, 1970b):

> [ME/CFS] was a very contentious condition, because it had this kind of, most people had read the McEvedy reports and thought it was sort of a psychological thing. (clinician/researcher, participant 2)

Another clinician/researcher maintained the view that ME/CFS 'is probably a psychological illness', going on to say that: 'Now the problem, one of the difficulties is that of course the vast majority of the people who have it don't like that' (clinician/researcher, participant 3). However, clinicians who had completed their medical education more recently suggested a slow shift away from the legacy of historical ME/CFS thought styles due to the advent of Long COVID:

> I think it relates to that historical attitude towards ME/CFS which has been, this doesn't make sense – the tests are normal, this is all in your head, which a lot of professionals carry with them. And the fact that it's quite clearly happening to a large number of people after COVID is really challenging that belief that a lot of people still hold. And it's becoming clearer that this is a real illness, it's not a manifestation of a psychological issue, which is a valid thing in itself. (clinician, participant 17)

Another clinician suggests that the medical profession's 'psychological' thought style is changing over time due to the introduction of the ME/CFS clinical guidelines (Toulkidis, 2002). However, this interviewee claims that some psychiatrists, as a specific thought collective, retain the legacy thought style:

> [I]t's likely that people still harboured views to themselves that, you know, these people [with ME/CFS] are all a bit, you know, sort of 'psychiatric'. They wouldn't say that in public anymore, and their written communication with other doctors was a lot more circumspect and respectful and the patients didn't come back with the horror stories that they used to come with pre-guidelines. My colleagues, the younger graduates who are in the next generation since then, they seem quite happy to just incorporate chronic fatigue syndrome as yet another diagnosis that you make. (clinician/researcher, participant 2)

This same clinician/researcher further stated, 'I know that there are still people who don't have that view, you know, because the whole thing about medically unexplained symptoms and somatoform illness, it's still out there'. After further questioning about who still holds such views, they responded, 'psychiatrists'.

The above excerpts are illustrative of the medical profession's acculturation or informally learnt knowledges and behaviours of how to practise medicine. One clinician, who lives with Long COVID, highlights this when having informal discussions about Long COVID with their colleagues: 'we have got a chat group we still keep on, highlighting instances of medical professionals saying is [Long COVID] even a real thing?' (clinician, participant 18). Fox et al. (2003) provide an example of how negative perceptions of patients can be transmitted informally among medical professionals through the use of medical slang. Medical slang is a secret short-hand language between medical professionals learnt informally via peers and seniors. Examples relevant to those with ME/CFS and Long COVID include: 'TATT' (tired all the time), 'OAP' (overanxious patient or parent) and 'heart sink' (frequently attending patients for whom the physician has little to offer).

The idea of the heart sink patient is frequently used by the clinicians, either explicitly or implicitly, as illustrated in the following comment:

> There's definitely a lot of scepticism about ME/CFS among the medical community, and I don't think I ever really bought into that. And so my

> perception was, it's definitely real, just don't understand, and probably felt quite helpless about what to do. And I guess the same with Long COVID, it kind of had that heart sink feel to it. (clinician, participant 17)

Other clinicians mention heart sink patients in the context of the continuing scepticism about ME/CFS as 'real' among the medical profession, and how these historical thought styles are now influencing medical perspectives about those with Long COVID. Such sentiments have been foreseen in the social science literature, highlighting the dismissive and stigmatising attitudes of professionals towards those with ME/CFS and similar contested illnesses. The literature also demonstrates how these thought styles can become institutionalised and internalised, in part, through lack of formal training and the acquisition of informal knowledges (for example, Stenhoff et al., 2015), or culturally transmitted thought styles. These perpetuate negative and biased attitudes that are reified as 'fact' both within the medical profession and the wider public: due, in part at least, to the prestigious and authoritative status that medical practitioners still hold within society.

The scepticism shown towards those with contested chronic illnesses is illustrated by a clinician/researcher's response to a question about what it means when people characterise Long COVID as real. This participant's comment illuminates the difficulties medical professionals face working within an EBM philosophy, and how striving towards standardisation and certainty can lead to lack of support for those suffering from symptoms that are not currently captured in the EBM framework. It also highlights the significance of knowledge acquired through lived experience:

> So, before I had Long COVID, real is something you can demonstrate by, you know, objectively, something you can tangibly show exists. Post COVID, I am more likely now to utilise the scientific philosophy of 'just because you didn't detect it, doesn't mean it's not there'. So, and I'm more likely to believe a patient experience than I did before [...] so the shift in my mindset is more around critiquing the evidence than critiquing the patient, if you know what I mean? So, what is reality is now something that I understand a lot of moral judgement comes

> into it. Because it implies a lot of bias within how I think and how clinicians and doctors and patients and that whole interaction is full of power dynamics and shifts. Particularly with the sort of the concept of we have power of knowledge, the knowledge is biased, it's faulty, it's not designed to generate that information. Anyway, so I'm beginning to be a bit more analytical and critical of research output. But what is real to me is what is real to the patient now, that's how I see it. (clinician/researcher, participant 8)

Conclusion

People living with ME/CFS and Long COVID, as contested chronic illnesses, continue to face dismissal, prejudice and denial of their lived realities (Spandler & Allen, 2018; Wild et al., 2024;). The research presented in this chapter has demonstrated that it is vitally important for those living with contested chronic illnesses to know how biomedical knowledges are created: particularly who is involved and what counts as evidence. The impacts of the continuing uncertainties and biases they encounter include difficulties receiving a diagnosis, lack of funding for research into pathophysiology, lack of suitable treatments, lack of financial support, and prejudice towards invisible illnesses whose causation is yet to be explained biomedically (Au et al., 2022; Spandler & Allen, 2018).

The participants' comments around the development of biomedical knowledges for ME/CFS and Long COVID in Australia succinctly demonstrate the varied influences on the development of knowledges for illnesses that are contested. These include political influences, both at a government level and within the medical profession, and the biases that are legacies of 'psychological' ways of thinking which are reproduced primarily through culturally transmitted thought styles. The multifaceted factors overlaying how contested illnesses are framed and created further highlights the need for the lived experience to be incorporated as credible evidence in biomedical knowledge production. Finally, it is hoped that this research raises awareness for both politicians and the medical profession to understand some of the barriers to support and treatments for those with contested chronic illnesses. It is crucial that these powerful contributors to thought styles and thought collectives acknowledge the need for reflexivity and new ways of conceptualising Long COVID and ME/CFS to assist in moving beyond the biological/psychological binary with the aim of providing much needed support for those living with these debilitating long-term illnesses.

Acknowledgements Kathy Anderson is supported by an Australian Government Research Training Programme (RTP) Scholarship. The author would like to thank all the research participants who took the time to participate in this study.

Note

1. The terminology of ME/CFS is used in this chapter, as this is the term often favoured by those living with the condition (Emerge Australia, 2022).

References

Ankeny, R. A., & Mackenzie, F. J. (2016). Three approaches to chronic fatigue syndrome in the United Kingdom, Australia, and Canada: Lessons for democratic policy. In S. Dodds & R. A. Ankeny (Eds.), *Big picture bioethics: Developing democratic policy in contested domains* (pp. 227–243). Springer International Publishing.

Aronowitz, R. A. (1998). *Making sense of illness: Science, society, and disease.* Cambridge University Press.

Au, L., Capotescu, C., Eyal, G., & Finestone, G. (2022). Long COVID and medical gaslighting: Dismissal, delayed diagnosis, and deferred treatment. *SSM. Qualitative Research in Health, 2.* https://doi.org/10.1016/j.ssmqr.2022.100167

Barker, K. K. (2005). *The fibromyalgia story: Medical authority and women's worlds of pain.* Temple University Press.

Blease, C., & Geraghty, K. J. (2018). Are ME/CFS patient organizations "militant"?: Patient protest in a medical controversy. *Journal of Bioethical Inquiry, 15*(3), 393–401. https://doi.org/10.1007/s11673-018-9866-5

Braun, V., & Clarke, V. (2022). *Thematic analysis: A practical guide*. Sage.

Broom, A., & Adams, J. (2012). A critical social science of evidence-based healthcare. In A. Broom & J. Adams (Eds.), *Evidence-based healthcare in context: Critical social science perspectives* (pp. 1–19). Routledge.

Brown, P., Zavestoski, S., McCormick, S., Mayer, B., Morello-Frosch, R., & Gasior Altman, R. (2004). Embodied health movements: New approaches to social movements in health. *Sociology of Health & Illness, 26*(1), 50–80. https://doi.org/10.1111/j.1467-9566.2004.00378.x

Callard, F., & Perego, E. (2021). How and why patients made long Covid. *Social Science & Medicine, 268*. https://doi.org/10.1016/j.socscimed.2020.113426

Carruthers, B. M., Jain, A. K., De Meirleir, K. L., Peterson, D. L., Klimas, N. G., Lerner, A. M., Bested, A. C., Flor-Henry, P., Joshi, P., Powles, A. C. P., Sherkey, J. A., & van de Sande, M. I. (2003). Myalgic encephalomyelitis/chronic fatigue syndrome: Clinical working case definition, diagnostic and treatment protocols. *Journal of Chronic Fatigue Syndrome, 11*(1), 7–115. https://doi.org/10.1300/J092v11n01_02

Dumes, A. A. (2020). *Divided bodies: Lyme disease, contested illness, and evidence-based medicine*. Duke University Press.

Emerge Australia. (2022, November). *ME/CFS—What's in a name?* https://www.emerge.org.au/mecfs-whats-in-a-name/

Epstein, S. (2008). Patient groups and health movements. In E. J. Hackett, O. Amsterdamska, M. E. Lynch & J. Wajcman (Eds.), *The handbook of science and technology studies* (3rd ed.) (pp. 499–539). MIT Press.

Fleck, L. (1979). *Genesis and development of a scientific fact* (F. Bradley & T. J. Trenn, Trans.) University of Chicago Press. (Original work published 1935).

Fox, A. T., Fertleman, M., Cahill, P., & Palmer, R. D. (2003). Medical slang in British hospitals. *Ethics & Behavior, 13*(2), 173–189. https://doi.org/10.1207/S15327019EB1302_04

Grue, J. (2016). Illness is work: Revisiting the concept of illness careers and recognizing the identity work of patients with ME/CFS. *Health, 20*(4), 401–412. https://doi.org/10.1177/1363459315628044

Hunt, J., Blease, C., & Geraghty, K. J. (2022). Long COVID at the crossroads: Comparisons and lessons from the treatment of patients with myalgic encephalomyelitis/chronic fatigue syndrome (ME/CFS). *Journal of*

Health Psychology, 27(14), 3106–3120. https://doi.org/10.1177/135910532 21084494

Jason, L. A., & Richman, J. A. (2007). How science can stigmatize: The case of chronic fatigue syndrome. *Journal of Chronic Fatigue Syndrome, 14*(4), 85–103. https://doi.org/10.3109/10573320802092146

McEvedy, C. P., & Beard, A. W. (1970a). Royal free epidemic of 1955: A reconsideration. *British Medical Journal, 1*(5687), 7–11. https://doi.org/10.1136/bmj.1.5687.7

McEvedy, C. P., & Beard, A. W. (1970b). Concept of benign myalgic encephalomyelitis. *British Medical Journal, 1*(5687), 11–15. https://doi.org/10.1136/bmj.1.5687.11

Medina-Aedo, M., Günther, M., Arauz, I., Domancic, S., Diaz-Menai, S., Gregorio, S., León-García, M., Santero, M., Pardo-Hernadez, H., & Alonso-Coello, P. (2024). Incorporating postmenopausal women's perspectives into osteoporosis clinical guidelines: A systematic review. *Journal of Clinical Epidemiology, 173*. https://doi.org/10.1016/j.jclinepi.2024.111468

Millen, N. T., Peterson, C. L., & Woodward, R. (1998). A sociological analysis of chronic fatigue syndrome and the impact on family support structures. *International Journal of Sociology and Social Policy, 18*(7/8), 127–147. https://doi.org/10.1108/01443339810788470

Mullard, J., Mir, G., Herbert, C., & Evans, S. (2024). 'You're just a guinea pig': Exploring the barriers and impacts of living with long COVID-19—A view from the undiagnosed. *Sociology of Health & Illness, 46*(8), 1602–1625. https://doi.org/10.1111/1467-9566.13795

Spandler, H., & Allen, M. (2018). Contesting the psychiatric framing of ME/CFS. *Social Theory & Health, 16*(2), 127–141. https://doi.org/10.1057/s41 285-017-0047-0

Spence, N. J., Russell, D., Bouldin, E. D., Tumminello, C. M., & Schwartz, T. (2023). Getting back to normal? Identity and role disruptions among adults with long COVID. *Sociology of Health & Illness, 45*(4), 914–934. https://doi.org/10.1111/1467-9566.13628

Stenhoff, A. L., Sadreddini, S., Peters, S., & Wearden, A. (2015). Understanding medical students' views of chronic fatigue syndrome: A qualitative study. *Journal of Health Psychology, 20*(2), 198–209. https://doi.org/10.1177/1359105313501534

Timmermans, S., & Angell, A. (2012). Evidence-based medicine, clinical uncertainty, and learning to doctor. In A. Broom & J. Adams (Eds.), *Evidence-Based healthcare in context: Critical social science perspectives* (pp. 23–41) Routledge.

Toulkidis, V. (2002). Chronic fatigue syndrome, clinical practice guidelines. *Medical Journal of Australia, 176*(S9), S17–S55. https://doi.org/10.5694/j.1326-5377.2002.tb04499.x

Ware, N. C. (1992). Suffering and the social construction of illness: The delegitimation of illness experience in chronic fatigue syndrome. *Medical Anthropology Quarterly, 6*(4), 347–361. https://doi.org/10.1525/maq.1992.6.4.02a00030

White, K. (2017). *An introduction to the sociology of health and illness* (3rd ed.). Sage.

Wild, C., MacLean, A., Nettleton, S., Hunt, K., & Ziebland, S. (2024). The double invisibility of Long COVID in children. *Social Science & Medicine, 347*. https://doi.org/10.1016/j.socscimed.2024.116770

5

Long COVID Services Between Medical Clinics and Healing Rituals: A Case Study in Switzerland

Marjolaine Viret and Francesco Panese

Introduction

Even as the world strives to move on from SARS-CoV-2 and the COVID-19 pandemic, each wave of infection leaves behind individuals who develop post-acute sequelae, often colloquially referred to as 'Long COVID'. Long COVID represents the intrusion of an entity that has not yet been stabilised in terms of nosology, aetiology, symptomatology; and, not least, therapeutics. Patients are then often faced with an erratic

M. Viret (✉)
Faculty of Law, Criminal Sciences and Public Administration, Centre of Comparative, European & International Law, University of Lausanne, Lausanne, Switzerland
e-mail: Marjolaine.viret@unil.ch

F. Panese
Faculty of Social and Political Sciences, Institute of Social Sciences, University of Lausanne, Lausanne, Switzerland

Faculty of Biology & Medicine, Institute of Humanities in Medicine, University of Lausanne, Lausanne, Switzerland

D. Lupton (ed.), *Long COVID and Society*,
https://doi.org/10.1007/978-981-96-9168-5_5

journey towards a diagnosis. Because of this rather unusual medical situation, due to the conditions of emergence of the pathology of Long COVID and the pandemic context, patients' illness narratives usually developed outside a 'therapeutic dialogue' with a health professional who would 'make sense of their illness and construct a healing narrative, helped by continuity of the clinical relationship over time' (Rushforth et al., 2021). Where the narrative was not constructed in complete isolation, dialogue about this new illness initially occurred almost exclusively among patients (Rushforth et al., 2021). Long COVID has therefore been described as the first illness made through patient communities finding themselves on social media (Callard & Perego, 2021).

This exceptional configuration certainly testifies to the dynamics of tension and negotiation of the clinical and social integration of Long COVID as a novel entity that we can observe in the development of dedicated consultations. Patients' voices and increasing epidemiological evidence have been the main 'vectors of observability' of the 'ecological niche' (Hacking, 1998, pp. 5 and 86), allowing the development of specialised support for Long COVID as an attempt to reintroduce a component of patient-doctor interaction into the experience of this 'new illness'. In Switzerland, university hospitals, private clinics, or practitioner networks, have set up specialised Long COVID services. In these services, since Long COVID's manifestations vary from one patient to another, and since its aetiology is considered incurable, the condition is approached through its symptomatic expressions and their impact on the lives of the patients concerned. Thus, insofar as Long COVID is regarded as a 'disease of symptoms', its medical management is based primarily on identifying the elements on which action can be taken to transform patients so that they can cope to the extent possible with the new condition. This is what we observed in the case of the two Swiss Long COVID services we studied.

Inspired by field (self-)observations, we conducted a critical analysis of documentary resources (published between 2020 and June 2024) from two Long COVID services established by two university hospitals in the French-speaking part of Switzerland. We supplemented this documentation with Swiss press articles relating to these services, both of which attracted media attention. These sources are important to consider because patients, who are often at a loss, turn to a variety of information sources to find ways to alleviate their problems. In our analysis, we have also drawn on scientific publications where available.

The first example ('Service 1') offers on-site consultations and has developed a publicly accessible online information platform, including an AI-driven chatbot tool, for patients, their relatives, and health professionals. This platform is available in English, and we analysed the English-language version. The second ('Service 2') has also set up on-site Long COVID care, including a website and various documents given to patients referred for rehabilitation. These documents were available in French only, and the extracts quoted in this chapter are our translation into English. It should be noted that, in the context of university hospitals, which are both clinical and research institutions, these two services would seem characterised by a greater capacity than other care structures of proposing experimental therapies and prescribing off-label treatments whose efficacy cannot be considered sufficiently established in the context of standard medical practice. This approach is justified by their research mission.

The analysis of the documentation, discourses, and attitudes of the professionals involved in these medical services specialising in Long COVID, which cannot be based on any stabilised anatomopathological standards, is hence performed under uncertainty. The analysis reveals what could be described as a fumbling clinical trial-and-error process, with the aim of dialogically adapting the patients to their situation of suffering, and the course of which can hardly be prognosed, and which can be likened to a chronic condition. We suggest that this adaptation takes place in what should be seen as *extended healing rituals* that influence the patients' experience, reshape their identity, and take on broader psychosocial roles, for the community of health professionals, the patients' social environment, and society at large.

Assuming that rituals are universal components of healing (Dow, 1986), even in (bio)medical[1] settings (Kaptchuk, 2011; Meza, 2019), we hypothesised that, in the specific context described, healing rituals further fulfil meaning-making and power functions for communities (Kirmayer, 2004). These are particularly relevant for afflictions that disrupt the social order, as Long COVID does, and appear to be key to the constitution of a moral economy (Fassin, 2009) that shapes professionals', patients', and collective moral principles around work, health, and social responsibility, overwhelmed by the illness.

Rituals as Integral Part of Long COVID Medical Services

Western medicine is said to 'spurn' ritual (Trotter, 2012). Indeed, much of biomedical doxa revolves around distinguishing the placebo effect—and thus assumed ritual/symbolic efficacy—from the 'real' efficacy of treatments. Though biomedicine may struggle to overcome its aversion to placebo (Apud & Romaní, 2020), several authors argue that biomedicine and ritual healing are not mutually exclusive. Ritual models of healing apply to every community, including modern Western societies (Farmer, 1988). Biomedical interventions contain a significant ritual dimension (Kaptchuk, 2011) which, despite their supposed 'official elimination', gives biomedical procedures an 'additional charged "symbolic" power': 'Despite the scientific ethos, for patients and perhaps for physicians, biomedicine goes beyond technical expertise and retains aspects of a healing ritual albeit with a secular mythos' (Kaptchuk, 2011, p. 1854). Given the transformative effects of this 'symbolic' power on patient subjects, our observation and experience of the Long COVID services was a reminder of Meza's reflections: 'I found a consistent structure for healing rituals discussed by many anthropologists; I realized that the clinical encounters of Western medicine follow this same structure' (Meza, 2019, p. 114).

We also find this structure in Long COVID services, even though they operate in university hospitals, which can be assumed to stand firmly rooted in the biomedical paradigm. In a process presumably reinforced by the lack of robust evidence-based clinical guidelines, their discourses and practices incorporate features of healing rituals that articulate an experience shared between clinician and patient, an interpretation of the experience that the clinician returns to the patient, and ideally shared expectations about the changes that the influences promoted by the ritual will bring about in the patient's illness (see e.g. Kirmayer, 2004,

p. 33). However, it is important to note that the situation is generally not symmetrical, in that clinicians use clinical and, when available, scientific knowledge to diagnose problems, and then persuade patients to jointly focus on a specific 'diagnostic narrative' directed at having patients accept a treatment plan linked to the diagnosed condition (see Meza, 2019, p. 116). The major drawback in the case of Long COVID is that the plan essentially takes the form of hypothetical meliorative advice aimed, it is said, at adapting patients to a condition that pervasively alters their lives:

> Post-COVID symptoms have a major impact on quality of life (social, personal and professional). Some people with long-term symptoms are unable to resume their normal activities or work because they have fluctuating symptoms of unpredictable duration. (Service 1 platform—Social impact and return to work).

As a ritual, the consultation thus has performative effects at various levels (see e.g. Dow, 1986, p. 56), which take the form in Long COVID services of a psychological and social refashioning of the patient's 'objective-self' (Dumit, 2003) and techniques to adapt daily life to the disease. Among these techniques is the 'activity pacing' proposed to patients to help them manage their symptoms and energy, discussed below.

Recognising a Condition Despite Uncertainty

Accounts of medical consultations often focus on a supposedly immediate interaction within the care encounter. In the case of the patient materials studied, the entry point proposed to patients is virtual (for those whose first contact is through the Service 1 platform) or at least supported by written documentation (for those who receive documentation at their on-site visit at Service 2). Patients are offered the opportunity to initiate a care encounter through generic information, on the one hand in a traditional way and on the other in the form of a chatbot, whose credibility is rhetorically produced through its overt belonging to university hospital institutions.[2] Despite their provisional nature, due of course to the considerable uncertainty surrounding Long COVID, these initiatives are attempts to combine different objectives.

The first declared objective is clearly the *recognition of the pathology* for patients often lost in therapeutic errands to 'legitimise [their] concerns about a new and unfamiliar disease and, at the same time, optimise their care' (Service 1 press release, 8 December 2020). According to the originators of the Service 1 platform:

> [the] main goal is to answer the increasing demand for information and communication on post–COVID-19 in a time of limited knowledge and limited resources for both children and adults. (Nehme, Schneider et al., 2023)

This recognition also takes the form of advice such as this:

> Advice - 1. Acknowledge and accept the fact that this is a proven illness, well recognized by the World Health Organization. […] Once we know what is affecting us, we can prepare ourselves better to deal with it. (Service 2 documentation)

Long COVID services therefore help to establish the 'truth of the disease' so that patients can claim it in the eyes of their private and professional *entourage*:

> If it's not clear to your relatives, don't hesitate to explain the disease to them and ask them to look it up on the internet. Understanding support from family and colleagues is essential, especially as the symptoms are not visible. (Service 2 documentation)
>
> Communication between employers and employees is important to facilitate an adapted return to work, avoiding relapses and potentially long-term disabilities. […] Employers must be made more aware of post-COVID symptoms. These symptoms affect every aspect of life, including the professional sphere, and should be considered in adapting the workplace. (Service 1 platform—Social impact and return to work)

Long COVID services, in their public expression, go even beyond the immediate social environment of the patients, seeking to strengthen and extend the recognition of the pathology to other bodies on which they depend; specifically *social security*:

> [Patients] should be supported through social insurance schemes, with the help of occupational health specialists, human resources departments and their primary care physicians, as well as post-COVID specialists, to determine whether professional reorientation is an option or whether they will require long-term disability benefits. (Service 1 platform—Social impact and return to work)

By doing so, Long COVID services take on an advocacy role for the recognition of the condition within society, and for both relational and economical support of the sufferers. These actions promote a process of mediation between the patient who has become unfit for social functions and society, together with supporting the creation of communities among patients (for example, links to patient associations and support groups).

Acknowledging and Sharing Uncertainties

Another aim of Long COVID services is to provide relevant information while acknowledging uncertainty. The strategy is then to mimic a one-to-one medical consultation and the process of healthcare encounters by featuring an 'ideal patient' who asks 'good' questions and aims to be representative of an entire patient community. The virtual meeting thus has a question-and-answer format, where the exchange is opened by an imaginary patient in search of a diagnosis (*What is it I have?*), followed by an attempt at identifying the aetiology (*Where does it come from?*) in order to subsume his or her experience under a biomedical perspective, and finally by the description of a 'treatment' which is more akin to an adaptative management plan (*What can I do* ?) (Service 2 documentation). Indeed, the answers to the questions remain vague and marked by the uncertainty that is shared with patients, as in the following information provided by the Service 1 platform:

> *How long do the symptoms last?* Post-COVID symptoms usually improve, although they may fluctuate over time. It is impossible to predict the duration of post-COVID condition.
> *What mechanism triggers post-COVID condition?* The pathophysiology and mechanisms behind persistent symptoms after a SARS-CoV-2 infection are still under investigation. [...] All these hypotheses are still being studied and have yet to be proven.
> *What test should I do to find out if I have post-COVID condition?* There is no specific test for diagnosing post-COVID condition.
> *How can I protect myself against post-COVID condition?* At present, there is no treatment for post-COVID condition and there are no measures that can prevent it.

Although the diagnostic phase is at the heart of the stated aims of recognition conveyed by these online encounters, it remains rather superficial, consisting mainly of naming the disease in a way that links it to a triggering event (SARS CoV-2 infection), while at the same time expressing the lack of a solid biomedical aetiology (unknown, unproven mechanisms, etc.) and the absence of proven treatments—in short, considerable biomedical uncertainty. A specific section of the Service 1 platform is even devoted to 'uncertainties around post-COVID [condition]', again in the form of questions and answers, focusing mainly on the pathophysiology of the disease and its causes. There is, then, a palpable tension between the stated aim of improving patients' experience of the disease through information, on the one hand, and the irreducible lack of knowledge on the part of the medical profession, on the other.

In their own way, these communications partake of preparing patients for the difficulties they will face in the subsequent stages of their care pathway, which can only be individualised and largely based on their own commitment to adapting to the disease under the guidance of clinicians:

> In most cases, it is impossible to determine how long the symptoms will persist. For all these reasons, Long COVID is like a chronic disease that needs to be treated specifically over the long term, in collaboration

> with the doctors treating the patient. The Long COVID service therefore meets a need. (Service 2 press release, 11 November 2021)

In these Long COVID services, uncertainty thus extends to all aspects of the traditional clinic: diagnosis, disease mechanisms, treatments, and prognosis. This has important consequences for the different strategies that emerge to deal with these deficits, with the adaptive restructuring of patients' lives as a key component of the medical advice.

Adaptive Restructuring of Patients' Lives

Despite these challenges, Long COVID services cannot entirely leave aside the definition of the 'effectiveness' of the limited patient care they can provide, the question of 'what counts as a good outcome' (Kirmayer, 2004, p. 42). Usually, what constitutes the legitimate outcome of a treatment is determined by shared standards of a 'correct prescription' defined within the biomedical paradigm. However, in the instable and fuzzy case of Long COVID, we observe a shift in the centre of gravity of care from disease to illness, towards the fact that 'disease makes the person unfit for social functions' (Meza, 2019, p. 117).

Long COVID services, therefore, involve the patient in a ritual process that combines knowledge and ignorance, advice, and prescription. These are all performative elements designed to ensure the social transformation of the patient's life, in a tangled tension between granting the sufferer 'the social legitimation of the sickness role' (Kaptchuk, 2011, p. 1853), and the obligation to properly assume the responsibilities of this role despite the powerlessness of medicine to bring about recovery. In this context, the terms of the therapeutic contract remain poorly defined, and therapeutic goals are equally tainted by uncertainty. For instance, these services offer 'rehabilitation advice [...] to help you manage your symptoms as effectively as possible throughout the day, in the hope that this will have a positive effect on your condition in the medium and long term' (Service 2 documentation), or recommend 'rehabilitation within a person's energy limits, and while avoiding post-exertional malaise' (Service 1 platform). This strategy has become a standard published in the 'Post-COVID recommendations for primary care physicians—Switzerland',[3] who are also encouraged to refer patients to specialised Long COVID services:

> The intervention is a self-management education in which the occupational issues are addressed with mainly compensatory and supportive elements. In the early disease stage, assessment sessions with initial brief information and tips are important. In a later stage when patients have more experience of the symptoms and a better understanding of their impact on daily activities, and they have started to accept that the prognosis regarding recovery and healing might be uncertain, a structured energy management education (individual or group) is needed. (Nehme, Diem et al., 2023, p. 24)

The most emblematic illustration of inducing patients to adapt to their new condition as part of their daily routine is 'pacing', which has been defined as 'an active self-management strategy whereby individuals learn to balance time spent on activity and rest for the purpose of achieving increased function and participation in meaningful activities' (Jamieson-Lega et al., 2013). This self-management strategy can be viewed as situated at the crossroads of biomedical culture and knowledge, and of culture-specific norms, values, and practices. From the biomedical side, it is proposed based on an analogy between Long COVID and myalgic encephalomyelitis/chronic fatigue syndrome (ME/CFS), a multisystem disease triggered, in particular, by viral infections and largely unknown in the general medical community (Davis et al., 2023). It was originally for ME/CFS patients that the pacing strategy had been specifically developed:

> Benefits of pacing' included short-term benefits, such as establishing baselines, improved symptom management and psychological well-being. Longer-term benefits included developing routines and setting goals to incorporate meaningful/desirable activities to improve quality of life. Pacing encouraged a modification of self-expectations/beliefs about activities, a reduction in fear of symptoms/activities, less boom–bust cycling and improved cumulative activity levels. Pacing could enable a sense of

choice and control over activities and allow for planned events due to more predictable symptoms. (Antcliff et al., 2019, p. 338)

Among the documents provided to Long COVID patients are detailed 'activity pacing' plans structuring the parts of the day down to the minute, with invitations to self-evaluation (Service 2 documentation). An example showing suggestions for 2 days at either end of the week is shown in Table 5.1:

While one would assume that these 'activity pacing' plans are negotiated with patients and can be adapted to individual preferences, the fact remains that their elaboration and implementation calls into question cultural and social norms and values intrinsic to the tool itself and to the examples of 'desirable' activities listed. Pragmatically, this strategy tends to exclude people with low literacy and reflexivity skills, those with socioeconomic circumstances that do not permit these adaptations (for example, access to remote work or supportive childcare), as well as those who are too severely affected to have any daily activity management compatible with pacing. More generally and critically, according

Table 5.1 Example of activity pacing from a Long COVID service

Monday *Morning*	wake up affirmations breakfast stretching (10 min) meditation (30 min) painting (15 min) lunch	...	***Sunday*** Morning	wake up affirmations breakfast walk (10 min) meditation (30 min) drawing (15 min) lunch
Afternoon	Rest wash hair work emotions breathing/rest TV (40 minutes) dinner	...	*Afternoon*	Rest visit friends/family (1hour) relaxation dinner
Evening	reading (15 minutes) gratitude yoga nigra	...	*Evening*	reading (15 minutes) gratitude yoga nigra
Remarks	Writing down my emotions in a diary helps me a lot	...	*Remarks*	Next time, make my parents' visit a little shorter

to Risør and Lillevoll (2021), who carried out an ethnographic study of ME/CFS sufferers who were given the same type of advice to improve their symptom management (namely 'pacing'), this kind of tool related to self-management could

> contribute [...] to the constitution of a particular personhood, precipitating an agency that places individuals in a moral dilemma between the social rules of their everyday lives and the rules of self-care. (Risør & Lillevoll, 2021, p. 432)

Although our current data on Long COVID services do not allow us to verify this highly critical interpretation, we can nevertheless agree with them that we are faced with 'a transfer of responsibility from the health professional to the patient, who became enacted as a particular, self-governing person who could do what was needed to recover' (Risør & Lillevoll, 2021, p. 440). Facing this burden of responsibility also leads these services to advise sharing with peers so as to feel understood by people going through similar experiences, to share information, and to work together to develop resources for coping with difficulties. Biosociality (Rabinow, 1996) and biosolidarity (Bradley, 2021) are therefore encouraged, either by creating new patient communities or by joining existing patient associations and/or psychologist-led discussion groups.

Intervention in Long COVID is then not simply a palliative action to mitigate the burden of illness within the psycho-social spheres of patients' agency, behaviours, and relations. Nor do the Long COVID services propose an intervention that is akin to biomedical research; that is, whose modalities and endpoints are to be understood in molecular, biological, or physiological terms. A mixed biosocial strategy of intervention (Harris & McDade, 2018) is deployed here as a healing ritual enacting a dual transformative move. The first dimension of this move transforms the impasse of biomedical institutions facing an unknown clinical entity into a therapeutic pathway linking social stratification, biology and health. Second, there is the strategy that turns the deteriorating psychological and social circumstances of Long COVID patients into the actionable determinants of their well-being.

In addition, the self-management strategy involves encouraging patients to make use of therapeutics outside biomedicine. Indeed, we observe an interesting shift from the *recognition of the systemic nature of the disease*[4] to *an ideal of holistic care*, resulting in a mosaic of practices that are far removed from biomedical clinical standards. Thus, paradoxically for university medical institutions, advice and prescriptions give prominence to alternative medicines and lifestyle interventions. On the Service 1 platform, 11 of the 20 symptom-specific sections propose a variety of non-conventional, non-pharmacological treatments (for example, tai chi, mindfulness meditation, (self-)hypnosis, pilates, yoga, acupuncture, biofeedback, various dietary supplements, aromatherapy, cardiac coherence breathing). The same applies to Service 2 documentation (for example, luminotherapy, various lifestyle changes, mindfulness meditation, vagus nerve stimulation, acupuncture, hypnosis, relaxing massage with essential oils, artistic creation). The bridging element between the biomedical paradigm and these interventions is a model of the disease in which the patients must seek to rebalance their central nervous system disturbed by the infection (hence the emphasis on 'calming' activities and rest, which are to activate the parasympathetic system).

Long COVID services are not completely abandoning their biomedical orientation, however. Patient referral platforms echo elements of the scientific literature. Furthermore, as part of the clinic, research groups revolving around the Long COVID services are experimenting, for example, with monitoring of heart rate variability, a technological tool increasingly used in sports, or the introduction of vagus nerve stimulation studies into a cohort of patients, or even a clinical trial on a monoclonal antibody (Temelimab). In the context of a non-stabilised entity, assessing the effectiveness of any intervention, but also defining what effectiveness would be, is not straightforward.

Mobilising Patients for Research

While the strikingly hybrid nature of Long COVID services may come as a surprise, one wonders whether they do not ultimately reflect all-encompassing research dynamics illustrative of the 'participatory turn in healthcare' (Prainsack, 2017) that seeks to mobilise the patients not only for the self-management of their symptoms, but also as a source of information that can potentially be incorporated into research and clinical experience. In this sense, the involvement of the patient in the services is also characterised by an epistemic dimension. Indeed, their founders emphasise that 'given the current state of knowledge [meaning ignorance], it is important to support the people concerned and to listen to them' (Service 1 press release, 8 December 2020). They add that acquisition of knowledge is a two-way process: the questions asked by patients become data for the ongoing training of the AI chatbot tool on the Service 1 platform, which could ideally become a means of assessing not only patients' needs but also the therapeutic strategies they adopt. It should be noted here that one of the key players in setting up this platform is very involved in the development of this type of technology in Switzerland (see Nehme et al., 2024).

Thus, perhaps at a modest level, the platform mobilises patient-generated health data (PGHD)[5] through 'lay questions'. Although patient responses often reflect experiential knowledge and expertise, they are processed as Long COVID-related information. The algorithm integrates so-called 'data collection through patient engagement'—or more critically, through 'invited and uninvited participation' (Weiner et al., 2023). These datasets potentially include symptoms, lifestyle choices, descriptions of (self-)therapies or (self-)care practices and their outcomes, and other self-reported information. In a research paper, the Service 1 study group explains that the use of the 'chatbot and platform was driven by the monthly thematic webinars as well as communication campaigns, with an average of 250 participants at each webinar' to address and discuss results of the 'chatbot regarding themes and requests', including some 20 post-COVID symptoms (Nehme, Schneider et al., 2023).

The involvement of patients and professionals in the information economy managed by the chatbot therefore also has a social dimension. In proposing quasi-social interactions through exchange of data, scientific knowledge, subjective experience, and advice, the platform contributes to the creation of an online community of users who begin to visit it ritually as they progress through their illness. One could even say that the efficiency of the tool is conditional on the interactive ritual in which it successfully enrols patients; and this enrolment has been undoubtedly facilitated by the widespread use of chatbots during the pandemic for emotional support in community contexts in response to isolation.

While we will have to wait to observe further research outcomes based on this specific strategy of data collection through patient engagement, clearly, the classical therapeutic contract is then disturbed. Instead of being a *knower*, the clinician is led to adopt the attitude of a 'learner' (learning from the patient) as well as acting as a 'carer'; even when little can be suggested for the patient's cure. This is probably one of the reasons why patient participation is so highly valued by the clinicians involved in these Long COVID services. Uncertainty therefore plays a dual role here: on the one hand, in justifying the need for Long COVID services' existence and in encouraging therapeutic research, and, on the other, in explicitly acknowledging the limits of their ability to cure because of the lack of scientific robustness of their prescriptions.

Between Recognition and Resignation

The Long COVID services established in Switzerland have claimed, and continue to claim, a critical role in negotiating the integration of the condition into society as a novel health entity. Beyond their biomedical foundation, they have distinct characteristics, with multifaceted dimensions that extend beyond the patient-carer nexus. Dealing with a novel health entity therefore has an impact not only on the individuals affected but also on a larger social context in a dynamic of mutual adaptation. As we have seen, one of the levers of this adaptation is the recognition of the patients' condition as 'real', providing a disease label to their suffering despite the non-stabilised character of Long COVID. This recognition is the starting point for leading patients through a process of 'modulation of expectations' (Kaptchuk, 2002), towards an injunction to engage into compliant meaning-making in the face of the illness. This phenomenon is compounded by the—explicit or implicit—assimilation of Long COVID into ME/CFS via the transposition of coping techniques ('pacing') developed in the context of an understudied disease with which most non-specialised health professionals are unfamiliar (Davis et al., 2023). In effect, this process amounts to layering uncertainty upon uncertainty rather than providing clarity or hope.

This situation represents a notable departure from classical biomedical treatment, in which the healer/carer is the 'impresario and guide' (Kaptchuk, 2011, p. 1853), 'whose powers are accepted by the patient' (Farmer, 1988, p. 36). Instead, emphasis is placed here on the role of the patient, through a process in which self-management is elevated to treatment, self-attention to a duty, and self-transformation to a desirable effect. Through the Long COVID services' insistence on the holistic approach needed for Long COVID (Service 2 documentation), and the central role assigned to 'pacing', patients' entire lives are converted into transformational spaces, into an embodied experience of the adaptive journey in which they are directed to go along with the illness rather than to fight it. Due to the absence of prognosis, there is only a fine line between enabling patient empowerment and demanding patient resignation. Through a discourse that emphasises acceptance justified through the need to avoid any additional disruption to the central nervous system, patients are gradually led to conform to social norms (McGuire, 1987) defining 'acceptable' Long COVID sufferers. Their psychological and spiritual attitudes, which are modulated by their ability or inability to cope with their illness for themselves and for their entourage, are integral to these norms.

The recognition of patients has also looping effect on the medical institution itself, which gains in positive moral recognition, despite ignorance and uncertainty, lacunary diagnostic and therapeutic strategies. Promoting the visibility of Long COVID and advocating it as an important ongoing problem serves to legitimise Long COVID services. This moral recognition seems even to be reinforced, albeit paradoxically, by a kind of 'epistemic generosity' evident in their trial-and-error approach. As we have seen, under the banner of a 'holistic approach', Long COVID services incorporate a wide range of recommendations which blur the lines between typical biomedical targets of treatment, on the one hand, and self-management and adaptation to illness identity, on the other hand. Moreover, knowledge gaps and uncertainty on the part of the health professional are reframed as a collaborative journey placing the patient at the centre of their own care, with the emphatic presence of the health professional, who learns along with the patient.

In contrast, ignorance in the face of uncertainty, confusion and lack of resources caused by the sudden emergence of Long COVID is a lever for promoting innovation, as demonstrated through the development of novel tools and technologies (for example, chatbots), experimenting with novel ways of generating medical encounter and initiating healing. This positions Long COVID services as 'specialised' and well-informed within the medical community and more widely in society, through the media, which are always very active on this dramatic topic.

Conclusion

The even wider resonance of Long COVID and its management should be assessed in further work beyond the scope of this chapter. Follow-up research should, in particular, assess the resonance, within the local health professional community, of the creation of Long COVID medical care services, and the manner in which their existence and composition modulates the interplay between medical specialties. It would also be interesting, and perhaps necessary, to examine the moral and legal responsibilities of these services, given that their stated aim goes beyond the strict biomedical sphere, claiming functions related to the reorganisation of the patient's social roles in relation to their entourage or employer, but also to the establishment of an authority in the health professional community by providing guidance to treating physicians. Further research is also needed to better understand the practices and dynamics of sociality and solidarity among patients who are encouraged to spread information about Long COVID to those around them in order to obtain adequate support, patients who are 'invited' in addition to get involved in creating and managing affected communities that other patients can join to share their new illness identity and their experiential knowledge and expertise.

As we have seen, Long COVID services enshrine elements of advocacy work, particularly with respect to socio-economic impacts of the disease, which are extensively thematised, to support calls for adapted work conditions and access to disability benefits. This political extension of Long COVID services role needs to be better understood: perhaps as a result of the failure of the biomedical approach to produce outcomes that restore the patient's full social capabilities, or as a consequence of the novel character of the disease and the general reluctance for society to consider SARS CoV-2 as an ongoing problem.

Though much remains to be done, we have attempted to explore the way in which specialised services dealing with Long COVID as a new health entity perform functions that pertain to the social order and treat society as well as the patient. We have done so by proposing the notion of *extended healing ritual* which, far from being a linear transformative process, takes the form of iterative and transformative loops in several nested registers. As epistemic practice, a ritual contributes to the dynamic looping of the production, transmission, incorporation and updating of knowledge between patients and professionals. It thus plays a role in the reflexive constitution of knowledge about Long COVID, which at minimum makes the uncertainties surrounding the condition manageable, and at best enables patients to partake in the knowledge-building process in which they participate.

These iterative loops extend the scope of the ritual into the clinic, where the care relationship, as we have seen, takes the form of a reciprocal trial-and-error process between patient and healthcare provider. The ritual then takes patients into a sometimes very extensive network of medical specialties and subspecialties, but also outside traditional biomedicine, and inscribes them in an activity and a temporality of self-monitoring of symptoms and clinical examinations that are integrated into and profoundly alter their daily lives. This care relationship spills over a broader social register insofar as its rituality transforms the identity of patients beyond the realm of healthcare, as well as their awareness of the illness. By extension and reciprocally, it is therefore a ritual that produces collective medical knowledge and social visibility for the disease. And this social extension of the ritual contributes to the differentiated recognition of Long COVID in the plurality of spheres involved, mainly work and social insurance, but also the health system and the specific investments made in the care of the condition. These aspects should be explored in greater depth than we have been able to do here, but it seems clear that Long COVID services, in their own way and to their own degree, contribute to shaping the moral economies of the pathology that are still being negotiated in a society that dreams of being post-COVID.

At the end of this investigation, we might ask whether this rituality is common in biomedicine. The answer, in line with Kaptchuk (2011) and (Meza, 2019), is undoubtedly yes. But it also seems that the density and centrality of this rituality are all the greater in the case of a novel and uncertain entity such as Long COVID. Just as traditional therapeutic rituals usually end with a clear diagnosis and adapted intervention ('treatment plan'), in the case of Long COVID—as in other particularly trying chronic illnesses—this rarely happens. Patients are then caught up in a ritual spiral of transformation and adaptation: sometimes for the better, sometimes for the worse.

Acknowledgements We wish to thank Dr Luca Chiapperino for his review of, and insightful comments on a first draft of this chapter; the Long COVID patients who, over the course of multiple discussions since 2020, have contributed to shaping our research questions; and finally, the medical institutions for granting us access to their patient documentation.

Notes

1. Here we distinguish between 'medicine', which focuses on the diagnosis, treatment, and prevention of epistemically and therapeutically stabilised diseases, and 'biomedicine', which is more research-oriented and seeks to understand the processes underlying

diseases to develop new treatments and diagnostic tools, including clinical data and observations. As our fieldwork is carried out in university hospitals, and although translational research on Long COVID is difficult, we use the term biomedical in this chapter.

2. Note that the diagnostic label is heterogeneous in terms of terminology, a sign of persistent instability. Both services refer to themselves as providing 'Long COVID' consultations. Service 2 uses the title 'post-COVID syndrome' for its resources, but then 'Long COVID' throughout the documentation. Service 1, on the other hand, avoids the term 'Long COVID', referring instead to 'post-acute sequelae of SARS CoV-2' or 'post-COVID condition or syndrome', mentioning only *en passant* that this is 'also known as Long COVID or the post-acute effects of SARS-CoV-2'.
3. This highly detailed 60-page document is also designed to 'guide primary care physicians to in the diagnosis and management of post-COVID condition' by a symptom-based approach. Without going here into the details of these diagnostic issues, we limit ourselves to what is offered to patients to alleviate their suffering on a pragmatic level.
4. 'Long COVID is a complex, multisystem disorder that affects nearly every organ system, including the cardiovascular system, the nervous system, the endocrine system, the immune system, the reproductive system and the gastrointestinal system' (Al-Aly et al., 2024, p. 2148).
5. For a technical description and the expected benefits of this strategy, see Khatiwada et al. (2024). For a more critical approach, but which does not include chatbot technology, see Augst et al. (2025).

References

Al-Aly, Z., Davis, H., McCorkell, L., Soares, L., Wulf-Hanson, S., Iwasaki, A., & Topol, E. J. (2024). Long COVID science, research and policy. *Nature Medicine, 30*(8), 2148–2164. https://doi.org/10.1038/s41591-024-03173-6

Antcliff, D., Keenan, A.-M., Keeley, P., Woby, S., & McGowan, L. (2019). Survey of activity pacing across healthcare professionals informs a new activity pacing framework for chronic pain/fatigue. *Musculoskeletal Care, 17*(4), 335–345. https://doi.org/10.1002/msc.1421

Apud, I., & Romaní, O. (2020). Medical anthropology and symbolic cure: From the placebo to cultures of meaningful healing. *Anthropology & Medicine, 27*(2), 160–175. https://doi.org/10.1080/13648470.2019.1649542

Augst, A., Lämmerhirt, D., & Schubert, C. (2025). Patient-generated data as interventions in doctor-patient relationships? Negotiating (un)invited participation in medical consultations. *Sociology of Health & Illness, 47*(2). https://doi.org/10.1111/1467-9566.13864

Bradley, B. (2021). From biosociality to biosolidarity: The looping effects of finding and forming social networks for body-focused repetitive behaviours. *Anthropology & Medicine, 28*(4), 543–557. https://doi.org/10.1080/13648470.2020.1864807

Callard, F., & Perego, E. (2021). How and why patients made Long COVID. *Social Science & Medicine, 268*. https://doi.org/10.1016/j.socscimed.2020.113426

Davis, H. E., McCorkell, L., Vogel, J. M., & Topol, E. J. (2023). Long COVID: Major findings, mechanisms and recommendations. *Nature Reviews Microbiology, 21*(3), 133–146. https://doi.org/10.1038/s41579-022-00846-2

Dow, J. (1986). Universal aspects of symbolic healing: A theoretical synthesis. *American Anthropologist, 88*, 56–69. https://doi.org/10.1525/aa.1986.88.1.02a00040

Dumit, J. (2003). Is it me or my brain? Depression and neuroscientific facts. *Journal of Medical Humanities, 24*(1), 35–47. https://doi.org/10.1023/A:1021353631347

Farmer, M. F. (1988). Ritual and healing—An anthropological point of view. *Journal of Physical Education, Recreation & Dance, 59*(9), 34–36. https://doi.org/10.1080/07303084.1988.10606313

Fassin, D. (2009). Moral economies revisited. *Annales. Histoire, Sciences Sociales, 64*(6), 1237–1266.

Hacking, I. (1998). *Mad travelers: Reflections on the reality of transient mental illnesses.* Harvard University Press.

Harris, K. M., & McDade, T. W. (2018). The biosocial approach to human development, behavior, and health across the life course. *The Russell Sage Foundation Journal of the Social Sciences, 4*(4), 2–26. https://doi.org/10.7758/RSF.2018.4.4.01

Jamieson-Lega, K., Berry, R., & Brown, C. A. (2013). Pacing: A concept analysis of a chronic pain intervention. *Pain Research & Management, 18*(4), 207–213. https://doi.org/10.1155/2013/686179

Kaptchuk, T. J. (2002). The placebo effect in alternative medicine: Can the performance of a healing ritual have clinical significance? *Annals of Internal Medicine, 136*(11), 817–825. https://doi.org/10.7326/0003-4819-136-11-200206040-00011

Kaptchuk, T. J. (2011). Placebo studies and ritual theory: A comparative analysis of Navajo, acupuncture and biomedical healing. *Philosophical Transactions of the Royal Society B, 366*(1572), 1849–1858. https://doi.org/10.1098/rstb.2010.0385

Khatiwada, P., Yang, B., Lin, J.-C., & Blobel, B. (2024). Patient-generated health data (PGHD): Understanding, requirements, challenges, and existing techniques for data security and privacy. *Journal of Personalized Medicine, 14*(3). https://doi.org/10.3390/jpm14030282

Kirmayer, L. J. (2004). The cultural diversity of healing: Meaning, metaphor and mechanism. *British Medical Bulletin, 69*(1), 33–48. https://doi.org/10.1093/bmb/ldh006

McGuire, M. B. (1987). Ritual, symbolism and healing. *Social Compass, 34*(4), 365–379. https://doi.org/10.1177/003776868703400404

Meza, J. P. (2019). *Diagnosis narratives and the healing ritual in Western medicine.* Routledge & CRC Press.

Nehme, M., Diem, L., Bassetti, C. L. A., & Guessous, I. (2023). Swiss recommendations for the diagnosis, management and follow-up of post-COVID condition in primary care medicine (2023). *Swiss Medical Weekly, 153*(9), Article 9. https://doi.org/10.57187/s.3468

Nehme, M., Schneider, F., Amruthalingam, E., Schnarrenberger, E., Tremeaud, R., & Guessous, I. (2024). Chatbots in medicine: Certification process and applied use case. *Swiss Medical Weekly.* https://smw.ch/index.php/smw/article/view/3954

Nehme, M., Schneider, F., Perrin, A., Sum Yu, W., Schmitt, S., Violot, G., Ducrot, A., Tissandier, F., Posfay-Barbe, K., & Guessous, I. (2023). The development of a chatbot technology to disseminate post-COVID-19 information: Descriptive implementation study. *Journal of Medical Internet Research, 25*. https://doi.org/10.2196/43113

Prainsack, B. (2017). *Personalized medicine: Empowered patients in the 21st Century?* NYU Press.

Rabinow, P. (1996). Artificiality and enlightenment: From sociobiology to biosociality. *Politix, 90*(2), 21–46.

Risør, M. B., & Lillevoll, K. (2021). Caught up in care: Crafting moral subjects of chronic fatigue. *Medical Anthropology, 40*(5), 432–445. https://doi.org/10.1080/01459740.2021.1883011

Rushforth, A., Ladds, E., Wieringa, S., Taylor, S., Husain, L., & Greenhalgh, T. (2021). Long COVID—The illness narratives. *Social Science & Medicine, 286*,. https://doi.org/10.1016/j.socscimed.2021.114326

Trotter, G. (2012). Why the West spurns medical rituals. In D. Solomon, R. Fan, & P. Lo (Éds.), *Ritual and the moral life: Reclaiming the tradition* (p. 75–86). Springer Netherlands.

Weiner, K., Henwood, F., Andrews, J., Will, C., & Williams, R. (2023). The logics of invited and uninvited material participation: Bringing blood pressure self-monitoring into the clinic. *Science & Technology Studies, 36*(2). https://doi.org/10.23987/sts.112027

Part IV

Biopolitics and Social Determinants

6

Long COVID and the Biopolitics of Pandemic Timings and Endings

Mark D. M. Davis

Introduction

Long COVID has troubled relations with the timings and so-called endings of the COVID-19 pandemic, with implications for knowledge about pandemics and the health of those who continue to be affected by the novel coronavirus SARS-CoV-2. Significantly, 'Long COVID' as a commonly used term contrasts with the biomedically orthodox 'post-COVID syndrome' (National Institute for Health & Care Excellence, 2024; World Health Organization, 2022), which is used to mark the phenomenon of protracted illness subsequent to a COVID infection. This tension of different pandemic timings—'long' and 'post'—suggests that science and politics place weight on normative understandings of pandemic time and that Long COVID disturbs these norms because it asks for a different way of understanding pandemics. As we will see

M. D. M. Davis (✉)
School of Social Sciences, Faculty of Arts, Monash University, Melbourne, Australia
e-mail: Mark.Davis@monash.edu

D. Lupton (ed.), *Long COVID and Society*,
https://doi.org/10.1007/978-981-96-9168-5_6

in what follows, even in the face of biological knowledge of the virus's persistence, endings have been sought out to contain the pandemic for biopolitical purposes.

For this chapter, I frame biopolitics as the assemblage of scientific knowledge, governmental reason and disciplinary subjectification for the purpose of securing the health and wealth of populations (Lemke, 2010). The biopolitics concept is based on the notion that scientific knowledge does not simply reveal the mechanisms of life, it exercises power over life. Biopolitics, served by the life sciences, produces identities, shapes conduct, provides reasoning for the allocation of resources and is crystallised in law and regulation. Scientific knowledge of life, therefore, is the basis by which populations are asked to govern themselves to protect and promote their health and generativity. Pandemic threats are arch examples of biopolitics. Scientific knowledge about the HIV virus, for example, has led to effective treatments and biomedical means of prevention that have saved many millions of lives. At the same time, however, effective HIV treatment and prevention require that individuals accept that they have HIV in their bodies or are at risk of infection and therefore undergo testing for the virus and appropriate treatment and prevention. The COVID pandemic is no less an example of biopolitics since it also has required that individuals accept new at-risk identities, carry out lockdowns and seek vaccination (Lupton, 2022).

Long COVID, however, is a distinctive turning in pandemic biopolitics. It has taken form and force through appropriating and resisting virological, immunological, epidemiological and other knowledges of pandemics and combining them with lived experience of Long COVID (Callard & Perego, 2021). Long COVID is a new biopolitical identity shaped by the action of affected individuals, their collective agency and the support of their carers and advocates (Löwy & Segata, 2025). Social media action using the #LongCovid hashtag helped to produce these effects (Callard, 2020), underlining the pandemic/social media conditions for recent turnings in public health (Lupton, 2020). Sometimes referred to as 'long haulers' (Weliver, 2022), affected individuals and groups have collectivised in the form of supportive networks to share information, help each other to find supportive clinicians, advocate for clinical research and establish Long COVID's legitimacy as a healthcare problem.

Experiential narratives shared by people with the syndrome have been central to this action on knowing the pandemic and how it could best be managed. These stories have travelled transnationally (Löwy & Segata, forthcoming), appearing in the Anglosphere in the UK and the USA as early as April 2020 among people who reported distressing symptoms that no-one had predicted. Prominent academics and journalists blogged and journaled about their own experiences, marking both the power of mediatised narratives and something of the existential threat posed by the emergence of the virus; and then, for some, its perpetuation in the body and mind.

Long COVID stands as an important example of epistemic injustices connected with the pandemic (Callard, 2020; Callard & Perego, 2021; Löwy & Segata, 2025). Typically, epistemic injustice is considered to be comprised of testimonial and hermeneutical injustices, which are thought to produce material and symbolic harms (Fricker & Jenkins, 2017). Testimonial injustice is said to arise in circumstances wherein the lived experience of individuals and groups is discounted. Hermeneutical injustice is thought to be constituted by political imperatives and prejudices that lead to the misrepresentation of lives, especially for those who experience disadvantage. Testimonial injustices have been regularly documented by people with Long COVID, including experiences of being turned away by medical practitioners (Weliver, 2022). These effects represent the derogation of patients who do not fit with hitherto accepted understandings of how a viral infection and therefore a pandemic comes and goes. These epistemic tensions are at play in the uses of the already noted 'long' and 'post' as different ways of marking pandemic time. The injustices of Long COVID are all the more significant when it is acknowledged that the experience is patterned by unequal access to the resources that can help to resist denialism. For example, Long COVID is more likely to be experienced among African and Hispanic US citizens than others (Jacobs et al., 2023). In the UK, citizens living in deprived areas were most likely to report Long COVID symptoms (Shabnam et al., 2023). There is much at stake in the generation of knowledge and action for Long COVID.

In what follows, I develop my argument regarding the troubling of Long COVID and pandemic timings and endings, to draw out an agenda for the promotion of just and more effective public health. My theory-building approach is framed by the biopolitics of Long COVID and applies the lens of epistemic (in)justice to selected fragments of text from Australian political speeches, a parliamentary inquiry report, public policy documents and commentaries and news media. In the next section, I explore how governments sought political closure of the COVID pandemic in ways that are not easy to reconcile with the realities of Long COVID. I then trace these tensions into scientific debate regarding herd immunity and other attempts to secure the pandemic's ending, with implications for understandings of Long COVID. I then consider how attempts to define Long COVID for research and clinical purposes would benefit from further engagement with testimonial and hermeneutical justice.

Against 'COVID Normal' and Other Pandemic Endings

Long COVID runs counter to an investment in the end of the COVID pandemic that has immense cultural and historical inertia. For instance, the canonical beginning-middle-end structure is a common sense-making narrative form through which events are understood for their individual, relational and ethical implications (Squire et al., 2014). This same structure is found in folk tale narratives that seek to instruct audiences of the moral nuances of conduct in times of crisis (Todd, 2023). Health is similarly narrated as a morality tale with a beginning, middle and end. Sociological functionalism explained the sick role (Parsons, 1975) in terms of the privileges and duties bestowed on the unwell individual who was expected to return to their normal social role once illness had passed (Cheshire et al., 2021). This expectation that illness passes is coded into the promissory discourse of modern medicine in the form of restitution narrative (Frank, 1995).

Unsurprisingly, then, pandemics are also commonly represented as an event in time. Graphic depictions often depict pandemics as waves that grow, peak and subside over time (see, for example, World Health Organization, 2017). This way of depicting pandemic time gives the impression of scientific insight into the natural, biological ordering of birth, proliferation and death. But it is vital to question the sufficiency of this method of knowing about pandemics so that helpful additions can be found, most particularly for Long COVID. Felicity Callard has pointed out that the narrative of pandemic emerging, unfolding and subsiding is co-constitutive of scientific knowledge of pandemics:

> Epidemiology—its epistemological frameworks and concepts—comes to provide the skeleton around which epidemic narratives are built and illness and suffering remembered. Epidemiology's driving motor has political force, too: such a historiography pulls particular actors into the foreground and keeps other actors out of sight. (Callard, 2020, p. 738)

While important for framing how policy could be coordinated over time, the World Health Organization phasic scheme helps to erase real-life experience, especially for those whose experiences are at odds with official pandemic timings and endings. Such hermeneutical effects can be construed to be unjust, not only in the sense of misrepresenting the lives of people with Long COVID but by placing them outside of orthodox pandemic time with consequences for the legitimacy of claims to treatment, care and support.

Alternative readings of the pandemic drama are, of course, possible. Drawing on her own experience of COVID, Callard (2020) has proposed a reordering of commonly accepted pandemic epistemology. She speaks of 'thinking from the sickbed' to direct attention to the lived experience of illness and its contrast with forms of knowledge generated in other contexts, such as laboratories, hospitals and epidemiological surveys. Most particularly, the Long COVID standpoint offers up different ways of understanding pandemic time that honour suffering.

Also offering a resistive COVID episteme, Corinne Squire (forthcoming) has addressed the 'flatten the curve' discourse that became prominent in the UK and elsewhere. With reference to the lived experience of people with HIV, Squire explored how 'flatten the curve' was both appropriated and resisted by individuals responding to the emerging threat of COVID. Importantly, 'flatten the curve' is an experiment in power/knowledge (Foucault, 1991) applied to the manufacture of the pandemic ending. It was very often presented to audiences as graphs of infections and deaths over time, contributing to the pandemic dramaturgy cum epidemiological understanding noted by Callard (2020). 'Flatten the curve' invited publics to help contribute to a collective project of bringing the pandemic to a close, though what to do was not always clear, as Squire noted (forthcoming). When flattening the curve in an absolute sense proved impossible, politicians and scientists recommended what Squire refers to as the normalisation of life under pandemic conditions. Similar effects have been associated with admonishments that publics should 'learn to live with the virus' (Davis, 2022; Lewis et al., 2025; Lupton, 2022).

Politicians seemed especially invested in talking up the pandemic's end (Lewis et al., 2025). The following example comes from a statement by the Australian Prime Minister to Parliament on 13 May 2020:

> We're fighting the virus; flattening the curve, as the Minister for Health set out earlier today in his ministerial statement; extending the economic lifeline connecting to Australians to help them cross that bridge to the other side, as the Treasurer set out yesterday in his ministerial statement; buying us much needed time so now we are able to reopen the economy and the society, based on the important protections that we have put in place. (Commonwealth of Australia, 2020)

Coming in the middle of the first 12 months of the pandemic, this statement expresses a political will to end the pandemic, at least in terms of its economic effects and somewhat pre-emptively as it turned out. The bridge metaphor supplies the way to an imagined post-COVID life. This way of representing the crisis is created on behalf of general publics, implying that some politicians see that their role is to bring an end to the pandemic as governmental exception.

Public health experts questioned the approach adopted by Australia in the first few months of the pandemic (Bowtell, 2021), in particular, for its mixture of sometimes effective and at other times complacent action on the virus and mistaken attempts to foretell of the end of the pandemic. For example, on 1 February 2020, the Federal government-imposed travel restrictions on China and on 20 March 2020 placed restrictions on travellers from any country (Parliament of Australia, 2023a). The first national lockdown of schools and workplaces commenced on 29 March 2020 (Commonwealth of Australia, 2024). These efforts at suppressing viral spread were mostly successful. Until January 2022, Australia had a low incidence of infection compared with, for example, Sweden and the United Kingdom (Mathieu et al., 2020). It is thought that this apparent success led to some complacency on the part of decision makers and delayed Australia's vaccination programme. Vaccination commenced on 21 February 2021 (Commonwealth of Australia, 2024), which was some months after Sweden, Singapore and the United Kingdom (Mathieu et al., 2020). Despite this delay, Australians complied with vaccination policies and by November 2021, 80 of the adult population had been vaccinated (Commonwealth of Australia, 2024).

It is at this point that policymakers proclaimed that the nation could 'transition to living with COVID-19' (Commonwealth of Australia, 2024, p. 9). This position assumed that vaccination would curb transmission and mitigate illness which meant that the virus could be accommodated rather than prevented. This situation was anticipated in news media where a government spokesperson was reported to have stated, 'The government here is working towards something called "COVID-normal", which is life while COVID-19 is around, and I think we're getting pretty close to that' (Snow, 2020). However, in December 2021, just as Australia was 'opening up', the Omicron variant entered, causing a huge increase in COVID cases and deaths (Australian Institute of Health & Welfare, 2022) and thereby contradicting the notion of COVID normal. It was discovered that the initial vaccines did not necessarily reduce transmission (Franco-Paredes, 2022) and as the incidence of Long COVID shows, chronic illness following acute infection had also emerged.

Seeking out the closure of COVID was also linked with some muddying of pandemic knowledge and expertise. In a news article entitled 'Living in COVID "fantasy land"' (Loziol, 2022), the journalist made reference to dissent regarding how to best manage the pandemic, claiming that 'there has always been a range of views in the medical fraternity about how to handle COVID' and that the uncertainties associated with Long COVID should not distract from the overall project of bringing the pandemic to closure. The article also developed the idea that those who propose the continuation of risk mitigation for Long COVID are invested in a fallacious notion of 'COVID zero': that is, that the viral risk can be eradicated. The journalist went on to quote a medical expert who argued that the COVID zero advocates had adopted the erroneous logic of anti-vaxxers:

> Though long-COVID is real [...] it has been misused by hard line COVID-zero advocates in the same way anti-vaxxers said they won't take the vaccine because they don't know its long-term effects.

This way of arranging identities—COVID zero advocates, people with Long COVID, anti-vaxxers—has ideological properties. It identifies those who advocate caution as zero COVID absolutists and demonises any calls for continued caution, that is, any sense in which the pandemic is to continue. Indeed, the article asserts that, 'many who want stronger action on COVID claim the government and media are covering up the true extent of the virus in the community'. This use of language aligns Long COVID precautions with conspiracy theory. Moreover, the alignment of zero COVID advocates with anti-vaxxers perpetrates a sleight-of-hand by providing no evidence that those who advocate for continued public health precautions also reject vaccination. This news discourse interweaved with the reported speech of a medical expert could be construed as hermeneutical injustice for those seeking to take action on Long COVID.

COVID Immunity and Its Others

Long COVID has also been subject to dissent over the value of immunity for managing the pandemic. Long COVID is closely aligned with immunity because some signs and symptoms are thought to reflect immune disfunction (Budge et al., 2016). Links have been made between Long

COVID and myalgic encephalomyelitis/chronic fatigue syndrome (ME/CFS) due to similar signs and symptoms such as fatigue (Komaroff & Lipkin, 2023), the possible transformation of Long COVID into this condition (Jason & Dorri, 2023) and the possible post-viral causes of ME/CFS (Hwang et al., 2023). Sharing knowledge and building alliances are also emerging with people affected by Long COVID and ME/CFS (Callard, 2020).

A key difference between Long COVID and ME/CFS, however, is the notion of herd immunity (Morens et al., 2022). Advocacy for sustaining precautions to inhibit new COVID infections and therefore reducing the chance of an increased Long COVID burden clashes with the theory of herd immunity—and through it, the means to end the pandemic. Herd immunity is a rather crude summary term for the biosocial conditions that reduce the transmission of a pathogen such that it ceases to pose a threat to the health of a population (Sridhar & Gurdasni, 2021). Herd immunity can be achieved when a sufficient proportion of individuals in a population acquire immunity from serious contagious disease. Immunity might be innate, acquired or produced through vaccination.

Advocacy for herd immunity as the way to end the pandemic has been controversial. A famous example of this controversy has been the contrasting views of the Great Barrington Declaration (GBD) (Kulldorf et al., 2020) and the John Snow Memorandum (JSM) (Alwan et al., 2020). In the GBD, Kulldorf, Gupta and Bhattacharya advocated for the relaxation of 'lockdown policies' because, according to them, '[a]s immunity builds in the population, the risk of infection to all—including the vulnerable—falls' (Kulldorf et al., 2020). The JSM was published in *The Lancet* by a large cohort of scholars and asserted that the achievement of herd immunity against COVID 'is a dangerous fallacy unsupported by scientific evidence' (Alwan et al., 2020). The GBD authors advocated for the cessation of social isolation due to worries about its efficacy and economic impact. They therefore advocated for herd immunity as the pathway for ending the pandemic, based on the assumption that humans would eventually develop immunity to the virus through mass infections. In contrast, the JSM authors argued that the cessation of social isolation was unethical due to the biomedical features of the virus and remaining uncertainties. Too many people would die and 'herd' immunity via infection was not likely to be achieved in any case. The JSM's rejection of herd immunity as the answer to ending the pandemic also implied that continued protection from infection is needed. The JSM mentioned the risks posed by Long COVID, advocating protection for those who might develop the condition if exposed to the COVID virus. Moreover, other researchers have argued that, for some of those already with Long COVID, there appears to be some increase in disease symptoms linked with further infections (Willyard, 2023). The effective management of Long COVID, then, stands in opposition to herd immunity and the related concept of 'COVID normal'.

These dissenting views with regard to herd immunity were also found in the news reports of the views and statements of politicians, medical experts and other commentators (Giritli Nygren & Olofsson, 2021). In an example from Australian tabloid news media entitled 'Panic now would be moronic' (O'Brien, 2021), published on 30 November 2021, the journalist reflected on the emergence of the Omicron variant of SARS-Cov-2 and argued against the need for further lockdowns. He claimed that: 'The people of this state are weary of endless lockdowns and social manipulation from this power-hungry mob'. The 'power-hungry mob' may have been a reference to the chief medical officer and the premier of the Australian state of Victoria, who together implemented lengthy lockdowns during 2020 and 2021 (Macreadie, 2022).

This example demonstrated the heated politics evident in the first two years of COVID that centred on how best to manage the pandemic. It also showcased how theories of virology and immunology could be deployed to support the relaxation of precautions, echoing the GBD-JSM debate. The journalist went on to quote a medical expert who was reported to have said:

> If this [Omicron variant] is milder than Delta, you actually want it to spread within your community […] You want it to outcompete Delta and become the predominant circulating virus.

This statement implied herd immunity was the means to enable the world to return to normal. The article ended with the advice that: 'We must not flinch now that the new strain has emerged, but continue to live with the virus in all of its variations'. The article, then, echoed the GBD claims and the more general search for an ending to the pandemic, but in ways, it seems, that were likely to imperil some and ignore the actuality of Long COVID.

One of the important features of this debate is the creation of a COVID immunity hierarchy where the possibilities of living a 'COVID normal' life for some are prioritised over those whose bodies and life chances do not make that possible. We can consider this immunity hierarchy to be a variation on hermeneutical injustice in the sense that it divides publics in such a manner as to enlarge the agency of the immune privileged whilst leaving behind those who are suffering. As *The Lancet* editors put it:

> Although vaccination has become the immediate focus of the pandemic response for many countries, patients with long COVID must not be forgotten or sidelined as countries begin to consider the end of the pandemic. (The Lancet, 2020, p. 1861)

Defining Long COVID

Another way of understanding epistemic justice and Long COVID is found in attempts to define the condition to support the development of research and clinical care. As we have seen, Long COVID is prone to some erasure in the drama-science of pandemic timings and endings. Some immunological assumptions about how to best find a way of life with COVID also fail to address the particular complexities and differences of people with Long COVID. In this final section, we will see that debate about how best to define Long COVID reveals much about its contested scientific and political status.

The example for this section is a Parliament of Australia Long COVID Inquiry, entitled *Sick and Tired: Casting a Long Shadow* (Parliament of Australia, 2023b). This Inquiry was conducted in 2022, involving consultations with 566 private individuals, policymakers, physicians, general practitioners, epidemiologists and immunologists. Among its

239 pages of deliberations and recommendations, the Inquiry report established the view that differing definitions of Long COVID were in use, which has created problems. As noted previously, authorities do acknowledge Long COVID but prefer to use the term 'post-COVID syndrome'. The WHO defines what it calls post-COVID syndrome as 'the continuation or development of new symptoms 3 months after the initial SARS-CoV-2 infection, with these symptoms lasting for at least 2 months with no other explanation' (World Health Organization, 2022). The UK's National Institute for Health and Care Excellence (NICE) uses a temporal schema to define Long COVID, as follows:

> Acute COVID-19: Signs and symptoms of COVID-19 for up to 4 weeks.
> Ongoing symptomatic COVID-19: Signs and symptoms of COVID-19 from 4 weeks up to 12 weeks.
> Post-COVID-19 syndrome: Signs and symptoms that develop during or after an infection consistent with COVID-19, continue for more than 12 weeks and are not explained by an alternative diagnosis. It usually presents with clusters of symptoms, often overlapping, which can fluctuate and change over time and can affect any system in the body. Post-COVID-19 syndrome may be considered before 12 weeks while the possibility of an alternative underlying disease is also being assessed. (National Institute for Health & Care Excellence, 2024, p. 6)

WHO and NICE make reference to 'Long COVID' but appear to see it as a common term for signs and symptoms that continue or develop after acute COVID infection, including ongoing symptomatic COVID-19 (from 4 to 12 weeks) and post-COVID-19 syndrome (12 weeks or more). Though these definitions vary somewhat, they share a commitment to viewing Long COVID as involving a period of 12 weeks after which signs and symptoms cannot be attributed to acute infection. The derivation of the 12-week timeframe is not explained in the inquiry report or in WHO or NICE guidance, but it appears to reflect practitioner and patient experience. For example, a Delphi study focused on Long COVID case definition consulted with 265 individuals, including patients (23%) and experts (52%) and found consensus among participants with regard to the 12-week timeframe for defining Long COVID (Soriano et al., 2022).

It is significant that this 12-week notion is derived from the professional and lived experience of experts and patients. Equally, however, the criterion is likely to reflect the need to find an agreed temporal frame for Long COVID (in contradistinction to acute infection), for the purposes of research and clinical governance. The criterion may have less to do with lived experience than it does with a scientific (and biopolitical) focus on pandemic timings and endings. It would be valuable, too, to have insight into how expert-patient dialogue on the 12-week criterion has been enacted to shed light on the potential for epistemic justice in the development of a useful case definition.

Importantly, submissions to the Australian Parliamentary Inquiry advocated for an agreed definition to help create an evidence base of Long COVID that would meet scientific standards for the comparison and aggregation of data. Notably, the Inquiry only reported on the views of researchers and medical practitioners with regard to Long COVID definitions, though the views of affected individuals were considered in other parts of the report that addressed experience of Long COVID treatment and care. The Inquiry concluded that a Long COVID database should be established for Australia to help create evidence to inform treatment and care. The inquiry committee further recommended that Australia's new Centre for Disease Control should be missioned to establish a definition in consultation with affected community members, among other sources of knowledge and advice.

The spirit of the Inquiry report was consultative and supportive of people affected by Long COVID, but the focus on an agreed definition also demonstrated an epistemic puzzle:

(i) It is difficult to define Long COVID in a manner that can be agreed by stakeholders, which is therefore suggestive of enduring tensions;
(ii) The views of people with Long COVID on how to define it appear to have been omitted;
(iii) An agreed definition has value for governments, science and clinical practice but may not reflect the needs and wants of affected individuals; and
(iv) data-based evidence is seen as a solution for these tensions, but such a data-base requires an agreed definition.

Another problem with deciding on how to define Long COVID without properly consulting affected individuals is that the evidence used to determine it is likely to be partial. In particular, the experiences, views and needs of people with Long COVID are, for the most part, ignored in an institutional practice of testimonial injustice. In 'thinking from the sick bed', Callard (2020) pointed out that research and clinical perspectives on Long COVID are derived from the most ill, hospital-based patients, while the experiences of those who have not attended hospital are likely to be missed. Callard noted that this epistemic problem is expressed in disputes over 'mild' COVID, where this is assumed to be the case for people who do not come into inpatient care. There are likely to be many reasons why ill patients do not come into hospital, particularly during the disruptions produced by the pandemic and exhortations to the public to protect health systems, as occurred in the UK (Backhouse, 2023). These and other perspectives underline the importance of the epistemic justice lens on the production of meaningful and useful long COVID knowledge.

Conclusion

Long COVID is an important disruption of the biopolitics of COVID era public health. The stories crafted and shared by people experiencing illness in ways that were not predicted took form around the #LongCovid hashtag, marking the new conditions for public health agency during the early years of the pandemic. These narratives encode ways of securing legitimacy and effective care and support under conditions where these did not appear to be guaranteed. Long COVID storytelling reflects the short history of the pandemic and how knowledge about it can be shaped dialogically and through the participation of affected people.

As we have seen, political, science and media investments in bringing the pandemic to a close, perhaps mostly as a political problem, were in tension with the experience of people with Long COVID. Assumptions that pandemics form narrative arcs comprised of beginnings, middles and ends led into post-pandemic imaginaries of crossing the bridge, flattening the curve, learning to live with the virus and COVID normal. Long COVID, among other features of SARS-Cov-2, revealed these post-pandemic imaginaries to have political meaning because they did not accommodate the biological realities of the pandemic. Long COVID stories have proved vital for building more sophisticated ways of generating knowledge about pandemics.

The cultural investment in pandemic endings can be traced into the use of the term post-COVID syndrome. Long COVID has arisen out of the agential practices of affected individuals and importantly accommodates uncertainty about the timing of the pandemic and its effects. Post-COVID syndrome adopts a different stance because it pushes infection, and therefore the pandemic, back in time. These are different COVID epistemes, one fashioned from lived experience in dialogue with emerging knowledge of the pandemic, the other aligned with normative and political understandings of pandemic endings.

Epistemic (in)justice is a useful frame for these Long COVID troubles. It draws attention to the ways in which Long COVID testimonies have been ignored, but also to the powers that they have in the making of biopolitical identities and alliances that can force change. More inclusive approaches to immunity and its importance for pandemics are one possible Long COVID legacy. The participation of people with Long COVID in the science and public health that affects them is endorsed but remains in its nascent stages. There is much to be gained through the further development of, for example, ways to define Long COVID that promote research, effective clinical care and preserve epistemic justice. The legacy of Long COVID hopefully will be to make testimonial and hermeneutical injustices less possible for the continuing COVID pandemic and the pandemics forecast to arise in the future.

References

Alwan, N. A., Burgess, R. A., Ashworth, S., Beale, R., Bhadelia, N., Bogaert, D., & Ziauddeen, H. (2020). Scientific consensus on the COVID-19 pandemic: We need to act now. *The Lancet, 396*(10260). https://doi.org/10.1016/S0140-6736(20)32153-X

Australian Institute of Health and Welfare. (2022). *Australia's Health 2022: Data insights*. https://www.aihw.gov.au/reports/australias-health/australias-health-2022-data-insights/data

Backhouse, M. (2023). *'Stay at home, protect the NHS, save lives': A critical discourse analysis of UK Government COVID-19 press conferences* (MSc dissertation, LSE).

Bowtell, W. (2021, July 7). Morrison's 'new deal' for a return to post-COVID normal is not the deal most Australians want. *The Conversation.* https://theconversation.com/morrisons-new-deal-for-a-return-to-post-covid-normal-is-not-the-deal-most-australians-want-163889

Budge, S. L., Thai, J. L., Tebbe, E. A., & Howard, K. A. S. (2016). The intersection of race, sexual orientation, socioeconomic status, trans identity, and mental health outcomes. *The Counseling Psychologist, 44*(7), 1025–1049. https://doi.org/10.1177/0011000015609046

Callard, F. (2020). Epidemic time: Thinking for the sickbed. *Bulletin of the History of Medicine, 94*(4), 727–743. https://doi.org/10.1353/bhm.2020.0093

Callard, F., & Perego, E. (2021). How and why patients made Long COVID. *Social Science & Medicine, 268*,. https://doi.org/10.1016/j.socscimed.2020.113426

Cheshire, A., Ridge, D., Clark, L. V., & White, P. D. (2021). Sick of the sick role: Narratives of what "recovery" means to people with CFS/ME. *Qualitative Health Research, 31*(2), 298–308. https://doi.org/10.1177/1049732320969395

Commonwealth of Australia. (2020, 13 May). House of representatives. Questions without notice. COVID-19: Morrison Government.

Commonwealth of Australia. (2024). *Commonwealth Government COVID-19 response inquiry: Summary. Lessons for the next crisis*. Canberra.

Davis, M. (2022). 'Live with the virus' narrative and pandemic amnesia in the governance of COVID-19. *Social Sciences, 11*(8), 340. https://doi.org/10.3390/socsci11080340

Foucault, M. (1991). Right of death and power over life. In P. Rabinow (Ed.), *The Foucault reader* (pp. 258–272). Penguin.

Franco-Paredes, C. (2022). Transmissibility of SARS-CoV-2 among fully vaccinated individuals. *The Lancet Infectious Diseases, 22*(1), 16. https://doi.org/10.1016/S1473-3099(21)00768-4

Frank, A. (1995). *The wounded storyteller: Body, illness and ethics.* The University of Chicago Press.
Fricker, M., & Jenkins, K. (2017). Epistemic injustice, ignorance, and trans experiences. In A. Garry, S. A. Khader, & A. Stone (Eds.), *The Routledge companion to feminist philosophy* (pp. 268–278). Routledge.
Giritli Nygren, K., & Olofsson, A. (2021). Swedish exceptionalism, herd immunity and the welfare state: A media analysis of struggles over the nature and legitimacy of the COVID-19 pandemic strategy in Sweden. *Current Sociology, 69*(4), 529–546. https://doi.org/10.1177/0011392121990025
Hwang, J.-H., Lee, J.-S., Oh, H.-M., Lee, E.-J., Lim, E.-J., & Son, C.-G. (2023). Evaluation of viral infection as an etiology of ME/CFS: A systematic review and meta-analysis. *Journal of Translational Medicine, 21*(1), 763. https://doi.org/10.1186/s12967-023-04635-0
Jacobs, M. M., Evans, E., & Ellis, C. (2023). Racial, ethnic, and sex disparities in the incidence and cognitive symptomology of long COVID-19. *Journal of the National Medical Association, 115*(2), 233–243. https://doi.org/10.1016/j.jnma.2023.01.016
Jason, L. A., & Dorri, J. A. (2023). ME/CFS and post-exertional malaise among patients with Long COVID. *Neurology International, 15*(1), 1–11. https://doi.org/10.3390/neurolint15010001
Komaroff, A. L., & Lipkin, W. I. (2023). ME/CFS and Long COVID share similar symptoms and biological abnormalities: Road map to the literature. *Frontiers in Medicine, 10*,. https://doi.org/10.3389/fmed.2023.1187163
Kulldorf, M., Gupta, S., & Bhattacharya, J. (2020). *The Great Barrington Declaration.* https://gbdeclaration.org/
Lemke, T. (2010). Beyond Foucault: From biopolitics to the government of life. In U. Brockling (Ed.), *Governmentality: Current issues and future challenges* (pp. 165–184). Routledge.
Lewis, M., Govender, E., & Skogerbø, E. (2025). 'Living with COVID' government narratives: South Africa, Australia, and Norway. In S. Camporesi, S. Mulubale, & M. Davis (Eds.), *Crisis, inequity and legacy: Narrative analyses of the COVID-19 pandemic* (pp. 59–82). Oxford University Press.
Löwy, I., & Segata, J. (2025). Storytelling through Long COVID: Shaping a disease with patient testimonies in the US, UK, and Brazil. In S. Camporesi, S. Mulubale, & M. Davis (Eds.), *Crisis, inequity and legacy: Narrative analyses of the COVID-19 pandemic* (pp. 247–262). Oxford University Press.
Loziol, M. (2022, 29 May). Living in COVID 'fantasy land. *The Sun Herald.*

Lupton, D. (2020). A more-than-human approach to bioethics: The example of digital health. *Bioethics, 34*(9), 969–976. https://doi.org/10.1111/bioe.12798

Lupton, D. (2022). *COVID societies: Theorising the coronavirus crisis*. Routledge.

Macreadie, I. (2022). Reflections from Melbourne, the world's most locked-down city, through the COVID-19 pandemic and beyond. *Microbiology Australia, 43*(1), 3–4. https://doi.org/10.1071/MA22002

Mathieu, E., Ritchie, H., Rodes-Guirai, L., Appel, C., Giattino, C., Hasell, J., & Ortiz-Ospina, E. (2020). Coronavirus pandemic (COVID-19). https://ourworldindata.org/coronavirus

Morens, D. M., Folkers, G. K., & Fauci, A. S. (2022). The concept of classical herd immunity may not apply to COVID-19. *The Journal of Infectious Diseases, 226*(2), 195–198. https://doi.org/10.1093/infdis/jiac109

National Institute for Health and Care Excellence. (2024). COVID-19 rapid guideline: Managing the long-term effects of COVID-19. https://www.nice.org.uk/guidance/ng188/resources/covid19-rapid-guideline-managing-the-longterm-effects-of-covid19-pdf-66142028400325

O'Brien, S. (2021, 30 November). Panic now would be moronic. *Herald Sun*.

Parliament of Australia. (2023a). *Report 494: Inquiry into the Department of Foreign Affairs and Trade's crisis management arrangements*. Joint Committee of Public Accounts and Audit.

Parliament of Australia. (2023b). *Sick and tired: Casting a long shadow. Inquiry into Long COVID and repeated COVID infections*. https://www.aph.gov.au/Parliamentary_Business/Committees/House/Health_Aged_Care_and_Sport/LongandrepeatedCOVID/Report

Parsons, T. (1975). The sick role and the role of the physician reconsidered. *Health and Society, 53*(3), 257–278.

Shabnam, S., Razieh, C., Dambha-Miller, H., Yates, T., Gillies, C., Chudasama, Y. V., & Islam, N. (2023). Socioeconomic inequalities of Long COVID: A retrospective population-based cohort study in the United Kingdom. *Journal of the Royal Society of Medicine, 116*(8), 263–273. https://doi.org/10.1177/01410768231168

Snow, D. (2020, 12 September). Living in limbo. *Sydney Morning Herald*.

Soriano, J. B., Murthy, S., Marshall, J. C., Relan, P., & Diaz, J. V. (2022). A clinical case definition of post-COVID-19 condition by a Delphi consensus. *The Lancet Infectious Diseases, 22*(4). https://doi.org/10.1016/S1473-3099(21)00703-9

Squire, C. (2025). Curves and numbers: Dominant and counteracting narratives of the early COVID-19 UK pandemic. In S. Camporesi, S. Mulubale, & M. Davis (Eds.), *Crisis, inequity and legacy: Narrative analyses of the COVID-19 pandemic* (pp. 37–59). Oxford University Press.

Squire, C., Davis, M., Esin, C., Andrews, M., Harrison, B., Hyden, L., & Hyden, M. (2014). *What is narrative research?* Bloomsbury Academic.

Sridhar, D., & Gurdasni, D. (2021). Herd immunity by infection is not an option: Difficult lessons are learned from a largely uncontrolled COVID-19 epidemic in Manaus, Brazil. *Science, 371*(6526), 230–231.

The Lancet. (2020). Facing up to long COVID. *The Lancet, 396*(10266). https://doi.org/10.1016/S0140-6736(20)32662-3

Todd, K. L. (2023). Remembering a Goan folktale in the midst of a global pandemic. In A. Eizadirad & N. N. Wane (Eds.), *The power of oral culture in education: Theorizing proverbs, idioms, and folklore tales* (pp. 211–227). Springer International Publishing.

Weliver, P. (2022). Long COVID patient narratives: Part 1. https://thepolyphony.org/2022/07/15/long-covid-patient-narratives-part-1/

Willyard, C. (2023). Are repeat COVID infections dangerous? What the science says. *Nature, 616*, 650–653. https://doi.org/10.1038/d41586-023-01371-9

World Health Organization. (2017). *Pandemic influenza risk management: A WHO guide to inform and harmonize national and international pandemic preparedness and response.*

World Health Organization. (2022, 7 November). *Post COVID-19 condition (Long COVID), Fact sheet,* https://www.who.int/europe/news-room/fact-sheets/item/post-covid-19-condition, accessed 8 September 2024.

7

The Profound Societal Impacts of Long COVID and Pandemic Non-interventionism

Pantea Javidan

Introduction

Global Long COVID prevalence indicates a transformative historical moment in which Long COVID disrupts established societal structures and the broader social order, requiring systemic adaptations to achieve stability and equity. Non-intervention in the face of such profound negative changes predicts greater inequities and harms. For the first time in history, the global population exceeds 8 billion people, with rampant international travel, high frequency and volume of indoor crowding, and 90% of human life spent indoors (International Air Transport Association, 2024; Mannan & Al-Ghamdi, 2021; United States Census Bureau, 2023). Inadequate containment and mitigation measures during the COVID pandemic have permanently changed the conditions of human life. People now risk continual exposure to a multi-systemic infectious

P. Javidan (✉)
Department of Psychiatry and Behavioral Sciences, School of Medicine, Stanford University, Stanford, CA, USA
e-mail: pjavidan@stanford.edu

D. Lupton (ed.), *Long COVID and Society*,
https://doi.org/10.1007/978-981-96-9168-5_7

disease known to cause brain damage and immune dysregulation simply through daily interpersonal interactions, particularly in public indoor spaces, in which the bulk of human activity occurs (Davitt et al., 2022; Xu et al., 2022; K. Yin et al., 2024). Humans share indoor air, inhaling potentially pathogenic aerosols that can linger long after the passage of a contagious person (Smith et al., 2020; Wang et al., 2021).

Long COVID presents significant socioeconomic problems, with prevalence rates that are alarming regardless of whether at the lower or higher ends of estimates. Based on 2022 estimates, WHO has recently reported that approximately 200 million people previously experienced or are currently experiencing Long COVID (Torrance et al., 2024, p. 78). Regions such as the Eastern Mediterranean and Turkey report up to 63–64.7% rates of Long COVID among those infected with COVID (Kohn et al., 2024; Silver et al., 2025). Vaccines reduce Long COVID risk by about 20.9%, necessitating more comprehensive public health interventions to encourage vaccine uptake to address the ongoing crisis (Centers for Disease Control and Prevention, 2024a). For example, even in a highly vaccinated population, approximately 20% of Western Australian adults who had tested positive for COVID in 2022 reported Long COVID symptoms, significantly impacting their work, education, and social lives (Woldegiorgis et al., 2024).

What are the implications of nearly all members of society across age groups being subjected to repeat COVID infections when the most commonly reported symptom of Long COVID is chronic fatigue and half of Long COVID survivors report problems related to brain function: typically cognitive deficits and memory impairment (Zürcher et al., 2022)? Venkatesh et al. (2024, p. 2) explain that the COVID pandemic has resulted in 'tremendous economic dislocation in labour markets, creating historically volatile employment and reduced labour force participation rates due to unprecedented occupational health stresses and work loss'. Despite market stabilisation in most nations, and even sustained periods of low unemployment, infections, hospitalisations and deaths from COVID continue to have socioeconomic impacts for a substantial proportion of people. The economic and health impacts of Long COVID are substantial, with chronic fatigue, cognitive impairments, dyspnoea (breathing difficulties) and psychiatric symptoms such as anxiety and depression diminishing workability and productivity (Venkatesh et al., 2024, p. 10). Moreover, there is no compelling evidence supporting the effectiveness of available treatments for Long COVID (Zeraatkar et al., 2024). These health impacts are occurring alongside decreased life expectancy since the COVID pandemic and increased age of retirement within regimes of economic austerity, even in wealthy countries deep cuts to social welfare and public services are redrafting the social contract (Organisation for Economic Co-operation and Development, 2021; Schumacher et al., 2024).

This chapter examines the profound societal impacts of Long COVID, particularly in education and employment, through the lenses of systemic inequities and social determinants of health. A wide range of biomedical studies were reviewed for this chapter, with a particular focus on those addressing occupational, psychosocial and health issues. These studies address symptom persistence, challenges to job seeking and return-to-work, healthcare access, mental health impacts and socioeconomic and demographic disparities. The analysis critiques the effects of government policies of non-interventionism, which prioritise economic interests over public health, exacerbate health disparities and undermine workforce sustainability. It demonstrates how Long COVID's cognitive, psychiatric and psychosocial effects disrupt individual productivity and educational outcomes, disproportionately affecting marginalised populations. Inadequate public health responses to Long COVID, combined with a lack of systemic support, have amplified socioeconomic inequalities. The chapter advocates for robust public health interventions that address these challenges and promote health equity to mitigate the long-term social and economic costs of Long COVID.

Well-Being, Social Structure and Political Contexts

Physical well-being is a multidimensional concept that pertains to health and vitality, encompassing the optimal functioning of the body and active engagement in behaviours promoting and maintaining physical health. It may be defined as a state of physical health characterised by the absence of diseases and adverse health conditions, the ability to perform daily activities with vigour, and decision-making and behaviours that promote and maintain these activities (World Health Organization, 2021). Functional capacity requires executing daily, physical tasks without undue fatigue or limitations, while disease prevention operates to maintain overall health through protective measures. Positive behaviours that maintain baseline health such as nutrition, exercise and adequate sleep are also crucial for physical well-being and are largely determined by socioeconomic factors. Physical well-being also depends heavily upon psychosocial well-being. Both contribute significantly to quality of life and capacity to thrive: that is, to engage productively in society and reach one's full potential. Psychosocial well-being, which includes positive outlooks and cognitive evaluations of life satisfaction, has a significant, protective effect on physical health (Hernandez et al., 2018).

Social structure refers to predictable patterns of relationships and interactions that organise social order, regulation and the distribution of resources, shaping individual and collective actions (Martin, 2009). Workplaces and schools are foundational components of social structure, as they organise economics, labour distribution and social norms (Manstead, 2018). Education and employment are central to identity formation, social status, and broader social roles. Schools are sites of knowledge transmission and socialisation, and key to socioeconomic mobility, fostering cultural cohesion and unifying social identities (Breen & Karlson, 2014). The interconnectedness of schools and workplaces with other social structures—such as kinship networks and government institutions—ensures that their functioning has broad societal implications. Long COVID and laissez-faire public health policies detrimentally impact social structure and disproportionately harm marginalised populations, exposing systemic gaps in healthcare and public health policy and further entrenching inequities, while creating new vulnerabilities (Javidan, 2023, 2024).

Systemic inequities refer to embedded and unjust features of societal systems, laws, policies and institutions which perpetuate inequitable treatment with disproportionate detrimental impacts on marginalised groups based on race, socioeconomic class, gender, generational order and other social determinants. The World Health Organisation defines social determinants of health as 'the conditions in which people are born, grow, work, live, and age, and the wider set of forces and systems shaping the conditions of daily life' (World Health Organization, 2025). These determinants can include factors such as socioeconomic status, education, neighbourhood of residence and physical environment, employment and social support networks, as well as access to healthcare. Economic class—defined by wealth, income and occupation—creates social stratification and inequality, perpetuated through exploitation and cultural practices that shape notions of belonging (Bourdieu, 1987b; Burawoy, 1979; Tonkiss, 2006). Social mobility—which involves shifts in socioeconomic status—tends toward downward than upward mobility, reflecting structural barriers to economic advancement (Bourdieu, 1987a; Connor & Storper, 2020; Lammert, 2021). Although absolute mobility has increased in industrialised societies, relative mobility remains stagnant as wealth is increasingly concentrated upwards (Connor & Storper, 2020). Cumulative effects of social immobility on health outcomes, in turn, increase socioeconomic disparities, particularly across critical life stages (Gugushvili et al., 2021).

A libertarian approach to matters of public interest, including public health emergencies, insists upon government non-intervention (laissez-faire), heavy reliance on private sector involvement, and voluntary compliance with essential services such as vaccination and infectious disease prevention. This approach is shown to exacerbate health disparities due to over-emphasis on individual responsibility and over-reliance on market mechanisms to fulfil societal needs. Libertarian policies of government non-intervention that require the prioritisation of market 'solutions' and personal responsibilisation for structural socioeconomic problems have produced higher levels of inequality and worse health outcomes across socioeconomic groups. As social policy requires coordination—the primary role of government, especially in emergencies—libertarianism is fundamentally at odds with public health (Powers & Faden, 2003).

Adult Workers

Long COVID Prevalence and Symptoms

Global estimates show millions of workers suffering from enduring symptoms of Long COVID, causing substantial economic loss due to work incapacity. Low recovery rates, high economic costs and lack of standardised diagnostic approaches point to urgency for research and resources to manage the long-term impacts of Long COVID. A significant portion of workers report chronic fatigue (40–75%), cognitive dysfunction (20–60%), and respiratory distress (15–50%) (Kohn et al., 2024; Venkatesh et al., 2024). Among working-age adults, prevalence estimates range from 10 to 50%, which depends on demographics, study design and co-morbidities (Lunt et al., 2024b; Venkatesh et al., 2024).

In the USA, nearly 11% of adults are reported to have Long COVID, impacting workforce participation, with one million workers reporting job abandonment or reduced work capacity as a result (Calfas & Overberg, 2024; Clearinghouse for Labor Evaluation and Research, 2024). More specifically, over 40% of US workers exhibit Long COVID three months post-infection, leading to greater work loss, especially for those living with multiple symptoms (Venkatesh et al., 2024). In the UK, about 1 in 13 people of working age are economically inactive due to chronic health conditions. This rate has doubled in just two to three years, suggesting a strong association with COVID infections (Lunt et al., 2024a; Office for National Statistics, 2023). The workforce burden of Long COVID is further exacerbated by demographic disparities. Certain groups such as US farm workers experience 62% prevalence, disproportionately affected by structural factors such as poor labour conditions and lack of healthcare access (Mora et al., 2024).

Neurological and Psychiatric Impacts

The psychiatric sequelae of Long COVID and the increasing focus on its neurocognitive effects (Premraj et al., 2022) indicate profound societal impacts, reshaping structures of education and employment. Anxiety, depression, post-traumatic stress disorder (PTSD) and cognitive impairments are the most prevalent COVID-induced psychiatric disorders. Prevalence rates for anxiety and depression range from 20 to 40%, while PTSD is reported in 10–25% of cases (Anderson et al., 2024; Kohn et al., 2024; Marques et al., 2024; Reuschke et al., 2024; Venkatesh et al., 2024). With Long COVID prevalence among working-age adults ranging from 10 to 50%, a substantial proportion of working people experience neurocognitive sequelae, presenting a substantial burden in high-exposure industries such as healthcare, education, and frontline, essential and public-facing services, in which higher rates of Long COVID and psychiatric effects are reported (Faux-Nightingale et al., 2024; Looker et al., 2024).

It has been estimated that 30–50% of workers experience cognitive impairments that lessen their ability to perform complex or sustained tasks (Krupa et al., 2024). Workers often report inability to focus, retain or recall information, or manage multiple tasks, which has resulted in extended sick leave or reduced work hours (Anderson et al., 2024). Healthcare workers frequently cite new cognitive limitations as a barrier to performing critical tasks requiring precision and skilled decision-making. Among those who manage to return to work, cognitive symptoms often reduce productivity due to making more errors, requiring more time to complete tasks, and struggling to meet deadlines. This is particularly concerning in the most impacted sectors, which are high-stakes environments such as healthcare, education and technology (Krupa et al., 2024; Marques et al., 2024).

In the UK, more than half of Long COVID survivors with cognitive dysfunction had reduced paid work hours or exited employment entirely, with average monthly income reductions of nearly 25% and steeper declines for those with Long COVID for more than two years (Kwon et al., 2024). The aggregate national productivity impact attributable to severe Long COVID is estimated to be 5.7 billion Euros, extrapolated from the study sample. Up to 50% productivity loss is reported in some workers due to Long COVID (Reuschke et al., 2024), as others find 35% of workers becoming unable to work and 40% struggling to work (Green et al., 2024). A dose-response relationship is observed between symptom burden and missed work days, in which those experiencing five or more symptoms are three times as likely to miss substantial amounts of work time (Venkatesh et al., 2024).

COVID not only causes new psychiatric conditions but also exacerbates preexisting ones (Zonglin et al., 2023). Many studies and scoping reviews show severe illness and increased mortality in individuals with mental disorders post-infection (De Hert et al., 2022). High prevalence of depression, anxiety, and PTSD are observed in COVID survivors months after acute infection, with about half of survivors experiencing a high burden of psychiatric sequelae typically, cognitive deficits and memory impairment—which tend to endure (Zürcher et al., 2022) and these affect functional status, mood and physical activity, with higher rates observed among women (Gramaglia et al., 2022). These psychiatric conditions severely impact employability, as workers cite mental health distress as a primary reason for prolonged sick leave or reduced work hours. For example, in the Brazilian population of workers, higher absenteeism is observed due to combined physical and psychiatric symptoms, and Belgian workers report challenges reintegrating into demanding professional workplaces (Kohn et al., 2024; Marques et al., 2024). Even among those reintegrating, neurocognitive symptoms such as anxiety and 'brain fog' result in substantial losses in productivity. For example, UK workers report reductions in productivity of up to 50% (Looker et al., 2024; Reuschke et al., 2024).

Impacts on the Economy, Productivity and Socioeconomic Disadvantage

Long COVID's impact on the macroeconomy is profound. It has been estimated that 10–20% of the 250 million SARS-CoV-2 infected individuals in the WHO European Region are experiencing lingering symptoms. In the USA, Long COVID accounts for up to 15% of job vacancies, with an estimated annual loss of $170 billion in wages, affecting around 4 million workers. These statistics emphasise the critical need for international cooperation to improve Long COVID management and integrate patient experiences into research and treatment strategies (Long COVID Europe). As mentioned earlier, one quarter of

US adult Long COVID survivors are unable to work, which has exacerbated labour shortages and reduced productivity. This has resulted in a persistent labour gap despite high demand for labour (NBC New York, 2022; Liberty Street Economics, 2022; Urban Institute, 2023; Brookings Institution, 2025). It has contributed to economic slowdown through decreased output, income loss and increased healthcare costs. COVID and its long-term effects also deter workforce participation, increasing unemployment and reducing full-time work to part-time among sufferers (Sheiner & Rendell, 2023; Perlis et al., 2023; Sheiner et al., 2025).

The unavailability of paid sick leave in the US exposes the socioeconomic inequities that pervade the workforce, which is exacerbated by Long COVID. As of March 2024, about 20–23% of US civilian workers (between 28 and 34 million Americans) lack access to paid sick leave (Bureau of Labor Statistics, 2024; Mehta & Milli, 2023). This is a significant gap in worker protections, which disproportionately affects lower-income workers: 41% in the lowest earnings quartile are denied paid sick leave, compared to 6% in the highest quartile (Bureau of Labor Statistics, 2024). The disparities are even more pronounced among the lowest earning tenth of workers, where paid sick leave is denied to 61% of workers in this category (Bureau of Labor Statistics, 2024). Service workers, who tend to earn lower wages than other occupations, have varied access to paid sick leave, further highlighting the socioeconomic divide. This is a systemic inequity whereby the most vulnerable workers face greater risks of financial instability, especially when grappling with chronic illness and disability such as Long COVID.

Furthermore, the pandemic has strained the US education system, with nearly half of public schools reporting vacancies by early 2022, many due to COVID or Long COVID, affecting key teaching roles and leading to larger class sizes and reduced services (National Center for Education Statistics). Efforts to counteract this, such as wage increases, are often unreliable and not sustained.

As Long COVID continues to afflict millions, the lack of universal paid sick leave contributes to socioeconomic disparities and underscores the critical need for policies that ensure equitable access to health and financial protections for all workers, irrespective of their income level or job type. But instead the Centers for Disease Control and Prevention's (CDC) 2024 update to its guidance, essentially eliminating the requirement for an isolation period following a COVID diagnosis, will significantly deepen disparities (Centers for Disease Control and Prevention, 2024b). It places workers without access to paid sick leave (disproportionately those in lower-income brackets and service occupations) at a stark disadvantage. With no mandated isolation period, employees feeling pressured to work despite a COVID diagnosis may face difficult choices between safeguarding their health (and that of others) and their financial stability. This situation is especially precarious for workers who lack paid sick leave, compelling them to either risk losing income or attend work while ill, thereby increasing the risk of virus transmission. For Long COVID survivors, the absence of isolation requirements without adequate sick leave protections will cause more severe health outcomes and prolonged recovery times. Rather than comprehensive sick leave policies that protect all workers, public health guidance is effectively penalising the most vulnerable populations.

Sociodemographic Disparities

Demographic factors such as race, ethnicity, socioeconomic status, gender and age greatly affect Long COVID prevalence and impact, due to individual and structural factors, including poverty, health-seeking behaviours, institutional mistrust and cultural incompetence in healthcare (Islamoska et al., 2021; Khanijahani et al., 2021; Saarinen et al., 2022; Shabnam et al., 2023; Mkoma et al., 2024). By amplifying health disparities, reducing workplace productivity and widening structural inequities, Long COVID profoundly disrupts economic class stability and stagnates socioeconomic mobility. Burdening workers with debilitating symptoms such as chronic fatigue and cognitive impairments result in reduced working hours, prolonged absences, and greater risks of permanent withdrawal from employment—all of which cause immediate income loss and downward mobility, particularly for those lacking financial safety nets. The inability of workers to return to cognitively-demanding roles limits career progression, diminishes occupational prestige, and compounds structural and long-term disadvantages. Long COVID jeopardises absolute and relative mobility by reducing household incomes, contributing to factors that perpetuate intergenerational poverty, and obstructing career trajectories, particularly for those in high-exposure roles such as healthcare and education.

Black and Hispanic workers in the US are disproportionately affected by severe Long COVID symptoms due to higher rates of reinfection and systemic inequities in resources and healthcare access (Khullar et al., 2023; Subramanian et al., 2022). Lower socioeconomic status and poor work-life conditions exacerbate these disparities, as seen in Brazil and India, where financial instability and lack of paid sick leave compound Long COVID symptoms like chronic fatigue and cognitive impairments (Anderson et al., 2024; Reuschke et al., 2024). Gender disparities are also evident, with women, particularly in healthcare, education and caregiving roles, facing higher rates of chronic fatigue, anxiety, and depression caused by increased exposure and psychosocial burdens (Gemma et al., 2024; Kohn et al., 2024; Lunt et al., 2024a, 2024b; Marques et al., 2024). Additionally, age-related trends show that younger workers report more cognitive impairments, while older workers experience more physical symptoms, challenging the assumption that younger age is protective against Long COVID (Marques et al., 2024; Masahiko et al., 2024; Shang et al., 2024; Subramanian et al., 2022). These intersecting vulnerabilities, particularly among women of colour in low-income caregiving roles, intensify hardships related to health, productivity, and workability, underscoring the need to address social determinants of health and improve infection control measures (Mkoma et al., 2024; Venkatesh et al., 2024).

Protective factors for Long COVID—which mitigate its development and negative productivity—include vaccination, early medical intervention, equitable workplace policies and proactive psychosocial support (Landry et al., 2022; Mkoma et al., 2024; Shang et al., 2024). Personal protection measures, such as well-fitted high-filtration respirators (masks) and indoor air quality (IAQ) management, are most effective in reducing exposure and subsequent Long COVID prevalence (Bland et al., 2023). Supportive workplace policies, including flexible labour arrangements, phased return-to-work programs and paid sick leave, are essential to alleviating symptoms and promoting recovery (Bland et al., 2023; Green et al., 2024; Lunt et al., 2024a).

Conversely, systemic failures in workplace safety measures—such as inadequate personal protective equipment (PPE) and poor air quality—exacerbate Long COVID risks, particularly in high-stress sectors like healthcare and education, where emotional labour and burnout increase Long COVID severity (Bland et al., 2023; Torrance et al., 2024). Socioeconomic factors such as delayed healthcare access and financial instability force lower-income workers to return to work prematurely, worsening symptoms and prolonging recovery. The strained context in which these changes occur predicts its harms. For example, due to financial strain, over half of educators in California struggle to cover healthcare costs due to high out-of-pocket expenses, with 37% having skipped or delayed medical care, even while possessing 'good' health insurance (California Teachers Association, 2025).

Children and Adolescents

Long COVID Prevalence and Symptoms

Paediatric Long COVID shares key characteristics with adult Long COVID but presents some distinct symptoms and impacts uniquely affecting children and young people. Recent studies show paediatric Long COVID prevalence ranging from approximately 23–40% of those who have had COVID (Huynh Ngoc et al., 2024; Looker et al., 2024; Y. Yin et al., 2024). These children experience prolonged symptoms that most commonly include chronic fatigue, headaches and learning difficulties. These conditions disrupt educational attainment, critical development milestones, and social participation, which significantly diminishes a child's quality of life. Paediatric COVID also presents psychiatric effects, including anxiety, depression, mood dysregulation and social withdrawal (Huynh Ngoc et al., 2024; Krupa et al., 2024; Torrance et al.,

2024). Psychiatric symptoms are particularly concerning for their disruption of academic achievement, athletic activity and peer relationships, which risk impeding developmental progress during critical life stages.

Neurological and Psychiatric Impacts

Paediatric COVID most commonly presents chronic fatigue and cognitive impairments, including learning impairments, attention problems and difficulties with recall and retention (memory), attention and executive functioning (Huynh Ngoc et al., 2024; Looker et al., 2024). Unlike adults, who primarily experience diminished work productivity, Long COVID diminishes children's capacities during key life stages of development, learning and socialisation, with negative consequences for their life chances through poorer academic performance. The cognitive deficits that paediatric COVID presents also compromise strategic thinking and coordination, which impact athletic skills and can limit participation in extracurricular activities (Ludvigsson, 2023). Long COVID often impairs social functioning, causing children to struggle to interpret social cues and maintain friendships, which can lead to isolation, declining self-esteem and psychological distress (Abrams, 2024).

Implications

The profound impacts of unmitigated COVID transmission in educational settings, communities and households can be demonstrated through the percentage of US children infected with SARS-CoV-2 and the range that develop Long COVID, according to the most recent studies. Nearly all US children have been infected with SARS-CoV-2. As of December 2022, 92% of US children had antibodies indicating a previous COVID infection, a percentage which can reasonably be expected to have increased since then, and it likely does not capture children who do not seroconvert following infection (Vahratian et al., 2023). Applying the percentage of children who develop Long COVID based on 2024 studies, which ranges between 23 and 40%, to the estimate that at least 92% of US children have been infected with SARS-CoV-2, it can be suggested that approximately 21–37% of US children likely have developed or will develop Long COVID. This represents an alarming estimate of the Long COVID burden on US children, but a more reliable one than those presenting lower estimates. The 2024 studies provide more comprehensive, diverse and statistically robust data, incorporating broader symptom criteria, longitudinal data and clinical findings, compared to those which use more restrictive definitions or sample only hospitalised children, which risks underestimation.

Furthermore, the paediatric Long COVID burden emerges in a national context in which a significant portion of the US child population has underlying conditions that place them at high risk of severe outcomes from COVID or death. Using only a single factor, more than 40% of US children are either overweight, obese or severely obese, thus putting a major portion of the child population at high risk unless commensurate institutional or familial awareness and action are implemented (National Institute of Diabetes and Digestive and Kidney Disease, 2025). This does not include other high-risk conditions among children, such as cancers, chronic diseases including asthma and diabetes, disabilities and mental health conditions. Moreover, physical inactivity is listed as a high-risk factor. According to data from 2023 to 2024, the vast majority of US children and adolescents (between 72 and 80%) do not meet the recommendation for daily physical activity (Centers for Disease Control and Prevention, 2024c, 2025).

Higher body mass index risks increased inflammation, reduced immune response, cardiovascular and respiratory inefficiency and higher probabilities of requiring intensive care during acute illness (Ferreira et al., 2021; Singh et al., 2022). Reinfections increase cumulative risk for long-term health consequences, whereby more infections increase the likelihood of developing severe or lasting symptoms, increasing risk of severe illnesses and complications (Bowe et al., 2022). Given that children with obesity comprise such a large percentage of the population, many risk worse and longer-lasting Long COVID symptoms, as obesity exacerbates conditions such as fatigue and cognitive and respiratory difficulties. Compounding conditions and co-morbidities may lead to a vicious cycle of each hampering recovery from the other. Strained healthcare systems under austerity regimes are ill-equipped to provide increasing resources required for long-term management of chronic conditions.

Societal impacts of paediatric Long COVID include chronic school absenteeism, which has doubled among US students since the pandemic (Attendance Works, 2024). In 2024, as new studies showed alarming paediatric Long COVID prevalence rates, an alarming one-third of public-school students in the US became chronically absent. This is largely attributed to direct effects of COVID itself (infections, illness and Long COVID) particularly in the poorest districts, which are hardest hit by COVID (Attendance Works, 2024). A chronically ill youth population requires accommodations in school and future workplaces in a political economy unwilling to even acknowledge the existence of this problem, but which will nonetheless experience productivity loss, increased disability claims and economic strain. Health inequities are worsening health outcomes, as obesity and Long COVID disproportionately impact children from lower socioeconomic backgrounds with less access to vaccinations, preventive healthcare, and early interventions to remedy either condition (Ayala-Marín et al., 2020; Davison et al., 2021; Jin & Jones-Smith, 2015; Oliveira et al., 2022; Singh, 2017; Tran et al., 2024). Obesity and Long COVID exacerbate depression, anxiety and reduce overall well-being and may persist into adulthood with potential effects on long-term mental health.

Current and foreseeable impacts of unmitigated COVID transmission among US children in ongoing reinfection cycles amidst near-ubiquitous exposure of US children ensure a significant public health problem and the persistence of societal burdens, including strained healthcare and education systems. The combination of high rates of infection, obesity and Long COVID increases demand for healthcare services while paediatric clinics and hospitals are already strained and need for long-term care increases. Impacted children will require continual health monitoring, rehabilitation, psychological supports and specialist medical care in overburdened healthcare systems. Higher rates of depression, anxiety and suicide observed among US children increase demand for psychiatric services, particularly as they become adults with chronic health conditions. The social costs of such psychological strain will be absorbed by families, communities, and depleted public health systems.

Similar to adults, children and young people in low- and middle-income countries and those in lower-income communities in wealthy nations contend with compounded risks from inadequate preventive measures and healthcare access, poor nutrition and baseline health and overcrowded living conditions, which risk over-exposure to SARS 2 and greater Long COVID severity and duration. Public health policies that include robust infection prevention measures and vaccination programs have resulted in lower paediatric Long COVID complications, while weaker ones have led to higher post-infection burdens for children (Bland et al., 2023; Kohn et al., 2024; Mkoma et al., 2024; Salci et al., 2024; Torrance et al., 2024).

The common response of retributive policies enforcing presenteeism and increasing academic pressures on teachers and students to correct 'learning loss' is failing to achieve its stated aims because it avoids the major root causes—unmitigated infectious disease and attendant Long COVID risks—while placing greater pressure on overburdened children and families, particularly since educational pressures exacerbate Long COVID effects in children and young people (Y. Yin et al., 2024). Contrary to the entrenched myth that COVID risks are negligible for young children, they are particularly vulnerable to Long COVID's disruption of critical stages of cognitive and social development, which magnify long-term impacts (Huynh Ngoc et al., 2024; Looker et al., 2024). COVID hospitalisation rates among infants less than 6 months old are higher than rates among any other age group, except adults over 75 years of age, and are comparable to rates among adults aged 65–74 years old (Havers et al., 2024). Studies from 2024 show that the greatest risk factors for paediatric Long COVID are socioeconomic disparities, severe initial COVID infections (the risks of which increase with rampant reinfections) and pre-existing vulnerabilities, which are far more prevalent than commonly understood or reflected in policy (Huynh Ngoc et al., 2024; Mkoma et al., 2024; Salci et al., 2024). Infection prevention measures such as universal masking and improved ventilation in schools and healthcare settings are highly effective protections, especially when systematically implemented (Bland et al., 2023; Howard et al., 2024; Torrance et al., 2024). The abandonment of PPE protocols, even during periods of high transmission that contribute to chronic absenteeism, and lack of IAQ management in these major transmission hubs predict poor outcomes for the health and life chances of children and youth.

Conclusion

The consequences of non-intervention in the ongoing pandemic are profound and far-reaching. The isolation that Long COVID survivors experience from their communities and workplaces contribute to social disconnection, alienation and lack of support, especially where workplace accommodations are inadequate. Weakened social cohesion among marginalised communities as well as high-risk professions deepen socioeconomic inequities. Persistent health problems, diminished earnings and precarity have significant negative effects on socioeconomic participation and quality of life, particularly as demands increase for long-term medical care and rehabilitation services under regimes of austerity inherently resistant to systemic adaptations to meet growing needs. Increased healthcare expenditures amidst rising job insecurity risk economic instability on personal and societal levels.

By prioritising free-market individualism to the exclusion of coordinated and inclusive public health measures, health disparities are predictably exacerbated and met with a disinterested polity. Laissez-faire policies eradicate awareness and competence regarding COVID and obfuscate its substantial role in increasing chronic illness and socioeconomic problems. This non-policy worsens health outcomes while undermining economic stability, as persistent health issues contribute to diminished productivity, chronic absenteeism, and reduce labour force and educational participation. Inadequate healthcare and lack of structural supports for workers and students further entrench socioeconomic inequities, deepening cycles of poverty, disability and reduced quality of life. Failure to implement coordinated policies based on scientific consensus, empiricism and commitment to public health to mitigate Long COVID impacts and prevent further transmission widens inequalities, threatens workforce sustainability and overburdens healthcare, educational and social systems along with workers and students contributing their labour and efforts to a system that is abandoning them. Long COVID in both children and adults clearly requires early intervention, ongoing screening and integrated care, which healthcare systems, especially in the US, are ill-equipped to provide (Marques et al., 2024; Venkatesh et al., 2024). Policy solutions emphasising workplace and educational setting accommodations, protective measures and infrastructural adjustments are essential to improving outcomes and sustaining workforce viability, as seen in countries with robust support systems (Hoerger, 2023a, 2023b; Solomou et al., 2024).

References

Abrams, Z. (2024). The reality of pediatric long COVID. *Monitor on Psychology, 54*(3). https://www.apa.org/monitor/2023/04/pediatric-long-covid

Anderson, E., Hunt, K., MacLean, A., Wild, C., Ziebland, S., & Nettleton, S. (2025). Episodic disability and adjustments for work: the 'rehabilitative work' of returning to employment with Long COVID. *Disability and Society, 40*(5), 239–1261. https://doi.org/10.1080/09687599.2024.2331722

Attendance Works. (2024). *Stemming the surge in chronic absence: What states can do.* https://www.attendanceworks.org/wp-content/uploads/2019/06/Policy-Brief-2024-062524.pdf

Ayala-Marín, A. M., Iguacel, I., Miguel-Etayo, P. D., & Moreno, L. A. (2020). Consideration of social disadvantages for understanding and preventing obesity in children. *Frontiers in Public Health, 8*. https://doi.org/10.3389/fpubh.2020.00423

Bland, D., Evans, R., Binesmael, A., Wood, S., Qureshi, S. P., Fearnley, K., Small, A., Strain, W. D., & Agius, R. (2023). Post-acute COVID-19 complications in UK doctors: Results of a cross-sectional survey. *Occupational Medicine, 74*(1), 99–103. https://doi.org/10.1093/occmed/kqad120

Bourdieu, P. (1987a). *Distinction: A social critique of the judgement of taste*. Harvard University Press.

Bourdieu, P. (1987b). What makes a social class? On the theoretical and practical existence of groups. *Berkeley Journal of Sociology, 32*, 1–17.

Bowe, B., Xie, Y., & Al-Aly, Z. (2022). Acute and postacute sequelae associated with SARS-CoV-2 reinfection. *Nature Medicine, 28*(11), 2398–2405. https://doi.org/10.1038/s41591-022-02051-3

Breen, R., & Karlson, K. B. (2014). Education and social mobility: New analytical approaches. *European Sociological Review, 30*(1), 107–118.

Brookings Institution. (2025). New data shows long Covid is keeping as many as 4 million people out of work. *Brookings*. Retrieved from https://www.brookings.edu/articles/new-data-shows-long-covid-is-keeping-as-many-as-4-million-people-out-of-work/

Burawoy, M. (1979). *Manufacturing consent: Changes in the labor process under monopoly capitalism*. University of Chicago Press.

Bureau of Labor Statistics. (2024). *Percent of U.S. civilian workers with access to paid sick leave by occupation*. https://www.bls.gov/ebs/factsheets/paid-sick-leave.htm

Calfas, J., & Overberg, P. (2024, August 26). Long COVID knocked a million Americans off their career paths. *The Wall Street Journal*. https://www.wsj.com/health/wellness/long-covid-knocked-a-million-americans-off-their-career-paths-48926445

California Teachers Association. (2025). *The state of California's Public Schools*. https://www.cta.org/document/the-state-of-ca-public-schools

Centers for Disease Control and Prevention. (2024a). *Long COVID: Household pulse survey. National center for health statistics*. https://www.cdc.gov/nchs/covid19/pulse/long-covid.htm

Centers for Disease Control and Prevention. (2024b). *CDC updates and simplifies respiratory virus recommendations* https://www.cdc.gov/media/releases/2024/p0301-respiratory-virus.html

Centers for Disease Control and Prevention. (2024c). *Physical activity facts*. https://www.cdc.gov/physical-activity-education/data-research/facts-stats/index.html

Centers for Disease Control and Prevention. (2025). *People with certain medical conditions and COVID-19 risk factors*. https://www.cdc.gov/covid/risk-factors/index.html

Clearinghouse for Labor Evaluation and Research. (2024). *Rapid evidence review: Long COVID and the workforce*. https://clear.dol.gov/sites/default/files/documents/files/44696_CLEAR_Rapid_Review_Synthesis_Long_COVID_and_the_Workforce_v4_03112024_508.pdf?

Connor, D. S., & Storper, M. (2020). The changing geography of social mobility in the United States. *Proceedings of the National Academy of Sciences of the United States of America, 117*(48), 30309–30317. https://doi.org/10.1073/pnas.2010222117

Davison, G. M., Fowler, L. A., Ramel, M., Stein, R. I., Conlon, R. P., Saelens, B. E., Welch, R. R., Perri, M. G., Epstein, L. H., & Wilfley, D. E. (2021). Racial and socioeconomic disparities in the efficacy of a family-based treatment programme for paediatric obesity. *Pediatric Obesity, 16*(10). https://doi.org/10.1111/ijpo.12792

Davitt, E., Davitt, C., Mazer, M. B., Areti, S. S., Hotchkiss, R. S., & Remy, K. E. (2022). COVID-19 disease and immune dysregulation. *Best Practice and Research Clinical Haematology, 35*(3). https://doi.org/10.1016/j.beha.2022.101401

De Hert, M., Mazereel, V., Stroobants, M., De Picker, L., Van Assche, K., & Detraux, J. (2022). COVID-19-related mortality risk in people with severe mental illness: A systematic and critical review. *Frontiers in Psychiatry, 12*. https://doi.org/10.3389/fpsyt.2021.798554

Dorfman, D., & Wolff, J. L. (2023). Approving workplace accommodations for patients with long COVID. *New England Journal of Medicine, 389*(14), 1291–1293. https://www.nejm.org/doi/full/10.1056/NEJMp2302676

Faux-Nightingale, A., Saunders, B., Burton, C., Chew-Graham, C. A., Somayajula, G., Twohig, H., & Welsh, V. (2024). Experiences and care needs of children with long COVID: a qualitative study. *BJGP Open, 8*(1). https://doi.org/10.3399/BJGPO.2023.0143

Ferreira, M. E. R., de Andrade, A. V. S., Queiroz, A. A. F., Martins-Filho, P. R., de Aquino Neves, E. L., de Carvalho, F. O., de Souza Araujo, A. A., Silva, É. R., & Nunes, P. S. (2021). COVID-19 and obesity: A systematic review and meta-analysis on the pre-existing clinical conditions, COVID-19 symptoms, laboratory findings and clinical outcomes. *EXCLI Journal: Experimental and Clinical Sciences, 20*, 1610–1614. https://doi.org/10.17179/excli2021-4226

Gemma, T., Diana, P., Constanza, J.-A., Lucia, A. C.-R., Concepció, V., Tomás, L.-J., Veronica, R., Alba, M. C., Laura, M.-P., Israel, R.-G., & Anna, B. (2024). Characterisation, symptom pattern and symptom clusters from a retrospective cohort of Long COVID patients in primary care in Catalonia. *BMC Infectious Diseases, 24*(1), 1–16.

Gramaglia, C., Gattoni, E., Gambaro, E., Bellan, M., Balbo, P. E., Baricich, A., Sainaghi, P. P., Pirisi, M., Binda, V., Feggi, A., & Jona, A. (2022). Anxiety, stress and depression in COVID-19 survivors from an Italian cohort of hospitalized patients: Results from a 1-year follow-up. *Frontiers in Psychiatry, 13*. https://doi.org/10.3389/fpsyt.2022.862651

Green, C. E., Leeds, J. S., & Leeds, C. M. (2024). Occupational effects in patients with post-COVID-19 syndrome. *Occupational Medicine, 74*(1), 86–92. https://doi.org/10.1093/occmed/kqad118

Gugushvili, A., Bulczak, G., Zelinska, O., & Koltai, J. (2021). Socioeconomic position, social mobility, and health selection effects on allostatic load in the United States. *PLoS ONE, 16*(8), 1–22. https://doi.org/10.1371/journal.pone.0254414

Havers, F. P., Whitaker, M., Chatwani, B., Patton, M. E., Taylor, C. A., Chai, S. J.,…COVID-NET Surveillance Team. (2024). *Morbidity and Mortality Weekly Report: COVID-19–associated hospitalizations and maternal vaccination among infants aged. 6 months*. https://www.cdc.gov/mmwr/volumes/73/wr/pdfs/mm7338a1-H.pdf

Hernandez, R., Bassett, S. M., Boughton, S. W., Schuette, S. A., Shiu, E. W., & Moskowitz, J. T. (2018). Psychological well-being and physical health: Associations, mechanisms, and future directions. *Emotion Review, 10*(1), 18–29. https://doi.org/10.1177/1754073917697824

Hoerger, M. (2023a, August 23). U.S. SARS-CoV-2 wastewater levels, COVID-19 cases, and 3-week forecast: Report for August 23, 2023. Pandemic Mitigation Collaborative. https://pmc19.com/data/PMC_Report_Aug23_2023.pdf

Hoerger, M. (2023b, October 30). U.S. SARS-CoV-2 wastewater levels, COVID-19 cases, and 3-week forecast: Report for October 30, 2023. Pandemic Mitigation Collaborative. https://pmc19.com/data/PMC_Report_Oct30_2023.pdf

Howard, J., Cloeren, M., & Vanichkachorn, G. (2024). Long COVID and occupational medicine practice. *Journal of Occupational & Environmental Medicine, 66*(1), 1–5. https://doi.org/10.1097/JOM.0000000000002961

Huynh Ngoc, L., Nguyen The, T., Le Thi Minh, T., Nguyen Tu, L., Nguyen Thi To, U., Le Thanh Thao, T., Truong Thanh, N., & Doan Hoang, P. (2024). Prevalence and risk factors associated with long COVID symptoms in children and adolescents in a southern province of Vietnam. *Asian Pacific Journal of Tropical Medicine, 17*(3), 119–128.

Linh, H. N., Loan, N. T., Uyen, N. T. T., Trang, L. T. T., Nam, T. T., & Phu, D. H. (2024). Prevalence and risk factors associated with Long COVID symptoms in children and adolescents in a southern province of Vietnam. *Asian Pacific Journal of Tropical Medicine, 17*(3), 119–128. https://doi.org/10.4103/apjtm.apjtm_781_23

International Air Transport Association. (2024). *Industry statistics: Fact sheet.* https://www.iata.org/en/iata-repository/pressroom/fact-sheets/industry-statistics/

Islamoska, S., Petersen, J. H., Benfield, T., & Norredam, M. (2021). Socioeconomic and demographic risk factors in COVID-19 hospitalization among immigrants and ethnic minorities. *European Journal of Public Health, 32*(2), 302–310.

Javidan, P. (2023). The struggle to breathe: Pandemic years on Western frontiers. *Legalities: The Journal of Law and Society in Australia and New Zealand, 3*(1), 71–96. https://doi.org/10.3366/legal.2023.0046

Javidan, P. (2024). False divisions and dubious equivalencies: Children's right during the COVID-19 pandemic. In S. S. F. Regilme (Ed.), *Children's rights in crisis: Multidisciplinary, transnational, and comparative perspectives* (pp. 46–70). Manchester University Press.

Jin, Y., & Jones-Smith, JC. (2015). Associations between family income and children's physical fitness and obesity in California, 2010–2012. *Preventing Chronic Disease, 12*. https://doi.org/10.5888/pcd12.140392

Khanijahani, A., Iezadi, S., Gholipour, K., Azami-Aghdash, S., & Naghibi, D. (2021). A systematic review of racial/ethnic and socioeconomic disparities in COVID-19. *International Journal for Equity in Health, 20*(1), 248.

Khullar, D., Zhang, Y., Zang, C., Xu, Z., Wang, F., Weiner, M. G., Carton, T. W., Rothman, R. L., Block, J. P., & Kaushal, R. (2023). Racial/Ethnic Disparities in Post-acute Sequelae of SARS-CoV-2 Infection in New York: An EHR-Based Cohort Study from the RECOVER Program. *Journal of General Internal Medicine, 38*(5), 1127–1136.

Kohn, L., Dauvrin, M., Detollenaere, J., Primus-de Jong, C., Maertens de Noordhout, C., Castanares-Zapatero, D., Cleemput, I., & Van den Heede, K. (2024). Long COVID and return to work: A qualitative study. *Occupational Medicine, 74*(1), 29–36. https://doi.org/10.1093/occmed/kqac119

Krupa, V., Martina, R., Anna, S.-J., Elena, A., & Veena, K. (2024). Cognitive and mental health trajectories of COVID-19: Role of hospitalisation and long-COVID symptoms. *European Psychiatry, 67*. https://doi.org/10.1192/j.eurpsy.2024.7

Kwon, J., Milne, R., Rayner, C., Rocha Lawrence, R., Mullard, J., Mir, G., Delaney, B., Sivan, M., & Petrou, S. (2024). Impact of Long

COVID on productivity and informal caregiving. *The European Journal of Health Economics, 25*(7), 1095–1115. https://doi.org/10.1007/s10198-023-01653-z

Lammert, C. (2021). Dream a little American dream with me: Income inequality and social mobility in the United States. *Amerikastudien/American Studies, 66*(1), 111–115. https://doi.org/10.33675/AMST/2021/1/19

Landry, S. A., Subedi, D., Barr, J. J., MacDonald, M. I., Dix, S., Kutey, D. M., Mansfield, D., Hamilton, G. S., Edwards, B. A., & Joosten, S.A. (2022). Fit-tested N95 masks combined with portable high-efficiency particulate air filtration can protect against high aerosolized viral loads over prolonged periods at close range. *The Journal of Infectious Diseases, 226*(2), 199–207. https://doi.org/10.1093/infdis/jiac195

Liberty Street Economics (Federal Reserve Bank of New York). (2022). Long COVID appears to have led to a surge of the disabled in the workplace. https://libertystreeteconomics.newyorkfed.org/2022/10/long-covid-appears-to-have-led-to-a-surge-of-the-disabled-in-the-workplace/

Looker, K. J., McClenaghan, E., Judd, A., Pierotti, L., Downing, H., Phelan, J., Warren-Gash, C., Ngozi, K., Dawe, F., Relton, C., & Christensen, H. (2024). Acute and long-term outcomes of SARS-CoV-2 infection in school-aged children in England: Study protocol for the joint analysis of the COVID-19 schools infection survey (SIS) and the COVID-19 mapping and mitigation in schools (CoMMinS) study. *PLoS ONE, 19*(5). https://doi.org/10.1371/journal.pone.0303892&type=printable. https://doi.org/10.1371/journal.pone.0303892

Ludvigsson, J. F. (2023). Long COVID in children and adolescents: Mechanisms, symptoms, and outcomes. *Journal of Clinical Medicine, 14*(2). https://doi.org/10.3390/jcm14020378

Lunt, J., Hemming, S., Burton, K., Elander, J., & Baraniak, A. (2024a). What workers can tell us about post-COVID workability. *Occupational Medicine, 74*(1), 15–23. https://doi.org/10.1093/occmed/kqac086

Lunt, J., Hemming, S., Elander, J., Burton, K., & Hanney, B. (2024b). Sustaining work ability amongst female professional workers with long COVID. *Occupational Medicine, 74*(1), 104–112. https://doi.org/10.1093/occmed/kqad134

Mannan, M., & Al-Ghamdi, S. G. (2021). Indoor air quality in buildings: A comprehensive review on the factors influencing air pollution in residential and commercial structure. *International Journal of Environmental Research and Public Health, 18*(6). https://doi.org/10.3390/ijerph18063276

Manstead, A. S. R. (2018). The psychology of social class: How socioeconomic status impacts thought, feelings, and behaviour. *British Journal of Social Psychology, 57*(2), 267–291. https://doi.org/10.1111/bjso.12251

Marques, F. R. D. M., Laranjeira, C., Carreira, L., Gallo, A. M., Baccon, W. C., Paiano, M., Baldissera, V. D. A., & Salci, M. A. (2024). Illness experiences of Brazilian people who were hospitalized due to COVID-19 and faced Long COVID repercussions in their daily life: A constructivist grounded theory study. *Behavioral Sciences, 14*(1). https://doi.org/10.3390/bs14010014

Martin, J. L. (2009). *Social structures*. Princeton University Press.

Masahiko, O., Noriyuki, I., Sho, K., Ichiro, K., Kengo, N., Hideki, T.,…Koichi, F. (2024). Upper respiratory symptoms as Long COVID: Insight from a multicenter cohort study. *OTO Open, 8*(1). https://doi.org/10.1002/oto2.120

Mehta, S., & Milli, J. (2023). Millions of working people still don't have access to a single paid sick day. https://www.clasp.org/wp-content/uploads/2023/05/2023.5.31_Millions-of-Working-People-Still-Dont-Have-Access-to-A-Single-Paid-Sick-Day.pdf

Mkoma, G. F., Agyemang, C., Benfield, T., Rostila, M., Cederstrom, A., Petersen, J. H., & Norredam, M. (2024). Risk of long COVID and associated symptoms after acute SARS-COV-2 infection in ethnic minorities: A nationwide register-linked cohort study in Denmark. *PLoS Medicine, 21*(2). https://doi.org/10.1371/journal.pmed.1004280

Mora, A. M., Kogut, K., Sandhu, N. K., Ridgway, D., Patty, C. M., Renteria, M., Morga, N., Rodriguez, M. T., Romero, M., Valdovinos, J. M., & Torres-Nguyen, A. (2024). SARS-CoV-2 infection and Long COVID among California farmworkers. *Journal of Rural Health, 40*(2), 292–302. https://doi.org/10.1111/jrh.12796

National Institute of Diabetes and Digestive and Kidney Disease. (2025). *Overweight & obesity statistics*. https://www.niddk.nih.gov/health-information/health-statistics/overweight-obesity?

NBC New York (in partnership with CNBC). (2022, December 8) Long Covid is distorting the labor market–and that's bad for the U.S economy. CNBC / NBC New York. https://www.nbcnewyork.com/news/business/money-report/long-covid-is-distorting-the-labor-market-and-thats-bad-for-theus-economy/

Office for National Statistics. (2023). *Rising ill health and economic inactivity because of long-term sickness, UK: 2019 to 2023.* https://www.ons.gov.uk/employmentandlabourmarket/peoplenotinwork/economicinactivity/articles/risingillhealthandeconomicinactivitybecauseoflongtermsicknessuk/2019to2023

Oliveira, C. R., Feemster, K. A., & Ulloa, E. R. (2022). Pediatric COVID-19 health disparities and vaccine equity. *Journal of the Pediatric Infectious Diseases Society, 11*(Supplement_4), S141–S147. https://doi.org/10.1093/jpids/piac091

Organisation for Economic Co-operation and Development. (2021, 8 December 2021). Pensions protected during COVID-19 pandemic but ageing challenges persist, says OECD. https://www.oecd.org/en/about/news/press-releases/2021/12/pensions-protected-during-covid-19-pandemic-but-ageing-challenges-persist.html

Ottiger, M., Poppele, I., Sperling, N., Schlesinger, T. & Muller, K. (2024). Work ability and return-to-work of patients with post-COVID-19: A systematic review and meta-analysis. *BMC Public Health, 24.* https://doi.org/10.1186/s12889-024-19328-6

Perlis, R. H., Trujillo, K. L., Safarpour, A. et al. (2023). Association of post–COVID-19 condition symptoms and employment status. *JAMA Network Open, 6*(2), e2256152. https://doi.org/10.1001/jamanetworkopen.2022.56152

Powers, M., & Faden, R. (2003). Racial and ethnic disparities in healthcare: An ethical analysis of when and how they matter. In B. Smedley, A. Stith, & A. Nelson (Eds.), *Unequal treatment: Confronting racial and ethnic disparities in health care* (pp. 722–738). National Academies Press.

Premraj, L., Kannapadi, N. V., Briggs, J., Seal, S. M., Battaglini, D., Fanning, J., Suen, J., Robba, C., Fraser, J., & Cho, S. M. (2022). Mid and long-term neurological and neuropsychiatric manifestations of post-COVID-19 syndrome: A meta-analysis. *Journal of the Neurological Sciences, 434*. https://doi.org/10.1016/j.jns.2022.120162

Reuschke, D., Houston, D., & Sissons, P. (2024). Impacts of Long COVID on workers: A longitudinal study of employment exit, work hours and mental health in the UK. *PLoS ONE, 19*(6). https://doi.org/10.1371/journal.pone.0306122

Saarinen, S., Moustgaard, H., Remes, H., Sallinen, R., & Martikainen, P. (2022). Income differences in COVID-19 incidence and severity in Finland among people with foreign and native background: A population-based cohort study of individuals nested within households. *PLoS Medicine, 19*(8). https://doi.org/10.1186/s12889-024-19328-6

Salci, M. A., Carreira, L., Baccon, W. C., Marques, F. R. D. M., Höring, C. F., Oliveira, M. L. F. D., Milan, N. S., de Souza, F. C. S., Gallo, A. M., Covre, E. R., & Dixe, M. A. (2024). Perceived quality of life and associated factors in long COVID syndrome among older Brazilians: A cross-sectional study. *Journal of Clinical Nursing, 33*(1), 178–191. https://doi.org/10.1111/jocn.16618

Schumacher, A. E., Kyu, H. H., Aali, A., Abbafati, C., Abbas, J., Abbasgholizadeh, R., Abbasi, M. A., Abbasian, M., Abd ElHafeez, S., Abdelmasseh, M., & Abd-Elsalam, S. (2024). Global age-sex-specific mortality, life expectancy, and population estimates in 204 countries and territories and 811 subnational locations, and the impact of the COVID-19 pandemic: A comprehensive demographic analysis for the Global Burden of Disease Study 2021. *The Lancet, 403*(10440), 1989–2056. https://doi.org/10.1016/S0140-6736(24)00476-8

Shabnam, S., Razieh, C., Dambha-Miller, H., Yates, T., Gillies, C., Chudasama, Y. V., Pareek, M., Banerjee, A., Kawachi, I., Lacey, B., Morris, E. J. A., White, M., Zaccardi, F., Khunti, K., & Islam, N. (2023). Socioeconomic inequalities of Long COVID: A retrospective population-based cohort study in the United Kingdom. *Journal of the Royal Society of Medicine, 116*(18), 263–273.

Shang, H., Chang, T., Yang, W., Shi, L., Hu, S., Tian, L., Ren, J., Wang, T., Wang, J., Guo, J., & Cui, Y. (2024). Analysis of influencing factors on long COVID in COVID-19 patients infected with omicron variant three months after discharge: A cross-sectional study. *BMC Infectious Diseases, 24*(1), 1–9. https://doi.org/10.1186/s12879-023-08947-w

Sheiner, L., & Rendell, L. (2023, March 30). Where are the missing workers? Anticipated and unanticipated labor supply changes in the pandemic's aftermath. *Brookings Papers on Economic Activity*. https://www.brookings.edu/articles/where-are-the-missing-workers/

Sheiner, L., Wessel, D., & Asdourian, E. (2025, March). Recovering from COVID. *Brookings*. https://www.brookings.edu/articles/recoveringfrom-covid/

Silver, S. R., Li, J., Ford, N. D., Saydah, S. H., & Shi, D. (2025). Prevalence of COVID-19 and Long COVID by industry and occupation: Behavioral risk factor surveillance system 2022. *American Journal of Industrial Medicine, 68*(1), 26–52. https://doi.org/10.1002/ajim.23665

Singh, A. (2017). Women, wealth and law: Anglo-Hindu and Anglo-Islamic inheritance law in British India. *South Asia, 40*(1), 40–53. https://doi.org/10.1080/00856401.2017.1258612

Singh, R., Rathore, S.S., Khan, H., Karale, S., Chawla, Y., Iqbal, K., Bhurwal, A., Tekin, A., Jain, N., Mehra, I., & Anand, S. (2022). Association of obesity with COVID-19 severity and mortality: An updated systemic review, meta-analysis, and meta-regression. *Frontiers Endocrinolology, 13*. https://doi.org/10.3389/fendo.2022.780872

Smith, S. H., Somsen, G. A., van Rijn, C., Kooij, S., van der Hoek, L., Bem, R. A., & Bonn, D. (2020). Aerosol persistence in relation to possible transmission of SARS-CoV-2. *Physics of Fluids, 32*(10). 107108. https://doi.org/10.1063/5.0027844

Solomou, I., Nikolaou, F., Michaelides, M. P., & Constantinidou, F. (2024). Long-term psychological impact of the pandemic COVID-19: Identification of high-risk groups and assessment of precautionary measures five months after the first wave of restrictions was lifted. *PLOS Global Public Health, 4*(2). https://doi.org/10.1371/journal.pgph.0002847

Subramanian, A., Nirantharakumar, K., Hughes, S., Myles, P., Williams, T., Gokhale, K. M., Taverner, T., Chandan, J. S., Brown, K., Simms-Williams, N., & Shah, A. D. (2022). Symptoms and risk factors for long COVID in non-hospitalized adults. *Nature Medicine, 28*(8), 1706–1714. https://doi.org/10.1038/s41591-022-01909-w

Tonkiss, F. (2006). *Contemporary economic sociology: Globalisation, production, inequality*. Routledge.

Torrance, N., MacIver, E., Adams, N. N., Skåtun, D., Scott, N., Kennedy, C., Douglas, F., Hernandez-Santiago, V., & Grant, A. (2024). Lived experience of work and long COVID in healthcare staff. *Occupational Medicine, 74*(1), 78–85. https://doi.org/10.1093/occmed/kqad117

Tran, P. T. M., Amill-Rosario, A., & dosReis, S. (2024). Antidepressant treatment initiation among children and adolescents with acute versus long COVID: A large retrospective cohort study. *Child and Adolescent Psychiatry and Mental Health, 18*(1). https://doi.org/10.1186/s13034-024-00787-z

Urban Institute. (2023, July 20). *Employment and material hardship among adults with Long Covid in December 2022*. Retrieved from https://www.urban.org/research/publication/employment-and-material-hardship-among-adults-long-covid-december-2022

United States Census Bureau. (2023). *Global population estimates vary but trends are clear: Population growth is slowing*. https://www.census.gov/library/stories/2023/11/world-population-estimated-eight-billion.html

Vahratian, A., Adjaye-Gbewonyo, D., Lin, J.-MS., & Saydah, S. (2023). *Long COVID in children: United States, 2022. NCHS Data Brief, no 479.* NCHS Statistics. https://www.cdc.gov/nchs/products/databriefs/db479.htm?

Venkatesh, A. K., Yu, H., Malicki, C., Gottlieb, M., Elmore, J. G., Hill, M. J.,…Inspire Group. (2024). The association between prolonged SARS-CoV-2 symptoms and work outcomes. *PLoS ONE, 19*(7). https://doi.org/10.1371/journal.pone.0300947

Wang, C. C., Prather, K. A., Sznitman, J., Jimenez, J. L., Lakdawala, S. S., Tufekci, Z., & Marr, L. C. (2021). Airborne transmission of respiratory viruses. *Science, 373*(6558), eabd9149. https://doi.org/10.1126/science.abd9149

Woldegiorgis, M., Cadby, G., Ngeh, S., Korda, R. J., Armstrong, P. K., Maticevic, J., Knight, P., Jardine, A., Bloomfield, L. E., & Effler, P. V. (2024). Long COVID in a highly vaccinated but largely unexposed Australian population following the 2022 SARS-CoV-2 Omicron wave: A cross-sectional survey. *Medical Journal of Australia, 220*(6), 323–330. https://doi.org/10.5694/mja2.52256

World Health Organization. (2021). *World health statistics 2021: monitoring health for the SDGs, sustainable development goals.* World Health Organization. https://www.who.int/publications/i/item/9789240027053

World Health Organization. (2025). *Social determinants of health.* https://www.who.int/health-topics/social-determinants-of-health#tab=tab_1

Xu, E., Xie, Y., & Al-Aly, Z. (2022). Long-term neurologic outcomes of COVID-19. *Nature Medicine, 28*(11), 2406–2415. https://doi.org/10.1038/s41591-022-02001-z

Yin, K., Peluso, M. J., Luo, X., Thomas, R., Shin, M. G., Neidleman, J., Andrew, A., Young, K. C., Ma, T., Hoh, R., & Anglin, K. (2024). Long COVID manifests with T cell dysregulation, inflammation and an uncoordinated adaptive immune response to SARS-CoV-2. *Nature Immunology, 25*(2), 218–225. https://doi.org/10.1038/s41590-023-01724-6

Yin, Y., Yang, G., Wang, N., Zeng, M., Jiang, H., Yuan, S., Wu, J., Zhang, J., Cui, J., Zhou, G., & Yang, X. (2024). Exploring the prevalence and chest CT predictors of Long COVID in children: A comprehensive study from Shanghai and Linyi. *Frontiers in Pediatrics, 12.* https://doi.org/10.3389/fped.2024.1420196

Zeraatkar, D., Ling, M., Kirsh, S., Jassal, T., Shahab, M., Movahed, H., Talukdar, J. R., Walch, A., Chakraborty, S., Turner, T., & Turkstra, L. (2024). Interventions for the management of Long Covid (Post-Covid

Condition): Living systematic review. *BMJ*, *387*. https://doi.org/10.1136/bmj-2024-081318

Zonglin, H., Babatunde, A., & Wai-kit, M. (2023). Editorial: Psychosocial, behavioral, and clinical implications for public mental health during the COVID-19 pandemic. *Frontiers in Psychiatry*, *14*. https://doi.org/10.3389/fpsyt.2023.1274588

Zürcher, S. J., Banzer, C., Adamus, C., Lehmann, A. I., Richter, D., & Kerksieck, P. (2022). Post-viral mental health sequelae in infected persons associated with COVID-19 and previous epidemics and pandemics: Systematic review and meta-analysis of prevalence estimates. *Journal of Infection and Public Health*, *15*(5), 599–608. https://doi.org/10.1016/j.jiph.2022.04.005

8

Equity Amidst Uncertainty: A Comparative Critique of Multiple Stakeholder Perspectives About Health Equity for People with Long COVID

Danielle Hitch, Sam Wills, Sara Holton, Rebecca Corva, and Krishna Vakil

Introduction

Long COVID has emerged as a significant public health concern, posing unprecedented challenges for healthcare systems worldwide. It causes prolonged and debilitating symptoms which have a profound effect on people's health, well-being and ability to participate in daily life. It

D. Hitch (✉)
School of Health and Social Development and Institute of Health Transformation, Deakin University, Melbourne, VIC, Australia
e-mail: Danielle.Hitch@wh.org.au

S. Wills
Department of Allied Health, Western Health, Footscray, VIC, Australia

S. Holton
School of Public Health and Preventive Medicine, Monash University, Melbourne, VIC, Australia

R. Corva
The Institute for Mental and Physical Health and Clinical Translation (IMPACT), Deakin University, Melbourne, VIC, Australia

D. Lupton (ed.), *Long COVID and Society*,
https://doi.org/10.1007/978-981-96-9168-5_8

disproportionately affects disadvantaged groups, including people with disabilities, rural residents and Culturally and Linguistically Diverse (CALD) communities (de Leeuw et al., 2022). As the COVID-19 pandemic continues, growing evidence highlights worse outcomes for these groups compared to the general population. An equity-focused approach is urgently needed to ensure optimal care for everyone living with Long COVID.

This chapter critically examines the drivers of health inequities in Long COVID and strategies for equitable healthcare responses. Health equity ensures everyone has a fair opportunity for optimal health, regardless of social or economic circumstances (Peterson et al., 2021). It emphasises equitable access to resources, services and opportunities for wellbeing (Hoyer et al., 2022). By examining data from over 500 submissions to the Australian Federal Government Inquiry into Long COVID, this chapter discusses features of the national response to Long COVID, which potentially amplify or mitigate disadvantage for people with this condition.

The Health Equity Framework

The Health Equity Framework (HEF) (Peterson et al., 2021) underpins this chapter, systemically exploring how intersectional factors drive health inequities and highlighting pathways to equitable solutions. This justice-based model examines the complex interplay between individuals, environments and systemic factors to understand health disparities. Central to the HEF are three concepts: equity in health outcomes, multiple interacting influences and a historical life-course lens. By focusing on health equity, the HEF critiques public health approaches centred solely on individual behaviours and engages with structural determinants that limit resource access (Nakkeeran et al., 2021). It identifies four interdependent spheres of influence that shape health

---

K. Vakil
School of Medicine, Deakin University, Melbourne, VIC, Australia

outcomes: systems of power, relationships and networks, individual factors and physiological pathways (Peterson et al., 2021). These spheres interact dynamically as part of a complex system to either amplify or mitigate health inequities.

The HEF's historical perspective highlights how health inequities accumulate over time and generations. This approach addresses the root causes of inequities rather than simply addressing Long COVID symptoms. Therefore, this framework provides a valuable lens to examine disparities for people with Long COVID, showing how social and political determinants like economic disadvantage, limited healthcare and systemic biases impact their lived experience and health outcomes.

Sick and Tired: Casting a Long Shadow

The Australian Federal Government's Inquiry into Long COVID was initiated to address its individual, community and national impacts. The Inquiry was launched on 1 September 2022 by the House of Representatives Standing Committee on Health, Aged Care and Sport, following discussions with the Minister for Health and Aged Care (Parliament of Australia, 2023). The Inquiry's terms of reference examined lived experiences, healthcare responses, research and socio-economic impacts. It also explored repeated infections, vaccination effects and best practice guidelines for prevention, diagnosis and management. The Committee received 566 submissions from individuals with Long COVID, healthcare providers, academics, peak bodies, advocacy groups and other stakeholders. Public hearings and site visits occurred between October 2022 and February 2023 gathering diverse perspectives to inform recommendations for improving Australia's Long COVID response. The final report, entitled *Sick and Tired: Casting a Long Shadow*, was published in April 2023.

Exploring the Contribution of Health Equity Perspectives to the Inquiry

This chapter outlines a reflective thematic analysis of Inquiry submissions. Initially, 105 submissions were analysed with a priori codes based on HEF spheres of influence. These codes were reviewed by the first and second authors and applied as nodes in an automated analysis of all 566 submissions via NVivo (Lumivero, 2024). Extracts were reviewed against source material and developed into preliminary themes, finalised with illustrative quotes.

Most health equity-related content in the Inquiry submissions came from people with Long COVID, peak bodies and advocacy groups. Sentiment analysis revealed submissions were primarily 'negative' (43%) or 'very negative' (24%). Only 7% were described as 'very positive,' reflecting prevailing dissatisfaction, frustration and concern with Australia's Long COVID response. Three major themes related to health equity also reflected the negative nature of the submissions. The following text outlines the findings from the analysis of the submissions to the Inquiry. Verbatim quotes from the submissions have been included as examples to provide detail to the thematic findings, identified by submitter and their Inquiry registration number.

Polarisation, Fragmentation and Mistrust

> Long COVID—like almost every aspect of COVID-19—has become increasingly polarising in Australian health policy debate. (Professor Martin Hensher/175)

Long COVID has become a contentious issue in Australian health policy, marked by conflicting interests and little stakeholder consensus. The politically charged public health response to COVID-19 highlighted tensions between state and federal government responsibilities (Duckett, 2022), as disagreements arose over how Long COVID fits within the health system's acute, subacute and primary care sectors. Inquiry submissions described a fractured policy landscape, with governments, advocacy groups and healthcare professionals often at odds over priorities and support for managing Long COVID.

Political systems had a stronger influence on COVID policy more than usually found for health issues, as 'governments appear to be following political advice rather than medical advice' (Name withheld/494). While general reform targets had some agreement, progress was hindered by stakeholder veto power and a focus on differences over consensus (Contandriopoulos et al., 2018). As one person with Long COVID noted: 'Things do get misunderstood, distorted, hijacked and go off the rails in various other ways, especially in politically charged arenas' (Name withheld/499.1).

Inquiry submissions highlighted deep mistrust in political leadership and frustration with political inaction or poor responses to Long COVID. While political trust in Australia had declined over 15 years (Dassonneville & McAllister, 2021), it temporarily increased early in the pandemic (Goldfinch et al., 2021). However, Inquiry submissions suggest trust declined during the pandemic in comparison to the pre-pandemic baseline, reflecting global trends (Aassve et al., 2022; Murumba & Pashayan, 2024). As higher political trust is linked to lower COVID excess mortality (Farzanegan & Hofmann, 2022), these sentiments may have serious health consequences. These suspicions reflect broader concerns about Australia's pandemic response, regardless of political allegiances: 'I am one of many that no longer trust or have any faith or belief in our health care system or whatever political party is in power' (Scott Symington/065). Health professionals criticised political leaders for superficial solutions, with one stating: 'The idea that we can build our way out of the pandemic, that building more hospitals is the solution, is foolish. Politicians in high vis and hard hats are not the answer' (Dr Anita White/238). Submissions from people with Long COVID expressed strong feelings of betrayal, believing their struggles were ignored or underplayed: 'Just because politicians are bored with the pandemic doesn't mean it's over' (Adam Williams/029). Ironically, dissatisfaction with political systems' influence on responses to Long COVID was one of the few areas of stakeholder agreement.

A Lack of Resource Availability or Allocation

> Asking sick patients to wait up to a year for a consultation is inhumane. (Name withheld/400)

Systems of power can reduce health disparities through the equitable identification and allocation of resources, and Inquiry submissions highlighted this issue as especially critical for Australian healthcare. The pandemic placed unprecedented strain on global healthcare due to extreme demand, workforce shortages and public health order limitations (Williams & Karanikolos, 2021). Many Australians faced barriers to general and specialised care, particularly women/girls, culturally diverse people, those with disability or chronic illness, and regional or remote communities (Ivancic et al., 2022).

At the time of the Inquiry, Long COVID care was available through specialist clinics, GP-led respiratory clinics and Aboriginal Community Controlled Health Services (Bonning & Wyber, 2020; Luo et al., 2023). These services were mostly located in Victoria, focused on specific symptoms, and excluded children or adolescents (Luo et al., 2023). Variations in waitlists, care offerings and practices prompted calls for 'consistent expectations about the quality, thoroughness, staffing expertise' (Name withheld/233). COVID-19 services were treated as tertiary health services with limited integration into the broader system. People with Long COVID faced ad hoc service provision, with Australian Pathology/206 stressing the need for 'appropriate locations for testing sites and […] funding for rapid upscaling'. Many contributors to the Inquiry noted that they had endured financial hardship due to employment loss, in turn limiting their access to existing services: 'I don't know where to look or turn for information and don't have the money to try different options' (Name withheld/259). Developing Long COVID significantly reduced the financial resources they needed to access care and manage their health.

Australia's healthcare landscape has changed since the Inquiry, with all publicly funded Long COVID clinics now closed and no requirements for COVID testing or reporting. However, most resourcing issues identified in submissions are not unique to Long COVID but reflect pre-existing disadvantage and long-term resourcing shortfalls. Long COVID amplifies these negative effects. For instance, the impact of Long COVID for Aboriginal and Torres Strait Islander Peoples was 'compounded by inequitable resourcing to meet their specific needs' (Royal Australian and New Zealand College of Psychiatrists/176) alongside long-entrenched poorer health outcomes and lower life expectancy compared to non-Indigenous Australians. Healthcare leaders now advocate for intersectoral collaboration, recognising that consumer needs span health, social care, education and other sectors (Sorrell et al., 2023). However, Australia's political funding and service systems operate in independent 'silos' (Hussain et al., 2021), forcing people with Long COVID to navigate multiple systems and services to meet their needs.

Australia's hybrid public–private healthcare system includes numerous interfaces between services, systems, sectors and government levels. Some of the challenges around resourcing arise from the tension between the view of Long COVID as a singular, specialist area of care and a more expansive perspective that encompasses all social determinants of health. While some hoped the pandemic would enable transformative healthcare reform (Bhaduri, 2020; Bruen et al., 2024), the poorly integrated and fragmented system (Jackson & O'Halloran, 2021) remains a significant barrier to health equity for people with Long COVID.

Marginalisation and Social Exclusion of People with Long COVID

> At about the same time as I was floored by my diagnosis and disablement, Australia's Chief Health Officer declared, 'We're not seeing a major picture of long COVID.' [...] according to the Chief Health Officer's research and calculations and policy recommendations, I do not exist. (Name withheld/072)

Inquiry submissions on policy conflict and inadequate healthcare resourcing for people with Long COVID highlighted their marginalisation from mainstream Australian society, which was the most prevalent health equity-related theme in the submissions. Disengagement and reduced political participation by those with Long COVID exacerbate this marginalisation, but political activities require significant time and energy. Symptoms like fatigue and brain fog severely hinder civic and social participation, putting these Australians at high risk of being sidelined and unheard.

Cultural, geographic and resource barriers also contributed to marginalisation from Long COVID treatment and support, with many Inquiry submissions describing additional obstacles these Australians faced in obtaining care. Systemic gaps in service availability affected disadvantaged communities and priority groups the hardest (de Leeuw et al., 2022), and the existing Australian health system often lacks the inclusivity needed to adequately address diverse community needs.

> Referring to a metropolitan clinic poses challenges for clients who require supports/caregivers to travel to Adelaide and cost of travel and accommodation. (Aboriginal Health Council of South Australia/439)

Many people with lived experience described adapting to a new social reality shaped by Long COVID, marked by isolation, stigma and strained relationships. Social repercussions were often just as debilitating as physical and cognitive symptoms. Those staying 'COVID aware' by maintaining precautions, faced exclusion and ridicule, especially after mandates ended. They struggled to balance 'the potential risk of repeated COVID infections with normal, healthy family life' (Name withheld/031). Early public health messaging promoted altruism, but pushback against collective action reflects wider pandemic-related societal stress (Hanna et al., 2022). People with Long COVID had to defend their choices amid misunderstandings, leading to uncomfortable and sometimes aggressive interactions. Most Inquiry submissions from people with Long COVID withheld their names, suggesting that concerns about the personal implications of being identified with the condition are widespread.

People with Long COVID also avoided social situations with higher transmission risk, further isolating them from family and social life: 'We have chosen not to see family whose approach is riskier. Our social health and interaction with others is, and will continue to be, hampered' (Name Withheld/14). While uncertainty exists about subsequent COVID infections, concerns are not unfounded. Reinfections may cumulatively increase the risk of Long COVID (Boufidou et al., 2023), though the risk may be lower in later infections (Bosworth et al., 2023). These choices were seen by less COVID-aware people as 'self-imposed' or unnecessary, compounding isolation and marginalisation: 'In the absence of any serious public health campaign to explain why some people still need to mask, V has faced stigma and ostracism, particularly at school' (Name Withheld/117). Social isolation has a particularly high toll on personal health and wellbeing: 'Having a chronic/invisible illness is isolating. I don't even know where to begin in explaining the extreme feelings of isolation and guilt eating away at me' (Name Withheld/163). Research confirms people with 'invisible' conditions experience more isolation and loneliness than other disability groups due to the perceived mismatch between their appearance and functional ability (Ipsen & Repke, 2021), meaning people with Long COVID are especially at risk for this determinant of health.

The relaxation of public COVID measures by Australian federal and state governments from late 2021 sparked societal debate on personal responsibility versus collective safety. In their Inquiry submission, one person with Long COVID stated, 'This crap about personal responsibility enrages me. We make people wear seatbelts and have made drink driving illegal but refuse to ask them to protect others by isolating or wearing a mask' (Name Withheld/70). Others argued that emphasising personal responsibility in COVID management worsened social conflict, creating 'potential conflicts within families and on a personal and workplace level, as individuals try to do protective behaviours against the societal view that the risk is over' (COVID Safe Schools Inc/306). Attitudes towards personal responsibility in the broader community were described as strongly divided. Contributors argued that the choice to cease public health measures was deemed acceptable by most people. However, an individual choosing to continue to take precautions was not. As a result, those contributors to the Inquiry who viewed themselves as 'COVID aware' or 'COVID cautious' resented what they perceived to be collective inaction and its potential to jeopardise the health of vulnerable Australians.

Due to marginalisation, people with Long COVID who contributed to the Inquiry felt estranged from Australian society in general: 'I feel like I've been abandoned by the government, the medical profession, and many around me' (Name Withheld/28). A lack of official support and scepticism from health professionals intensified their struggle, as they could no longer rely on community and institutional help. For some, the absence of a formal diagnosis led to family and friends withdrawing support because 'patients are placed in the psychosomatic category without a diagnosis' (Name Withheld/12). Assumptions that symptoms were 'all in their head' undermined both the legitimacy of people's lived experiences and eligibility for social support.

People from higher socio-economic backgrounds or without prior health issues felt societal attitude shifts more acutely. Research on the experiences of healthcare professionals with Long COVID poignantly describes the experience of going from provider to patient. Qualitative studies found these 'wounded healers' viewed the shift as disappointing yet humbling, but believed it improved their empathy for those with invisible disabilities (Piredda et al., 2022; Taylor et al., 2021). However, the disability community noted such experiences are not unique to Long COVID: 'due to the neglect for post-infection disease, Long COVID patients are facing the same issues as people with ME/CFS [myalgic encephalitis/chronic fatigue syndrome]. Unnecessarily, the same assumptions and mistakes are being made' (Emerge Australia/67).

Recommendations for Inclusive Policy Reform to Reduce Health Inequity for People with Long COVID

Recommendations from Inquiry Contributors

Inquiry submissions comprehensively outlined the problems associated with Long COVID in Australia but offered few tangible recommendations. The only consensus was an urgent need for data-driven, evidence-based policymaking to counter short-term political decisions. Systems of power were 'building the plane while flying it' during the pandemic, simultaneously developing and implementing responses (McKenna et al., 2023). The evidence base for effective Long COVID treatments remains limited due to the novelty of SARS-CoV-2 and COVID.

People with Long COVID strongly advocated for science-based policymaking: 'I would like to see public health management based on the evidence and science instead of populist politics' (Name Withheld/326). They believed COVID-19 and Long COVID should be 'above politics' and not 'be political (or) undermined by the prioritisation of elections or corporate interests' (Name Withheld/162). Other stakeholders also supported data-driven decisions while recognising data is still being collected. Policy is crucial for addressing health equity in healthcare delivery and behaviour change, though its impact on structural determinants is limited (Fisher et al., 2016). Without a robust evidence base, policymaking will likely remain ad hoc and adaptive.

Addressing the 'information deficit' (Australian Long COVID Community Facebook Group/309.1) about Long COVID would enable more positive action. Many submissions called for better data collection, reporting, longitudinal analysis and use of evidence from related conditions like ME/CFS. Improving the evidence base requires a health equity focus to ensure inclusivity, such as 'linking COVID registries with social and demographic factors, such as occupation, geographical location, socioeconomic status and cultural background' (Australian Academy of Health and Medical Sciences and the Australian Academy of Science/165). Most Long COVID research includes high- and middle-income samples, with few studies on disadvantaged or culturally diverse communities (Taghrir et al., 2023). It is essential to collect representative data to ensure policies address the needs of all people with Long COVID.

Another consensus area (although less often mentioned) was the need for greater public awareness to reduce stigma and foster understanding through 'greater media attention on Long COVID without the stigma of it not being a "real disease"' (Name Withheld/152). The needs of people with Long COVID will remain unmet without societal attitudes recognising it as a legitimate, chronic and serious condition. Although mismatches between public health messaging and lived experiences are improving (Miyake & Martin, 2021), international public health campaigns about Long COVID are rare. Concerns include balancing hope with uncertainty about recovery (Bhogal et al., 2022; Mills et al., 2022) and avoiding a nocebo effect that could worsen symptoms (Vogt & Garner, 2023). Nonetheless, public health campaigns are vital to prevent new cases and improve Long COVID management.

Recommendations from the Inquiry Committee

The Inquiry's final report, released in April 2023, included seven recommendations from the Australian House of Representatives Standing Committee to address the challenges faced by Australians with Long COVID (Parliament of Australia, 2023). While health equity was not extensively addressed, all recommendations hold the potential to address inequity to some extent.

The first recommendation for a centralised database aims to consolidate COVID-19 data, enabling a more coordinated, evidence-based response. This could rebuild public trust, improve resource allocation, reduce polarisation, and address issues for people with Long COVID. While adopting WHO's term 'Post Acute COVID Condition' as per the second recommendation to standardise care, using 'Long COVID' would be more person-centred. However, involving people with Long COVID in developing practice guidelines, service design and policies could improve tiered care models and referral pathways, benefiting marginalised groups. Recommendation 3 proposes a nationally coordinated research program with inclusive practices targeting marginalised groups and continuous funding to address structural health equity issues. Recommendation 4 focuses on vaccination programs for marginalised groups but omits public awareness efforts about Long COVID. The fifth recommendation to improve antiviral access through increased involvement by pharmacists could benefit underserved communities where doctors are less accessible.

Recommendation 6's call for Long COVID management in primary care aims to create an integrated approach but relies on the provision of GP education to upskill the workforce. Expanding telehealth and outreach clinics addresses rural and remote access issues and could also benefit other excluded communities (Baker et al., 2021). Finally, improving indoor air quality, a critical factor in health disparities, would benefit vulnerable groups like children, older people and those with pre-existing conditions, extending its impact beyond COVID and Long COVID. The Inquiry therefore provided a foundation for addressing health inequities related to Long COVID, without any specific guidance on how to achieve change.

Response from the Australian Government

The Australian Government responded to the Inquiry on 26 February 2024, fully supporting two recommendations: Recommendation 2 (adopting WHO terminology and evidence-based guidelines) and Recommendation 4 (improving the COVID-19 vaccination communication strategy). Elements of the other five recommendations were supported, supported in principle or noted. Only one recommendation, regarding pharmacist-initiated antiviral prescribing, was not supported. Most supported recommendations align with ongoing or planned initiatives, reflecting an incremental rather than transformative policy approach to Long COVID.

While the government acknowledged the need for coordination, it largely deferred responsibility to state and territory governments or existing funding structures like Medicare. Given existing intergovernmental conflicts, this approach is unlikely to rebuild trust or reduce stakeholder polarisation described by contributors. Crucially, the government response offered few additional resources, aside from AUD50 million for Long COVID research and AUD4.7 million for CALD community engagement, focusing on existing systems rather than new targeted supports. While telehealth expansion was supported, aspects of this mode of care delivery can exacerbate health inequities (Kuziemsky et al., 2022), and it cannot fully address resource inequities highlighted in this analysis.

The government response does little to address social marginalisation and isolation. Adopting WHO terminology may alienate people with Long COVID by disregarding their role in identifying the condition. The only public awareness campaign focuses on vaccination, with no plans to improve general understanding of Long COVID. While the response includes some positive commitments, it is unlikely to significantly improve the lived experiences of people with Long COVID or reduce health inequity for this group.

Recommendations for Meaningful Policy Reform

We propose seven recommendations to support an equitable national response to Long COVID. Some build on the Australian Government's response, others fill policy gaps, and all should be enacted through the National Post-Acute Sequelae of COVID-19 Plan for a consistent, integrated approach to reducing health inequity.

Foregrounding Health Equity

A stronger focus on intersectional health equity in data collection is needed to complement the focus on priority groups. Equity-focused indicators should ensure marginalised communities are represented and disparities monitored. While health equity is implicitly present in the Inquiry's Final Report, it must become a more explicit element of national policy.

Improving Community Knowledge and Understanding

The National Post-Acute Sequelae of COVID-19 Plan (Australian Government Department of Health & Aged Care, 2024) highlights community education, but campaigns targeting both the general population and tailored to marginalised groups are needed to reduce stigma and misinformation about Long COVID. Culturally sensitive communication for CALD and Indigenous communities will ensure all Australians have the information they need for informed, evidence-based decisions about COVID risks.

Fair Access to Expert Care for All People with Long COVID

Re-establishing specialised Long COVID clinics with consistent care standards, alongside expanded telehealth, would improve access to high-quality support for marginalised communities. Primary care alone cannot provide the tertiary-level support needed for this complex condition. These clinics should include mobile outreach services for those unable or unwilling to use telehealth and could be co-designed with members of the community to ensure they are relevant and culturally appropriate for all Australians. Greater intersectoral collaboration across health, social care, community services and education is essential for creating seamless support systems for Long COVID patients. New Long COVID clinics could therefore include representatives from these sectors (such as welfare workers and cultural representatives) to provide a 'one stop shop' and reduce the need for patients to care coordinate for themselves.

Commitment to Investment to Support Economic Prosperity

People with Long COVID report severe financial distress, especially when unable to work. Those eligible for the National Disability Insurance Scheme (NDIS) should be allowed to access personalised support plans to enhance social and economic participation. Increased funding for multidisciplinary care teams, including mental health support, would address complex needs early and reduce deterioration while people remain on the waiting list for scarce specialist appointments. Given Long COVID's economic impact in Australia (Angeles et al., 2022) these investments would have lasting benefits.

Promoting Social Inclusion

People with Long COVID have formed informal peer support networks (predominantly online) which are recognised as an important, but imperfect source of support (Day, 2022). Australian governments and non-profits could foster community-based networks to reduce isolation and provide face-to-face alternatives. Returning to work is often challenging (Hitch et al., 2023), and the development of inclusive workplace policies, such as flexible hours, remote work, and extended sick leave, would support participation. National indoor air quality guidelines would also enable COVID-aware community members to engage more safely in civic life.

'Nothing About Us, Without Us'

The establishment of permanent patient advisory councils could ensure the lived experiences of people with Long COVID inform policy, service design and healthcare delivery. These councils should include representatives from marginalised communities and offer flexible participation options. In addition to advisory roles, they could lead co-creation of practice guidelines and service models providing tiered care, addressing symptom severity, and meeting the unique needs of vulnerable populations.

The COVID pandemic is far from over and has changed many Australians' lives forever. Despite the negativity, conflict, and fragmentation in this Inquiry analysis, opportunities exist for positive change locally, nationally and in communities. Structural change for health equity will take decades, but many quick improvements can build momentum. We know we can do better, and we know at least some of the ways this can be achieved.

Acknowledgements The authors acknowledge the Traditional Custodians of the unceded lands, skies and waterways on which this work was produced. We pay our deep respect to the Ancestors and Elders of Wurundjeri and Wadawurrung country in recognition of the deep history and culture of these lands.

References

Aassve, A., Capezzone, T., Cavalli, N., Conzo, P., & Peng, C. (2022). *Trust in the time of coronavirus: Longitudinal evidence from the United States.* Department of Economics and Statistics Cognetti de Martiis (Working Papers 202203). University of Turin.

Angeles, M. R., Wanni Arachchige Dona, S., Nguyen, H. D., Le, L. K., & Hensher, M. (2022). Modelling the potential acute and post-acute burden of COVID-19 under the Australian border re-opening plan. *BMC Public Health, 22*(1), 757. https://doi.org/10.1186/s12889-022-13169-x

Australian Government Department of Health and Aged Care. (2024). *National post-acute sequelae of COVID-19 (PASC) plan.* https://www.health.gov.au/resources/publications/national-post-acute-sequelae-of-covid-19-plan?language=en

Bhaduri, S. D. (2020). Post-COVID healthcare reform in India: What to expect? *Journal of Family Medicine and Primary Care, 9*(11), 5427–5431. https://doi.org/10.4103/jfmpc.jfmpc_1548_20

Baker, D. R., Cadet, K., & Mani, S. (2021). COVID-19 testing and social determinants of health among disadvantaged Baltimore neighborhoods: A community mobile health clinic outreach model. *Population Health Management, 24*(6), 657–663. https://doi.org/10.1089/pop.2021.0066

Bhogal, J. K., Mills, F., Dennis, A., Spoiala, C., Milward, J., Saeed, S., Jones, L. F., Weston, D., & Carter, H. (2022). The effects of messaging on expectations and understanding of Long COVID: An online randomised trial. *medRxiv*, 2022.2001.2018.22269467. https://doi.org/10.1101/2022.01.18.22269467.

Bonning, M. A., & Wyber, R. (2020). Respiratory clinics and rural and Aboriginal health. *The British Journal of General Practice, 70*(698). https://doi.org/10.3399/bjgp20/x712265.

Bosworth, M. L., Shenhuy, B., Walker, A. S., Nafilyan, V., Alwan, N. A., O'Hara, M. E., & Ayoubkhani, D. (2023). Risk of new-onset Long COVID following reinfection with severe acute respiratory syndrome coronavirus 2: A community-based cohort study. *Open Forum Infectious Diseases, 10*(11). https://doi.org/10.1093/ofid/ofad493.

Boufidou, F., Medić, S., Lampropoulou, V., Siafakas, N., Tsakris, A., & Anastassopoulou, C. (2023). SARS-CoV-2 reinfections and Long COVID in the post-Omicron phase of the pandemic. *International Journal of Molecular Sciences, 24*(16). https://doi.org/10.3390/ijms241612962.

Bruen, C., Burke, S., Parker, S., Schulmann, K., & Conghail, L.M. (2024). The politics of universal health system reform in the context of COVID-19. *European Journal of Public Health, 34*(Supplement 3). https://doi.org/10.1093/eurpub/ckae144.745.

Contandriopoulos, D., Brousselle, A., Larouche, C., Breton, M., Rivard, M., Beaulieu, M.-D., Haggerty, J. L., Champagne, G., & Perroux, M. (2018). Healthcare reforms, inertia polarization and group influence. *Health Policy, 122*(9), 1018–1027. https://doi.org/10.1016/j.healthpol.2018.07.007

Dassonneville, R., & McAllister, I. (2021). Explaining the decline of political trust in Australia. *Australian Journal of Political Science, 56*(3), 280–297. https://doi.org/10.1080/10361146.2021.1960272

Day, H. L. S. (2022). Exploring online peer support groups for adults experiencing Long COVID in the United Kingdom: Qualitative interview study. *Journal of Medical Internet Research, 24*(5). https://doi.org/10.2196/37674.

de Leeuw, E., Yashadhana, A., & Hitch, D. (2022). Long COVID: Sustained and multiplied disadvantage. *Medical Journal of Australia, 216*(5), 222–224. https://doi.org/10.5694/mja2.51435

Duckett, S. (2022). Public health management of the COVID-19 pandemic in Australia: The role of the Morrison government. *International Journal of Environmental Research and Public Health, 19*(16). https://doi.org/10.3390/ijerph191610400.

Farzanegan, M. R., & Hofmann, H. P. (2022). A matter of trust? Political trust and the COVID-19 pandemic. *International Journal of Sociology, 52*(6), 476–499. https://doi.org/10.1080/00207659.2022.2086729

Fisher, M., Baum, F. E., Macdougall, C., Newman, L., & McDermott, D. (2016). To what extent do Australian health policy documents address social determinants of health and health equity? *Journal of Social Policy, 45*(3), 545–564. https://doi.org/10.1017/S0047279415000756

Goldfinch, S., Taplin, R., & Gauld, R. (2021). Trust in government increased during the COVID-19 pandemic in Australia and New Zealand. *Australian Journal of Public Administration, 80*(1), 3–11. https://doi.org/10.1111/1467-8500.12459

Hanna, E., Martin, G., Campbell, A., Connolly, P., Fearon, K., & Markham, S. (2022). Experiences of face mask use during the COVID-19 pandemic: A qualitative study. *Sociology of Health & Illness, 44*(9), 1481–1499. https://doi.org/10.1111/1467-9566.13525

Hitch, D., Deféin, E., Lloyd, M., Rasmussen, B., Haines, K., & Garnys, E. (2023). Beyond the case numbers: Social determinants and contextual factors in patient narratives of recovery from COVID-19. *Australian and New Zealand Journal of Public Health, 47*(1). https://doi.org/10.1016/j.anzjph.2022.100002.

Hoyer, D., Dee, E., O'Leary, M. S., Heffernan, M., Gelfand, K., Kappel, R., & Fromknecht, C. Q. (2022). How do we define and measure health equity? The state of current practice and tools to advance health equity. *Journal of Public Health Management and Practice, 28*(5), 570–577. https://doi.org/10.1097/phh.0000000000001603

Hussain, R., Parmenter, T., Wark, S., Janicki, M., Knox, M., & Hayhoe, N. (2021). Mitigating the impact of the 'silos' between the disability and aged-care sectors in Australia: Development of a best practice framework. *Journal of Applied Research in Intellectual Disability, 34*(6), 1477–1488. https://doi.org/10.1111/jar.12890

Ipsen, C., & Repke, M. A. (2021). Reaching people with disabilities to learn about their experiences of social connection and loneliness. *Disability and Health Journal, 15*(1). https://doi.org/10.1016/j.dhjo.2021.101220.

Ivancic, L., Bond, D. M., & Nassar, N. (2022). Impact of the COVID-19 pandemic on access and use of health services by middle-aged and older Australians. *Australian Health Review, 47*(1), 100–109. https://doi.org/10.1071/AH22183

Jackson, C. L., & O'Halloran, D. (2021). Reforming our health care system: Time to rip off the band-aid? *Medical Journal of Australia, 215*(7), 301–303. https://doi.org/10.5694/mja2.51261

Kuziemsky, C. E., Hunter, I. M., Udayasankaran, J. G., Ranatunga, P. E. K. B., Kulatunga, G. G., John, S., John, O., Flórez-Arango, J. F., Ito, M., Ho, K., Gogia, S. B., Araujo, K., Rajput, V. K., Meijer, W., & Basu, A. (2022). Telehealth as a means of enabling health equity. *Yearbook of Medical Informatics, 31*(1), 60–66. https://doi.org/10.1055/s-0042-1742500

Lumivero. (2024). *NVivo (Version 15).* www.lumivero.com.

Luo, S., Zheng, Z., Bird, S. R., Plebanski, M., Figueiredo, B., Jessup, R., Stelmach, W., Robinson, J. A., Xenos, S., Olasoji, M., Wan, D. W. L., Sheahan, J., & Itsiopoulos, C. (2023). An overview of Long COVID support services in Australia and international clinical guidelines, with a proposed care model in a global context. *Public Health Review, 44*. https://doi.org/10.3389/phrs.2023.1606084

McKenna, K., Bouchoucha, S., Redley, B., & Hutchinson, A. (2023). "Building the plane while flying it" Reflections on pandemic preparedness and response; An organisational case study. *BMC Health Services Research, 23*(1), 940. https://doi.org/10.1186/s12913-023-09874-x

Mills, F., Bhogal, J. K., Dennis, A., Spoiala, C., Milward, J., Saeed, S., Jones, L. F., Weston, D., & Carter, H. (2022). The effects of messaging on Long COVID expectations: An online experiment. *Health Psychology, 41*(11), 853–863. https://doi.org/10.1037/hea0001230

Miyake, E., & Martin, S. (2021). Long COVID: Online patient narratives, public health communication and vaccine hesitancy. *Digital Health, 7*. https://doi.org/10.1177/20552076211059649

Murumba, R. N., & Pashayan, A. R. (2024). Political trust in the age of coronavirus: Experiences in Mukuru, Nairobi, Kenya. *Frontiers in Political Science, 6*. https://doi.org/10.3389/fpos.2024.1331229

Nakkeeran, N., Sacks, E., N Srinivas, P., Juneja, A., Gaitonde, R., Garimella, S., & Topp, S. M. (2021). Beyond behaviour as individual choice: A call to expand understandings around social science in health research. *Wellcome Open Research, 6*. https://doi.org/10.12688/wellcomeopenres.17149.1.

Parliament of Australia. (2023). *Sick and tired: Casting a long shadow*. Parliament of Australia. https://www.aph.gov.au/Parliamentary_Business/Committees/House/Health_Aged_Care_and_Sport/LongandrepeatedCOVID/Report

Peterson, A., Charles, V., Yeung, D., & Coyle, K. (2021). The health equity framework: A science and justice based model for public health researchers and practitioners. *Health Promotion Practice, 22*(6), 741–746. https://doi.org/10.1177/1524839920950730

Piredda, M., Fiorini, J., Marchetti, A., Mastroianni, C., Albanesi, B., Livigni, L., Carrabs, G., Zaghini, F., De Marinis, M. G., & Sili, A. (2022). The wounded healer: A phenomenological study on hospital nurses who contracted COVID-19. *Frontiers in Public Health, 10*. https://doi.org/10.3389/fpubh.2022.867826

Sorrell, T. C., Hensher, M., & Sanci, L. A. (2023). Long COVID in Australia: Achieving equitable access to supportive health care. *Medical Journal of Australia, 218*(10), 455–457. https://doi.org/10.5694/mja2.51950

Taghrir, M. H., Akbarialiabad, H., Abdollahi, A., Ghahramani, N., Bastani, B., Paydar, S., Razani, B., Mwangi, J., Asadi-Pooya, A. A., Roozbeh, J., Malekmakan, L., & Kumar, M. (2023). Inequity and disparities mar existing global research evidence on Long COVID. *Global Health Promotion, 30*(1), 63–67. https://doi.org/10.1177/17579759221113276

Taylor, A. K., Kingstone, T., Briggs, T. A., O'Donnell, C. A., Atherton, H., Blane, D. N., & Chew-Graham, C. A. (2021). 'Reluctant pioneer': A qualitative study of doctors' experiences as patients with long COVID. *Health Expectations, 24*(3), 833–842. https://doi.org/10.1111/hex.13223

Vogt, H., & Garner, P. (2023). 'Long COVID' and how medical information is causing illness: A philosophical issue affecting public health. *Journal of Evaluation in Clinical Practice, 30*(5), 838–841. https://doi.org/10.1111/jep.13934

Williams, G., & Karanikolos, M. (2021). Mobilizing human resources. *The European Journal of Public Health, 31*(Supplement 3). https://doi.org/10.1093/eurpub/ckab164.288

Part V

Lived Experience

9

We Will Not Be Silent: The Australia Long COVID Community Speak Out About the Role of Epistemic Injustice in Erasing Evidence of Long COVID in Australia

Robin Austin, Kirsty Yeates, Su Mon Kyaw-Myint, Ruth Newport, and Pippa Yeoman

Introduction

From the early months of the pandemic, those of us living with ongoing symptoms following a COVID-19 infection faced significant challenges on multiple fronts. We wake every day to a host of symptoms exacerbated by the simplest of tasks with no clear path to recovery. Many grieve the loss of independence that comes with good health and secure employment, and all yearn for social connections fading due to contractions in physical capacity. On leaving our homes, we must manage not

R. Austin (✉) · K. Yeates · S. M. Kyaw-Myint · R. Newport · P. Yeoman
Australia Long COVID Community, Melbourne, VIC, Australia
e-mail: lraustin@tpg.com.au

K. Yeates
Research School of Biology, College of Science and Medicine, The Australian National University, Canberra, ACT, Australia

P. Yeoman
The University of Sydney, Camperdown, NSW, Australia

D. Lupton (ed.), *Long COVID and Society*,
https://doi.org/10.1007/978-981-96-9168-5_9

only our symptoms but also the incomprehension of medical practitioners, complete strangers, and sometimes even those we know and love. This absence of understanding, often based in an unwillingness to see and hear, buttressed by silence in the public square, is driven by an unreflected-upon imperative to return to life as it once was.

This chapter is researched and written by members of the Australia Long COVID Community. We all live with, or care for someone with, Long COVID, and some of us are both patient and carer. Our group of now more than 5,000 members is one of many Facebook peer-support groups. We often feel alone, but we are alone-together. We are not the first, nor will we be the last. But what makes us different is the volume and reach of our collective voice enabled by online networks, and the growing financial impact of our absence in workplaces, communities and homes around the world.

As we struggled to make sense of our new reality, few of us would have described ourselves as having suffered an epistemic injustice. But all of us could describe the feeling of not being heard, of having the details of our lived experience—our testimony—blithely dismissed or cruelly denied. Testimonial injustice is a very personal thing. It refers to questioning the capacity of the knower to know (Fricker, 2007). Given many of us experience lower health-related quality of life than those living with diabetes and chronic cardiovascular conditions (Seeley et al., 2023), this failure to give credence to our lived experience is all the more damaging.

Ill health has made writing this chapter challenging, as has the emotional burden of bearing witness to the suffering of others. Our choice to persevere is fuelled by a determination to be heard and to preserve the evidence from member surveys carried out in preparation for submissions to Australian national inquiries into Long COVID and the wider COVID-19 pandemic. We write to amplify the voices of people like Joanne[1] who told us, 'I feel invisible. Forgotten by work. Forgotten by friends. Forgotten by family. Forgotten by society'. At the heart of this erasure sits another insidious form of epistemic injustice—hermeneutical or structural injustice—resulting from unfair treatment related to the production of knowledge and the practices of caring (Ireson et al., 2022; Kidd, 2017; Mullard et al., 2024; Plastina, 2025). When testimony is silenced, people with lived experience are excluded from decisions about what knowledge counts, and this impacts on definitions and diagnostic criteria, and the nature of care provided. Lived experience is always important, but it is crucial when dealing with an absence of evidence on which to base care.

When the Australia Long COVID Community responded to the Inquiry into Long COVID and Repeated Infections of COVID-19 by the Australian Parliament House of Representatives Standing Committee on Health, Aged Care and Sport (see Submission 309), our recommendations reflected our response to this sense of erasure. We asked the committee to see us, hear us, care for us, support us, partner with us and not dismiss us. In effect, we were asking the committee and the broader community to directly address testimonial injustice: to give us the space to be heard, to honour the credibility of our voices and to work with us to address the challenges we face. We hoped our voices might lead to positive action, but we failed to understand that culpability lies with the hearer (Fricker, 2007). This lack of listening, belief and subsequent erasure is not always conceptually recognised as epistemic injustice but it is something we share with those who have lived with myalgic encephalomyelitis/chronic fatigue syndrome (ME/CFS) (Bayliss et al., 2014; Blease et al., 2017), other post-infection associated chronic illnesses (Rebman et al., 2024), and the broader disability community as well (Ho, 2011; Porter et al., 2023).

In what follows, we draw on the findings of three surveys we conducted in 2022 and 2023 with members of the Australia Long COVID Community to inform responses to government inquiries. Across these surveys, we document the lived experiences of more than 1,200 respondents from a membership exceeding 4,500 by the time of the third survey. We add our experiences to the record in the hopes that what we have learned might contribute to slowing the rate at which our ranks swell.

Survey 1, September–October 2022

Administrators and members of the Australia Long COVID Community Facebook group developed an online questionnaire to capture members' experiences and share them with the Long COVID Inquiry. The survey was conducted in late 2022, following Australian federal and state governments' cessation of public health measures in December 2021 after having controlled the spread of the ancestral and Delta variants well in the first 2 years of the pandemic (Australian Institute of Health & Welfare, 2024). The survey ran from 30 September to 16 October 2022 and received 607 responses from a membership of 2,844 (21% response rate). The overwhelming majority (93%) were completed by people living with Long COVID, with a small portion completed on behalf of those aged under 18 years (5%) and carers of those too sick to complete the survey themselves. The survey focused on the lived experience of members. It included health, social, educational and economic impacts, highlighting the nature and impact of remitting, relapsing and often severely debilitating symptoms, and the cascade of poor outcomes as a result of inadequate access to appropriate medical, social and financial support.

Respondent Demographics

Our survey sample was broadly similar to other Long COVID studies at the time (Davis et al., 2021; Sawano et al., 2024; Torjesen, 2021), reflecting a predominance of middle-aged people (21% 30–39 years, 32% 40–49 years, 23% 50–59 years) and women (84%). However, there was a higher proportion of women and those aged 40–49 years compared with other studies (Robertson et al., 2023; Woldegiorgis et al., 2024), which likely reflects the demographics of Facebook users and the use of a non random sample.

Symptoms

Most respondents had at least two vaccinations and one infection (86%). As such, it is likely that most (84%) experienced breakthrough Omicron infections in 2022, with far smaller cohorts experiencing infections in 2020 (8%) and 2021 (8%). The predominance of Omicron infections over earlier variants reflects the lower incidence of infection in Australia due to public health measures compared with international cohorts (Sawano et al., 2024). Only 7% of our respondents developed Long COVID before the availability of COVID vaccines. A small number of participants (less than 2%) had developed Long COVID symptoms in response to vaccination rather than infection.

Prior to infection or vaccination, respondents were overwhelmingly healthy (92% reporting good, very good or excellent health), with very few (less than 1%) reporting pre-existing poor health. After developing Long COVID and at the time of completing the survey (October 2022), only 9% reported good health and 63% reported poor health. Sawano et al. (2024) found 54% of their respondents reported poor or fair health (on a five-point scale) with around 25% reporting excellent or very good health, with a tendency for poorer health with pre-Omicron index infections.

Our respondents reported a median of 22 symptoms with 12 severe symptoms, and those infected prior to the Omicron wave (16%) tended to have more symptoms categorised as severe, and fewer resolving symptoms (see Table 9.1). Davis et al. (2021) report an average of 56 symptoms in an unvaccinated pre-Omicron population in late 2020. We were unable to directly compare our data with other published resources due to the different categorisation methods. However, our analysis reflected findings that patients experience a wide range of symptoms across bodily systems with a high symptom burden and poor quality of life (Sawano et al., 2024).

Fatigue and post-exertional malaise, cognitive dysfunction, sleep disturbances, pain, weakness and dizziness are consistently reported as very common among people with Long COVID (Davis et al., 2021; Sawano et al., 2024). Our respondents widely reported fatigue and post-exertional malaise (PEM), which severely impacted their efforts to

Table 9.1 Ranking of the top 12 most severe symptoms reported and the overall prevalence of these symptoms (n varies from 570 to 594)

Symptom	% experiencing	% severe
Fatigue and post-exertional malaise (PEM)	98.3	68.3
Poor concentration	96.8	40.1
Sleep problems	90.5	37.7
Information processing problems	93.5	33.0
Working memory problems	94.0	33.0
Word finding problems	90.3	28.0
Muscle weakness	84.8	29.5
Breathlessness	87.3	28.9
Headaches	86.2	28.4
Anxiety	85.4	28.3
Muscle pain	83.3	27.9
Dizziness	83.7	21.8

recover from COVID or vaccination. Concentration, working memory and breathlessness also negatively affected our ability to gain a diagnosis and treatment. These symptoms are the most prevalent in other studies, although PEM is inconsistently captured (Sawano et al., 2024). In effect, the symptoms themselves operated as a barrier to diagnosis and treatment.

According to our respondents, diarrhoea, fainting, chest pain, nausea/vomiting were most likely to resolve (11–7%) while symptoms reported as severe were more likely to persist. Gastrointestinal symptoms were somewhat less prevalent than found by Sawano et al. (2024) with nausea/vomiting (33%), appetite loss (32%) and inability to eat (21%) reported in our survey. Analysis of symptoms over time (7 months) by Davis et al. (2021) also showed some gastrointestinal symptoms (diarrhoea, vomiting, appetite loss) as being more likely to resolve for some patients.

Our data corroborate other studies in demonstrating that while earlier SARS-CoV-2 variants resulted in more severe disease (Sawano et al., 2024), the range and severity of Long COVID symptoms in fully vaccinated populations remain highly debilitating irrespective of variant (Sawano et al., 2024). Many of us in the Australia Long COVID Community were first told by GPs or specialists that people spontaneously recover by 6 months, which then changed to 12 months, then 18 months and now 2 years. While some people recover, far too many have not. This raises questions about the nature of recovery from Long COVID and highlights that reduced care seeking, which many interpret as recovery, may in fact be a cessation of futile effort in the absence of supportive and meaningful care.

Employment and Study

Over three quarters of respondents (80%) were working prior to infection, a similar proportion to the study by Sawano et al. (2024) (85%). The development of debilitating symptoms led to 11% of our respondents ceasing employment altogether, with 8% experiencing the termination of employment. More than 50% were absent from work (with or without benefits), 40% worked reduced hours, and only 4% reported no impact on their employment. Davis et al. (2021) reported 27% of patients originally employed at infection were working full time and in a similar capacity, with around 50% working reduced hours and 23% not working at all. Similar to Davis et al. (2021), flexible working and reduced hours with more breaks were the most common workplace adjustments sought by our respondents, with 40% indicating they now had less responsibility at work. In the week prior to completing the survey, less than 1 in 5 respondents (19%) worked 30 hours or more, with a third working zero hours (32%). For respondents engaged in education, 33% had suspended their studies, 22% were studying remotely and 16% had discontinued. Almost half (46%) of those still attempting study reported Long COVID affected their studies every day, while 30% reported no impact on their studies. Sawano et al. (2024) did not collect data on the impact on work or study.

Impact on Activities of Daily Living

Debilitating impacts of Long COVID across all aspects of life were reported. Most people (96%) reported difficulty with basic housework, along with cooking and caring for others (90%). Many experienced a daily reduction in their capacity to shop (50%) or socialise (61%) and more than 60% reported feeling unsupported. This difficulty in completing activities of daily living, staying connected or social isolation and finding support was also reflected in Sawano et al. (2024).

Seeking Medical Care

Most respondents had experienced symptoms for more than 12 weeks (92%) and had been diagnosed with Long COVID by a GP (63%), with 30% self-diagnosing. We sought help from cardiologists (approximately 2 in 5 respondents), Long COVID clinics (21%), emergency departments (33%), psychologists (24%), physiotherapists (27%) and naturopaths (20%). Some people (12%) had been admitted to hospital. Despite actively seeking medical care, suitable care was often difficult to access. GPs had significant knowledge gaps regarding diagnosis and treatments. Around two-thirds of us experienced an unwillingness to diagnose and poor knowledge from medical professionals. This was often compounded by disbelief from medical professionals and the minimisation of symptoms in both their severity and their impact. The community widely reported the psychologisation of symptoms, with anxiety and or depression often diagnosed as the cause of our symptoms and our distress.

Access to Long COVID clinics was poor due to long waiting times, and 70% said they were not a helpful source of information. Respondents described significant variation in the quality of care they received, and many reported being offered little other than outdated treatments, such as incremental physical activity or graded exercise therapy (GET) and cognitive behavioural therapy (CBT). Post-exertional malaise (PEM) or an abnormal response to, and recovery from, exertion is the cardinal symptom of ME/CFS. Treatment in Australia for ME/CFS continues to recommend CBT and GET (RACGP, 2024) despite these therapies being withdrawn by the National Institute for Health and Care Excellence (UK) in 2021 and Centers for Disease Control (USA) in 2017 due to a lack of or poor-quality evidence (Haunhorst et al., 2024; Kingdon et al., 2022; Vink & Vink-Niese, 2022). While understanding of the overlaps in pathophysiology is developing, an estimated 68% of people with Long COVID meet the criteria for ME/CFS (Haunhorst et al,

2024). To know this in our bodies and find ourselves repeatedly offered 'help' in the form of exercise, with no effective screening or monitoring for PEM, resulted in deep distrust.

> The doctors we went to weren't really educated about Long COVID, they didn't see any connection to having COVID. My mum cried a lot because she couldn't find anyone that knew what was going on with my health [...] This is the worst part when you're struggling with your health and there's an obvious connection to the virus, but doctors minimise the symptoms and blame anxiety. Meanwhile you're stuck with debilitating symptoms that need treatment. I have been unable to attend school for months due to no access to specialist treatment in my area. (Chris)

When looking for trusted information, the hierarchy of sources consulted by respondents was as follows: social media (58%), GPs/medical specialists (45%) and research groups (34%). This reflects the key role of social media in establishing critical networks of information and establishing online communities crucial in learning to understand and manage our illness, based on shared experience (Callard & Perego, 2021; Turner et al., 2023; Yeoman, 2024). For many providers, despite the severity of symptoms and clear debilitating impact there appeared to be a lack of interest and resultant knowledge in this disease that compounded the challenges of surviving with Long COVID.

> I have been incapacitated for 4 months with severe neurological symptoms, pain and paraesthesia. Have been unable to work as an ED nurse, have exhausted all leave entitlements and have spent $5000 thus far looking for answers via GPs, neurologists and ED presentations to no avail. Shame on you all. Spark an interest into LC, the symptoms, treatment and care. Keep abreast of what is known in the UK and US. Stop hiding under a blanket and accept this is debilitating and real. (Donna)

Survey 2, February 2023

A short supplementary survey was conducted in February 2023 to address a gap in the first survey regarding the efficacy of treatments for Long COVID. It was open for six days and received 449 responses. As both surveys were confidential, we were unable to link responses from the two surveys. The five most common treatments or management strategies used by respondents were pacing (82%), anti-inflammatories (63%), Vitamin B (63%), H1 antihistamines (62%) and probiotics (58%).

It is worth noting the most used treatments were those we arrived at independent of the medical system, and this reflects the absence of basic medical support and the degree to which we rely on our own research and testing. A seminal patient-led review into Long COVID (Davis et al., 2023) noted that exercise is harmful for people with PEM and contained a list of potential treatments. However, in Australia, most require the support of a GP or specialist, and their absence or low usage in our survey indicates that these potential treatments were not available in Australia at the time of the second survey (see Table 9.2).

Table 9.2 Treatments tried, with corresponding reports of improvement (n varies from 375 to 401)

Treatments	% tried	% improved
Pacing	81.6	83.4
Anti-inflammatories	65.8	51.1
Vitamin B	62.7	39.5
H1 antihistamines	61.6	62.3
Probiotics	57.5	43.5
Coenzyme Q10	39.8	45.5
H2 antihistamines	37.1	58.2
Low dose Naltrexone	20.8	61.7
IV immunoglobulins	5.0	10.5
Vagus nerve stimulation	30.4	55.5
Paxlovid	10.4	40.0
Valacyclovir, famciclovir, valganciclovir and other antivirals	8.9	26.5
Apheresis	4.2	6.3
Sulodexide	5.1	0.0
Pycnogenol	4.3	0.0

Survey 3, December 2023

This survey was conducted in December 2023 to inform a submission to the Commonwealth Government's COVID-19 Response Inquiry (Commonwealth of Australia, 2024). Our submission focused on the impact of the government's COVID management policies on those living with Long COVID. From a membership of 4,500 at the time we received 619 responses, of which 91% were completed by people with Long COVID, with the remainder of responses from family members or friends on behalf of someone living with Long COVID. More than 75% were aged between 30 and 59 years, 1% had lived with symptoms for nearly 4 years, 18% for more than two years, 65% for between one and two years, and 16% for less than a year.

When asked to rate five broad pandemic control measures (vaccination, personal protective equipment (PPE), testing, quarantine and antivirals), plus data collection and research for all of which the federal government was responsible, less than half were deemed adequate. Data collection and research was overwhelmingly rated the poorest of the measures (Table 9.3).

Less than 50% of respondents rated general health messaging adequate, both to the public and to medical professionals. Nearly all

Table 9.3 Ranking of the Australian Government's high-level COVID-19 pandemic response (n varies from 595 to 607)

Control measure	Excellent (%)	Reasonably good (%)	Adequate (%)	Room for improvement (%)	Not appropriate (%)
Vaccination	6.6	18.5	19.6	42.2	13.2
PPE	3.9	12.4	22.2	47.7	13.8
Testing (PCR & RAT)	5.8	12.4	17.7	50.7	13.5
Quarantine	3.4	7.7	19.7	46.5	22.7
Antivirals	1.5	5.1	9.1	61.9	22.4
Data collection and research	0.8	3.5	7.8	60.2	27.7

(98%) rated messaging about Long COVID to the public and medical professionals as poor or very poor. The ratings of support services for those with ongoing Long COVID symptoms were similar. Both practical support and income support were rated poor or very poor by 98% of respondents, and mental health support was rated as poor or very poor by 94% of respondents (Table 9.4).

Major issues raised regarding support services were a lack of access to the Disability Support Pension (DSP) and the National Disability Insurance Scheme (NDIS). Long COVID has resulted in a wave of newly disabled, yet the eligibility criteria for existing support programs do not readily cover Long COVID and the government has largely failed to address this issue. This is a hermeneutical or structural injustice writ large. While the 2023 survey did not use the term epistemic injustice, many of the free-text responses described it with unerring accuracy. A high-level analysis of more than 3,000 free-text responses revealed that 52% referenced one or more issues that could be coded as epistemic injustice. In other words, of all the things survey respondents chose to say, the majority said they had been treated unjustly, and that the nature of this injustice was epistemic. When looking specifically at responses to 'Any final comments' alone, nearly two thirds of responses

Table 9.4 2023 survey responses related to government health messaging and support services (n varies from 539 to 614)

	Very good (%)	Good (%)	Adequate (%)	Poor (%)	Very poor (%)
General health messaging					
To the public	4.7	10.4	33.4	29.4	22.0
To medical professionals	2.6	8.7	32.5	31.7	24.5
Long COVID health messaging					
To the public	0.0	0.5	1.3	16.4	81.8
To medical professionals	0.0	0.2	1.5	24.3	74.0
LC support services					
Practical support	0.2	0.3	1.6	21.9	76.0
Income support	0.0	0.3	1.8	17.3	80.6
Mental health support	0.3	0.5	5.1	23.7	70.4

(64%) referenced an experience of epistemic injustice. As this question was open-ended, these responses are a good indication of the nature of people's primary concerns. In addition, when given the opportunity to offer comments about government health messaging, 100% of the 127 free-text comments detailed examples of epistemic injustice.

Many free-text comments raised the need to monitor the incidence of Long COVID in the present to deliver adequate care, and the need to include monitoring for post-infection syndromes in future pandemics. Identifying and monitoring adverse health outcomes is a foundation of justice in healthcare. Without visibility, the ill do not receive adequate care and the healthy are blind to the risks they face. Without information, knowledge and understanding, there can be no epistemic justice. Freya described living in this vacuum as follows:

> The government's intentional downplaying of the severity of COVID in light of its decision to force the 'back to normal' narrative instead of encouraging or mandating the very real mitigation strategies we have access to has ruined both my mental and physical health. Every day is a struggle to try and inform, educate and protect the people around me and myself who is now high risk. I feel completely abandoned by the government.

Combining all free-text responses to all questions in Survey 3, close to a third (29%) described experiences of epistemic injustice relating to government policy, responses and actions, and 3% were specifically about the science being ignored. The wording of the comments conveyed a strong view from the respondents that their personal experience was being erased and that governments were unwilling to act in the public interest despite growing evidence of the need to do so. It was seen not only as erasure but as a structural mass silencing, perpetuating the suffering of those living with Long COVID. It also added to Long COVID numbers due to an intentional strategic shift in which public health became a personal responsibility, with an absence of access to the most basic of information necessary to make informed decisions about personal mitigation strategies.

Over a quarter of respondents (27%) described inadequate, inappropriate or absent care and policies that might facilitate it. Amie told us her experience was 'extremely lonely and confusing. I wish there had been early briefing for GPs and better information about the risks of Long COVID'. Samantha described how 'Public Long COVID clinics seem to be flying in the dark—they just bounce you around from specialist to specialist with no treatment just doing test after test'. John called for 'more research and education to our local GPs. It's embarrassing how little they know'. And Jayson repeated a common theme: 'The government's messaging is trying to deny all dangers around COVID-19 and [they are] not willing to inform the general population about the actual known risks of infections'.

Nearly one in four respondents (23%) described the pain of not being heard or understood, of being ignored, abandoned or forgotten. Sarah pleaded: 'Take it serious again and stop sweeping [us] under the carpet'. Richard described his sense of abandonment with the aim of making sure that 'this medical condition is acknowledged and supported, so that people like me can at least feel more dignified in our existence and have some hope that our condition can be managed or may even improve with time and medical intervention.' Another Samantha, who has been bed and housebound for close to a year, is 'still waiting to access the Long COVID clinic'. And 4% of respondents specifically referenced being disbelieved: an example being Jess, who wrote 'Health professionals treating us like we are hypochondriacs is devastating'.

Testimonial injustice was most frequently experienced when consulting doctors dismissed concerns based on the absence of evidence using current testing, resulting in offers of treatment for anxiety or depression. As female sex is a risk factor for Long COVID, these experiences highlight the insidious consequences of medical paternalism. The refusal of the federal Health Minister or his staff to meet with us when requested was viewed as both a personal and a structural silencing. Hermeneutical injustices ranged from difficulty receiving a diagnosis due to an absence of diagnostic criteria, challenges accessing medical care due to an absence of care pathways and an inability to qualify for practical and financial support due to an absence of policy capable of dealing with poorly defined chronic illnesses or dynamic disabilities.

Mem lamented, 'The world moves on whilst we decline and remain housebound'.

Respondents consistently described an absence of urgency about Long COVID and its impacts on individuals and society. It was felt that very few people were taking Long COVID seriously, and fewer still chose to educate themselves adequately. This sentiment was borne out by government inaction in the development of a co-ordinated body of expertise in the emerging field of Long COVID, and reports from patient advocates whose attempts to communicate with local politicians made little to no impact, with the very really challenges of Long COVID continuing to be absent in public messaging and most people's day-to-day lives.

Employers and work colleagues were significantly ill-informed about the nature and incidence of Long COVID, with the result that they often failed to offer basic understanding and appropriate support. Sadly, many friends and family members were equally ill-informed, frequently unsympathetic, offering little to no support or worse, actively minimising or denying the challenges of living with Long COVID.

The impact of all this lack of recognition is captured in Kelly's words: 'This has been hell and if I didn't have the Long COVID Facebook page, I would have had nobody and nowhere to turn to. A disease not believed, often not recognised and not known how to treat. Jackpot!'

Conclusion, Where to from Here?

Long COVID has impacted every aspect of our lives. From working, to parenting, and relationships with partners, family and friends, our ability to participate in the most basic of daily activities has been deeply compromised, a situation compounded by inadequate care and an absence of financial or practical support. The social and financial fallout continues to reverberate throughout family units and social networks to this day. As one respondent told us:

> I'm so anxious about the future and what will happen when [my husband's] leave runs out. If he loses his job, it will be financial ruin for our family - we will not be able to pay our mortgage and will end up homeless with nothing. (Paula)

Those with lived experiences have had to learn the art of advocacy to access care in managing a raft of debilitating symptoms. This should not be so. In the words of one of this chapter's authors,

> I have never had any personal experience, or even significant contact with anything quite like this in my already long life. I am aware that such situations are not that uncommon, that our health and medical systems, while truly excellent in many ways, continue to fail many people, especially those with chronic conditions, for similar reasons. But to experience it for oneself and then to read repeatedly about similar and sometimes far worse experiences of so many others in this country has still been an extremely uncomfortable and very challenging revelation.

Despite the publication of the two government inquiries to which we submitted our survey findings, there has been an absence of government policy leading to a failure in the provision of appropriate medical, financial and practical support for people living with Long COVID. After 297 days, the Commonwealth Government issued a response to the Parliamentary Inquiry into Long COVID noting, but not acting on, a number of important recommendations, including a nationally co-ordinated research program, Long COVID education for primary care providers, funding for Long COVID clinics in regional and remote areas, establishing a multi-disciplinary advisory body for indoor clean air quality and reviewing eligibility for subsidised access to antivirals (Commonwealth of Australia, 2024). The lack of action on indoor air quality is particularly concerning due to the evidence demonstrating that clean indoor air is key in limiting the spread of COVID-19 (Bazant & Bush, 2021; Peng et al., 2022), and the current absence of Australian standards for indoor air quality (University of Wollongong, 2024).

Other recommendations given only in principle support included a nationally co-ordinated database for COVID-19 and Long COVID, nationally co-ordinated research from basic science through to trials, models of care, and health promotion to implementation science and a review of the pandemic response (Commonwealth of Australia, 2024). The recommendation to establish an Australian Centre for Disease Control did result in the establishment of an interim body in 2025 (Commonwealth of Australia, 2024). One recommendation supported without qualification was the production of evidence-based guidelines (Commonwealth of Australia, 2024), but while this is important it does little to address the social and financial impact of living with Long COVID for years. Most of the few recommendations that were fully supported could only be expected to offer minor improvements to the lives of people with Long COVID, due to poor funding and few significant changes in policy.

Long COVID and this chapter have been a journey from heartbreak to hope. The chapter offers a window into our lives. Unfortunately, in Australia, little has changed for us in the past five years. However, we are not alone. Many have faced such epistemic injustice before us. We are the latest and newest cohort living with a post-infection associated chronic disease. Our health system is flawed, humans are flawed and the road to understanding will be long and hard. Nonetheless, we live in hope that through continued advocacy the brave and understanding few will become the many and finally the great majority. We offer these findings as a contribution to that journey. We continue to live constrained lives and had not anticipated that our survey results would reach a wider audience. We are therefore grateful for the opportunity to contribute to the body of knowledge through this book. What happens next will depend on what readers with capacity will do with it. Our hope and our motivation for writing this chapter is that these final words will lead to ongoing dialogue and joint action to address this overwhelming epistemic injustice.

Acknowledgements We are indebted to every member of the Australia Long COVID Community who contributed to documenting the experience of living with Long COVID between 2020 and 2023: designing, creating, distributing, completing or analysing the surveys, giving permission to be quoted, helping to prepare or present submissions to government, as well as all those who provided details of their personal experience of epistemic injustice through other means.

Note

1. Some of our respondents wanted to keep their real first names in any reporting of findings, while others requested anonymity, and were therefore given pseudonyms.

References

Australian Institute of Health and Welfare. (2024). *Australia's health 2024: In brief*. https://www.aihw.gov.au/reports/australias-health/australias-health-2024-in-brief/summary

Bazant, M. Z., & Bush, J. W. M. (2021). A guideline to limit indoor airborne transmission of COVID-19. *Proceedings of the National Academy of Sciences—PNAS, 118*(17), 1–12. https://doi.org/10.1073/pnas.2018995118

Bayliss, K., Goodall, M., Chisholm, A., Fordham, B., Chew-Graham, C., Riste, L., Fisher, L., Lovell, K., Peters, S., & Wearden, A. (2014). Overcoming the barriers to the diagnosis and management of chronic fatigue syndrome/ ME in primary care: A meta synthesis of qualitative studies. *BMC Family Practice, 15*(1), 44–11. https://doi.org/10.1186/1471-2296-15-44

Blease, C., Carel, H., & Geraghty, K. (2017). Epistemic injustice in healthcare encounters: Evidence from chronic fatigue syndrome. *Journal of Medical Ethics, 43*(8), 549–557. https://doi.org/10.1136/medethics-2016-103691

Callard, F., & Perego, E. (2021). How and why patients made Long COVID. *Social Science & Medicine, 268*. https://doi.org/10.1016/j.socscimed.2020.113426

Commonwealth of Australia. (2024). *Commonwealth Government COVID-19 Response Inquiry Report*. https://www.pmc.gov.au/resources/covid-19-response-inquiry-report

Davis, H. E., Assaf, G. S., McCorkell, L., Wei, H., Low, R. J., Re'em, Y., Redfield, S., Austin, J. P., & Akrami, A. (2021). Characterizing long COVID in an international cohort: 7 months of symptoms and their impact. *EClinicalMedicine, 38*. https://doi.org/10.1016/j.eclinm.2021.101019

Davis, H. E., McCorkell, L., Vogel, J. M., & Topol, E. J. (2023). Long COVID: Major findings, mechanisms and recommendations. *Nature*

Reviews. Microbiology, 21(3), 133–146. https://doi.org/10.1038/s41579-022-00846-2

Fricker, M. (2007). *Epistemic injustice: Power and the ethics of knowing*. Oxford University Press.

Haunhorst, S., Dudziak, D., Scheibenbogen, C., Seifert, M., Sotzny, F., Finke, C., Behrends, U., Aden, K., Schreiber, S., Brockmann, D., Burggraf, P., Bloch, W., Ellert, C., Ramoji, A., Popp, J., Reuken, P., Walter, M., Stallmach, A., & Puta, C. (2024). Towards an understanding of physical activity-induced post-exertional malaise: Insights into microvascular alterations and immunometabolic interactions in post-COVID condition and myalgic encephalomyelitis/chronic fatigue syndrome. *Infection, 53*. https://doi.org/10.1007/s15010-024-02386-8

Ho, A. (2011). Trusting experts and epistemic humility in disability. *International Journal of Feminist Approaches to Bioethics, 4*(2), 102–123. https://doi.org/10.3138/ijfab.4.2.102

Ireson, J., Taylor, A., Richardson, E., Greenfield, B., & Jones, G. (2022). Exploring invisibility and epistemic injustice in Long Covid—A citizen science qualitative analysis of patient stories from an online COVID community. *Health Expectations, 25*(4), 1753–1765. https://doi.org/10.1111/hex.13518

Kidd, I. J. (Ed.). (2017). *The Routledge handbook of epistemic injustice*. Routledge. https://doi.org/10.4324/9781315212043

Kingdon, C., Lowe, A., Shepherd, C., & Nacul, L. (2022). What primary care practitioners need to know about the new NICE guideline for myalgic encephalomyelitis/chronic fatigue syndrome in adults. *Healthcare, 10*(12). https://doi.org/10.3390/healthcare10122438

Mullard, J., Mir, G., Herbert, C., & Evans, S. (2024). 'You're just a guinea pig': Exploring the barriers and impacts of living with Long COVID-19: A view from the undiagnosed. *Sociology of Health & Illness, 46*(8), 1602–1625. https://doi.org/10.1111/1467-9566.13795

Peng, Z., Rojas, A. L. P., Kropff, E., Bahnfleth, W., Buonanno, G., Dancer, S. J., Kurnitski, J., Li, Y., Loomans, M. G. L. C., Marr, L. C., Morawska, L., Nazaroff, W., Noakes, C., Querol, X., Sekhar, C., Tellier, R., Greenhalgh, T., Bourouiba, L., Boerstra, A., … Jimenez, J. L. (2022). Practical indicators for risk of airborne transmission in shared indoor environments and their application to COVID-19 outbreaks. *Environmental Science & Technology, 56*(2), 1125–1137. https://doi.org/10.1021/acs.est.1c06531

Plastina, A. F. (2025). Long COVID patients' reconstruction of medical gaslighting discourse in online epistemic communities. *Patient Education and Counseling, 134*. https://doi.org/10.1016/j.pec.2025.108665

Porter, T., Watson, N., & Pearson, C. (2023). Epistemic sabotage: The production and disqualification of evidence in disability benefit claims. *Sociology of Health & Illness, 45*(6), 1164–1186. https://doi.org/10.1111/1467-9566.13593

Rebman, A. W., Yang, T., & Aucott, J. N. (2024). Invalidation by medical professionals in post-treatment Lyme disease. *Scientific Reports, 14*(1), 19406–19410. https://doi.org/10.1038/s41598-024-70556-7

Robertson, M. M., Qasmieh, S. A., Kulkarni, S. G., Teasdale, C. A., Jones, H. E., McNairy, M., Borrell, L. N., & Nash, D. (2023). The epidemiology of long coronavirus disease in US adults. *Clinical Infectious Diseases, 76*(9), 1636–1645. https://doi.org/10.1093/cid/ciac961

Sawano, M., Wu, Y., Shah, R. M., Zhou, T., Arun, A. S., Khosla, P., Kaleem, S., Vashist, A., Bhattacharjee, B., Ding, Q., Lu, Y., Caraballo, C., Warner, F., Huang, C., Herrin, J., Putrino, D., Michelsen, T., Fisher, L., Adinig, C., … Krumholz, H. M. (2025). Long COVID characteristics and experience: A descriptive study from the Yale LISTEN Research Cohort. *The American Journal of Medicine, 138*(4), 12–720. https://doi.org/10.1016/j.amjmed.2024.04.015

Seeley, M.-C., Gallagher, C., Colman, F., & Lau, D. H. (2023). Impact of Long COVID on Australian sufferers: Implications for healthcare planning. *Heart, Lung & Circulation, 32*(10), 76–77. https://doi.org/10.1016/j.hlc.2023.09.002

Standing Committee on Health, Aged Care and Sport. (2023). *Sick and tired: Casting a long shadow. Inquiry into Long COVID and repeated COVID infections*. Parliament of Australia. https://www.aph.gov.au/Parliamentary_Business/Committees/House/Health_Aged_Care_and_Sport/LongandrepeatedCOVID/Report

The Royal Australian College of General Practitioners (RACGP). (2024). *Incremental physical activity for chronic fatigue syndrome/myalgic encephalomyelitis* (HANDI Interventions). https://www.racgp.org.au/clinical-resources/clinical-guidelines/handi/handi-interventions/exercise/incremental-physical-activity-for-cfs-me

Torjesen, I. (2021). COVID-19: Middle aged women face greater risk of debilitating long term symptoms. *British Medical Journal, 372*, 829–829. https://doi.org/10.1136/bmj.n829

Turner, M., Beckwith, H., Spratt, T., Vallejos, E. P., Coughlan, B. (2023). The longcovid revolution: A reflexive thematic analysis. *Social Science & Medicine, 333*. https://doi.org/10.1016/j.socscimed.2023.116130, https://www.sciencedirect.com/science/article/pii/S0277953623004872

University of Wollongong. (2024). *The impact of Indoor Air quality on the transmission of airborne diseases in public buildings*. https://www.chiefscientist.gov.au/sites/default/files/2024-08/Indoor%20Air%20Quality%20Report%202024.pdf

Vink, M., & Vink-Niese, A. (2022). The updated NICE guidance exposed the serious flaws in CBT and graded exercise therapy trials for ME/CFS. *Healthcare, 10*(5). https://doi.org/10.3390/healthcare10050898

Woldegiorgis, M., Cadby, G., Ngeh, S., Korda, R. J., Armstrong, P. K., Maticevic, J., Knight, P., Jardine, A., Bloomfield, L. E., & Effler, P. V. (2024). Long COVID in a highly vaccinated but largely unexposed Australian population following the 2022 SARS-CoV-2 Omicron wave: A cross-sectional survey. *Medical Journal of Australia, 220*(6), 323–330. https://doi.org/10.5694/mja2.52256

Yeoman, P. (2024). Knowledge, knowing, and the knower: A postdigital autoethnography of learning to live with Long COVID. In J. Lamb & L Carvalho (Eds.), *Postdigital learning spaces* (pp. 139–154). Springer. https://doi.org/10.1007/978-3-031-59691-9_8

10

Living with the Virus: An Autoethnography of Long COVID as Multilayered Traumatisation

Vivienne Matthies-Boon

Introduction

> The life I had before COVID is gone, and it will never return. […] Wounds of abandonment, societal abandonment, political abandonment. […] most of my interactions are behind a computer screen, like a window looking into a world that I am no longer part of. Seeing how life goes on without me. Long COVID feels like being buried alive under a rubble of negligence. (personal diary, 24 September 2023)

The above quote is taken from the diary that I started after my first COVID infection in January 2022, from which I never recovered. I, like the by now 400 million fellow sufferers (Al-Aly et al., 2024), developed Long COVID: a profoundly disabling disease that left me home-bound

V. Matthies-Boon (✉)
Department of Ethics and Political Philosophy, Faculty of Philosophy, Theology and Religious Studies, Radboud University, Nijmegen, The Netherlands
e-mail: vivienne.matthies-boon@ru.nl

D. Lupton (ed.), *Long COVID and Society*,
https://doi.org/10.1007/978-981-96-9168-5_10

for 1.5 years and bedbound in a semi-vegetative state for 6 months. Although Long COVID is a biomedical disorder, this chapter will not focus on its medical underpinnings, but rather on its existential impacts. More particularly, through an autoethnographic account, I argue that Long COVID entails a multilayered traumatic abandonment, entailing bodily incapacitation, medical neglect, psychologisation social isolation as well as political neglect. Hence, rather than having the existential effects of their physical illness alleviated through shared social, medical and political holding spaces, wherein the severity of suffering and disease can be recognised, patients face denial, indifference and even aggression that compounds the traumatic burden of their physical illness.

Importantly, as outlined in the first section of this chapter, I regard such traumatisation not as a psychological disorder as stipulated in the DSM, but instead, adopting a critical theoretical approach, as traumatic status subordination. Traumatic status subordination is a concept I developed (2022) by drawing on the philosophies of Jürgen Habermas, Nancy Fraser and Rahel Jaeggi explicitly, and entails a fundamental betrayal of the counterfactual presupposition of being treated as an equal human being. As the counterfactual presupposition of equal worth as a human being is severely damaged, the lifeworld crumbles, leading to traumatic alienation. The advantages of such a critical theoretical model are that it avoids the individualisation and cognitive psychologisation of trauma, grounding it in structures of social and political justice instead.

This chapter is personal: an autoethnographic account that draws on the Long COVID diary that I have kept since January 2022 as well as private conversations with other patients and the public statements of fellow patients. Autoethnography enables a deep reflection on the subjective existential experience of Long COVID that reaches beyond the level of philosophical intentionality to the underlying existential structures of Being (Ratcliffe, 2012, 2020). For example, it not only enables reflection on the 'I am angry at' but also on the ways in which such intentional emotions affect and are affected by one's Being in the world. Importantly, while the 'auto' component emphasises the researcher's subjective experiences, it places these in relation to social, political, medical and economic developments. Hence, following Chang (2016), autoethnography has three (interrelated) aims: (i) to testify through the articulation of a damaged self; (ii) to emancipate (giving voice to the voiceless) and (iii) to disrupt by destabilising dominant narratives. This chapter thus not only articulates my experience of my disrupted self, but in doing so gives voice to the physical and existential suffering of patients and disrupts the dominant discourse that COVID is 'nothing but a flu'.

A Critical Theory of Trauma: Trauma as Intersubjective Abandonment

Trauma is often equated with Post Traumatic Stress Disorder (PTSD). However, the conception of trauma as PTSD that gained dominance after its inclusion in the Diagnostic and Statistical Manual (DSM) of the American Psychological Association in the 1980s is problematic, since it remains stuck within a Philosophy of the Subject, and in doing so fails to sufficiently account for the social and political constitution of trauma (see Matthies-Boon, 2022). Although the concept of PTSD has been revised since its initial inclusion in the DSM, the standard conception of trauma as PTSD entails an (extraordinary) event that overwhelms the brain, resulting in symptoms such as hyper-alertness, avoidance, flashbacks, anxiety and stress (American Psychiatric Association, 2014).

This conception is epistemologically as well as ethically problematic. It is epistemologically problematic because while the aim of the DSM is to diagnose mental disorders on the basis of nosological observation of symptoms alone, trauma entailing its own aetiology in its definition (as it includes both the event as well as its effects) goes beyond the boundaries of nosological diagnosis (Alford, 2016; Kihlstrom, 2008; Matthies-Boon, 2022). After all, it is through an interpretative relation to an specific event or events that trauma is set apart from other psychological disorders such as anxiety or depression. Yet, this interpretive act that goes beyond the epistemic boundaries of nosological symptomology that the DSM was supposed to be based on.

Realising the thin epistemological ground on which trauma studies found itself, scholars have tried to seek epistemological refuge in neuroscience, which would surely provide firm empirical evidence. However, not only were the functional MRI scans used in trauma studies too imprecise to accord exact neurological functioning to them in the context of PTSD (Alford, 2016), but the causal relation to the event is still not empirically established through the observation of medical symptoms and facts. As Kihlstrom (2008) argued, rather than resolving this epistemological difficulty, all that has happened is the translation of psychological assumptions into the language of neuroscience.

The consequences of this arc significant, as trauma studies committed, I argue (2022), a classical category mistake: it moved trauma out of the realm of the realm of socio-normative rightenousness (concerned with issues of justice) and placed it in the realm of objective truth (concerned with medical facts), thereby reifying it as a medical objective fact located inside the individual mind or brain. This resulted in an individualist, cognitivist and eventist conception of trauma, with an undue focus on the cognitively overwhelming event (retrospectively conceived) rather than continuous chronic structures of social and political injustice. Hence, in addition to the epistemological difficulties, it resulted in the depoliticisation of (now individualist) trauma. This is also ethically problematic as it results in a double injury: namely those who already suffered an injustice are now also told that there is something wrong with their brain and are held responsible for its recovery through therapeutic interventions (Matthies-Boon, 2022).

And so, I argue for a critical theoretical understanding of trauma as broken intersubjectivity: namely as the violent betrayal of the counterfactual presupposition of being treated and regarded as having equal worth as a human being in relation to another.[1] This is not to say that we are always equal. We do for instance occupy different (unequal) roles in different situations and phases of our lives. However, the counterfactual presupposition of equality goes deeper than that: it is the presupposition that fundamentally as a human being, regardless of the different roles we occupy, we are in essence equal. It is precisely this fundamental presupposition that trauma breaks. As this fundamental presupposition ruptures, the lifeworld breaks down, and the victim is thrown into traumatic alienation. Importantly, trauma, grounded in an impairment of equal intersubjectivity, is thus less an issue of medical objective truth than socio-normative righteousness.[2]

Trauma is therefore a matter of grave injustice. It may have subjective effects but cannot be reduced to an individual cognitive problem. For in trauma, one suffers traumatic status subordination: the equal intersubjective value of an individual or a group is reduced by another individual or group through the imposition of violence (see Matthies-Boon, 2022). Such traumatic status subordination may occur through the active infliction of violent events and structures but actually also through radical inactivity or neglect, including abandonment—wherein the value of the other is reduced. Importantly, although unpleasant, not all forms of injustice are traumatic. An injustice becomes traumatic when the capacity to speak back at the inflicted injustice is destroyed. Hence, whether injustice is traumatic cannot be established a priori but rather has to be established empirically, on a case-based analysis.

Long COVID, I propose, is traumatic because patients suffer multiple levels of abandonment wherein they suffer traumatic status subordination *vis a vis* others. This means that Long COVID patients are robbed of the capacity to intersubjectively manifest themselves in the world, and as they are increasingly pushed into the margins of society, lose the capacity to speak back at the injustice inflicted. The resolution of such injustice does not lie in individual therapeutic interventions but rather in re-establishment of relations of care through institutionalised solidarity wherein the suffering and risk of post-viral chronicity is recognised (Matthies-Boon and Sharon, 2025).

Physical Traumatisation

The first level of traumatic abandonment that Long COVID patients experience is the physical abandonment of their body through severe bodily incapacitation following a SARS-CoV-2 infection. In my case, I developed Long COVID in January 2022, just a few days after my second COVID Pfizer vaccination. This immunological double load basically left me chronically impaired and profoundly disabled. For the first 1.5 years, I was home- and largely bedbound. From the (northern hemisphere) autumn of 2022, I suffered severe deterioration of my physical state, as a result of which I was bedbound in a semi-vegetative state for approximately 6 months. I continue to suffer from severe immune dysregulation, cardiovascular issues, gastrointestinal difficulties and haematological problems. I have a progressive immune disease of the white blood cells (mast cell activation syndrome [MCAS]) but also elevated auto-antibodies and inflammatory markers, as well as a reactivation of the herpes zoster virus. The essential amino acids eucine, isoleucine and valine are furthermore almost entirely depleted, and I suffer from muscle atrophy that gravely undermines my mobility. My eyes are often painful and blurry, I have difficulty breathing and suffer from random trembling. In the absence of a medical solution, I retain semi-functionality through immune suppressive, mast cell stabilising medication as well as blood thinners.

Long COVID throws one's entire life into disarray. As bodily functionality is seriously impaired, a deep sense of physical abandonment results. Such physical abandonment is not specific to Long COVID but often occurs in severe and chronic illness. As the body ceases to smoothly operate in the world, it not only enters into our awareness as an (alien) object, but we often feel abandoned by it as it appears to us as problematic malfunctioning object. As Havi Carel (2016) explains, severe and chronic illness therefore often challenges our fundamental assumptions about the trajectory of our lives, our sense of space and time as well as the self. Suddenly confronted with vulnerability and the possibility of mortality not as an abstract entity but as a more immediate possibility, our perception of our life changes: we no longer assume the functionality of our body but rather contemplate its (chronic) demise. In Long COVID, I argue this confrontation is severe because as a multisystemic disorder it affects not just a part of the body but throws the entire body into disarray.

The most profound experience of these challenges is post-exertional malaise (PEM), which entails an aggravation of symptoms after the slightest physical, cognitive or emotional exertion (such as taking a shower or even being exposed to the sound, touch or light). PEM entails a complete incapacitation of the body as it disappears into a dark tunnel of exhaustion and pain—of non-being. It is therefore referred to by patients as a state of 'living death' (Mannix, 2023). As I wrote in my diary:

> Came out the shower, lifeless body, apathetically hanging, unable to move. Crawling over the floor. Now slumped on the chair, bed is probably better, but I don't know how to get there. Breathing costs all energy I have. Apathetically gazing into space. Unable to even think. Like my body is taken away from me, no longer my own. Frustration [….] I am hungry, which further aggravates my helpless exhaustion. I cannot move my limbs, let alone make dinner. Reduced to nothingness. Arms have weights on them. Vision is blurred, or surreal, it is as if I see from behind a see through curtain. Nothing is real. I am in my head, yet no longer there either. Trying my best to type this but it is hard. Hard to think, to describe, but above all very hard to move my fingers on the keyboard. My arms rest on my table, I keep my body still, my head hanging slightly to the left side. I do not move, because movement costs too much. Heavy nothingness has descended over me. Unable to act. Mouth open, breathing. Easier to let everything hang. Blurred feeling in head, but also chest and stomach. Am sitting cross legged but it is hard to move one leg away from other. Takes 10 seconds to get my will to move my leg, for it to then be moved like a heavy log. Everything is heavy. Everything hangs. Gazing into nothingness. Breathing automatic pilot. My sense of self has been reduced, evaporated. I am suffocated by this heaviness. Even my will to will cannot be in this state. Instead, willing itself is too exhausting. I am lifeless matter, alive merely through open mouth breathing. Being without being. My head is heavy, a band is around my ears and eyes, and a nauseated turning in my stomach as exhaustion overtakes my entire being. High pitched ringing in my ears confirms the takeover, my submission. I sit, unmoving. Just breathing. Everything else is too much. My body feels alien, my legs no longer my own, my hands and my arms so heavy I cannot reach them inside. My will to will is absent. I lean against the back of the chair, in a state of non-being. Apathetic. Shaking inside, small vibrations, even doing nothing costs too much energy. I am disappearing into a state of non-being. (personal diary, 20 September 2022)

In PEM, bodily capacity is entirely impaired. Hence, PEM poses an extreme challenge to our most fundamental assumptions and beliefs through which we normally orient ourselves in the world. As I wrote in my diary, Long COVID fundamentally ruptures one's notion of self—that is, the idea of the self as a relatively autonomous actor capable of manifesting itself in the world. By contrast, I realised that:

> [T]his illness entails nothing less than submission. The submission to a force or an authority so great, that one does not stand a chance. Incapacitation. Utter nullification of the will, until the storm is over. No idea when it will end, or indeed if it will end. The fear that it might never end. My will does not stand a chance against the brute force of the body. It is utterly dependent on and crushed by the body. I normally live under the illusion of the will leading one's way through life. I made choices, thought that I was 'in control', partook in certain actions [...b]ut illness breaks through that illusion. The will is void, or rather small, not as big as one thought it was. Rather, it lies here in bed, broken, hurt and in tatters as I stare into space. For the will, or even the will to will, has the well-functioning abled body as its precondition. And when the body gives up or caves in, the will is forced to follow. Illness is submission. (personal diary, 5 September 2023)

Hence, given the severity as well as unpredictability of this illness, a deep existential struggle arises as the will feels abandoned (by a body that has ceased to function well). It is thus not surprising that many patients often complain of being 'imprisoned in their body', as they find themselves trapped in a body that no longer functions.

Medical Traumatisation

The experience of entrapment in a malfunctioning body is made worse by a lack of medical solutions and also particularly of medical care, leaving patients feeling abandoned and fending for themselves (in their broken bodies). Not only are proper Long COVID clinics often few and far between, and the waiting lists enormous (often lasting months and even years), but the quality of care also differs significantly between countries and even between these clinics.[3] Given the complexity of their illness, Long COVID patients are not unfrequently described as difficult time-consuming patients by professionals who should be responsible for their medical care.[4] In the absence of medical abnormalities detectable in standard medical testing, the illness remains perceived by such physicians as psychosomatic, despite the growing evidence to the contrary. Hence, the problem of medical stigmatisation amongst Long COVID patients is grave (Schomerus, 2024). Especially since 'standard' medical tests (such as MRI scans, EKG and ordinary blood tests) do not reveal medical abnormalities, patients have been routinely accused by medical professionals from whom they seek help of 'making it up' (Ärzteblatt & Redaktion Deutsches, 2023). Subsequently, the relation of medical care is withdrawn, or even violated, as patients are subjected to treatment (such as graded exercise therapy or cognitive behavioural therapy) that will often make their physical situation much worse.

This epistemic injustice, wherein the lived experiences of patients are not taken seriously by their physicians, stands in a long and unfortunate tradition of the psychologisation of post-viral and post-bacterial illnesses, and particularly myalgic encephalitis/chronic fatigue syndrome (ME/CFS) but also AIDS (Geraghty & Blease, 2019; Ware, 1992; Wasonga, 2014). And while most medical professionals would now regard HIV infection and AIDS as biomedical issues (as treatment developed due to patient activism), people living with other post-viral disorders such as ME/CFS have been far less fortunate. Here, the controversial PACE trial (Kindlon, 2011), which turned out to be methodologically deeply flawed, played an important role in the psychologisation of ME/CFS. It institutionalised the belief that the cause of post-viral and post-bacterial syndromes was 'unhelpful thoughts' by patients who were malingering in their attempt to reap 'illness gains'. Moreover, it ascribed exercise intolerance to a lack of willingness rather than physical incapacitation and deterioration. This resulted in a variety of abusive practices, including depriving patients of food and drink (which was placed at such a distance they had to get out of bed to reach them, despite their physical inability to do so) and the forced removal of children from their parental homes. This treatment often resulted in a physical deterioration, sometimes even up to the point of death (Smith, 2024). Psychologisation is an epistemic injustice with profound physical but also psychological damage: it also led many patients to internalised guilt. Many started to believe that they had themselves to blame for the fate that had befallen them (Vink & Vink-Niese, 2022).[5]

Moreover, the psychologisation of post-viral illness resulted in a decreased incentive to invest in biomedical research. After all, if the origins were to be found in the mind or brain, no further biomedical investigation was necessary. This not only gave rise to the self-fulfilling logic of psychologisation, as the opportunities to prove psychologisation wrong decreased, but also meant that biomedical research on post-viral illnesses is still lagging behind—to the detriment of current Long COVID and other post-viral patients. I argue therefore that post-viral illness is situated within a structural process of medical abandonment: namely the withdrawal of appropriate medical relations of care through psychologisation and the lack of biomedical research and development, wherein specific doctor-patient encounters (marked by disinterest, or a lack of care and even stigmatisation) are manifested (Schomerus, 2024).

Personally, I have been relatively lucky, in that the psychologisation I experienced has been minimal when compared to that of others: my GP and specialists in Germany believed that there was something physically (rather than psychologically) wrong with me. However, given the long-term shortage of biomedical research into such illnesses, there was nothing much they could do. And so, even in those cases where patients are not subjected directly to the harm of psychologisation (but rather had their physical complaints taken seriously), they do suffer from the broader indirect effects of the psychologisation of postviral illnesses—namely, medical negligence through a the lack of medical knowledge, biomedical research and treatment of post-infectious illnesses.

The upshot of this neglect is that, desperate as they mostly are for improvement, patients become personally responsible for trying to find their way to potential relevant expertise. More often than not, they not only have to pay for these appointments and prescribed treatments out of pocket (as in the absence of sufficient medical evidence, health insurers often do not pay) but these consultations also often deliver meagre results. Hence, like many other patients, I have a vast trail of medical specialists behind me (including a cardiologist, pulmonologist, neurologist, endocrinologist, haematologist, gynaecologist, gastroenterologist, ophthalmologist, immunologist as well as an rheumatologist), most of whom could not really help. It also meant that I spent at least a quarter of my salary on potential treatments. The consequences for the patient, both physical and existential, are very real. As I wrote in my diary:

> So on the XXth of February, I have an appointment with Dr XXX. And I am not sure what to think anymore. I am too tired by all these appointments, the anticipation, the hope that 'maybe, just maybe, this can help a little bit', only to find yourself out of the door 15 min later, 500 euros poorer with nowhere to go and turn. This illness honestly feels like being dropped in a never-ending, resource depleting labyrinth, filled with a growing number of other zombie-like guests or patients, each of whom is trying to find their own way out. And often, the moment they shout 'Eureka!', when they claim that they have found a way out, they fall right back in—either through a reinfection or an autoimmune flare up. It truly is a dark horrific nightmare without end. (personal diary, 14 January 2025)

This absence of medical care not only results in (potentially dangerous) self-experimentation by patients with supplements and medicine but also means that the worst affected, namely those who are entirely bedridden, remain deprived of care at all. And those who are excluded are of course also those who are not well-off, who would not have the means to bear these costs. Hence, within patient communities, stories abound of bedbound patients (adults and children) often in severe pain, in darkened rooms for years on end without any medical care or attention. They have been and continue to be medically abandoned.

Another form of medical abandonment patient experience is the lack of protection inside medical facilities, which leads to care avoidance out of fear of COVID reinfections. For instance, I was prescribed with Maraviroc, a HIV medication, in December 2024 by an immunologist, which, due to the overactivation of my white blood cells, went horribly wrong. I suffered a cytokine storm that directly affected my heart. It meant I had to be admitted to hospital. Except I could not be admitted as the doctors deemed the risk of a nosocomial COVID reinfection to be too great. Such a reinfection, the doctors agreed, would only make my situation much worse. The lack of preventive measures within medical facilities is another layer of medical abandonment of Long COVID patients. And the feeling of not being able to access acute medical care in a safe manner, just adds to the traumatic layering of Long COVID—to the feeling of traumatic abandonment.

Social and Political Traumatisation

Bodily and medical traumatisation is compounded by social and political abandonment. As with any trauma, the bodily and medical traumatisation of Long COVID patients could in principle be alleviated through social and political holding spaces wherein their suffering is recognised and the urgency of biomedical research and treatment underscored. But rather than receiving such social and political support, Long COVID patients find themselves neglected at best and being subjected to social and political stigmatisation, aggression and ridicule at worst.

One of the reasons for this absence of social and political recognition and support is the political failure to institutionalise structures of solidarity at the time Long COVID emerged as an increasing medical, social and political problem. Referring to the Netherlands, Matthies-Boon and Sharon (2024) argued that while in the early years of the pandemic there was considerable spontaneous solidarity between citizens, when this started to dwindle as the crisis endured, the government did not institutionalise solidarity: for instance, through the free supplies of protective equipment, facilitating flexible (online) work and educational modes, and investing in clean air through HEPA filters and ventilation, as well as emphasising the chronic health risks of COVID 19 infections to all citizens. Rather, like many other governments, the Dutch government withdrew from taking responsibility for the public health of their citizens. Indeed, the Dutch Ministry of Health directly admitted that in face of the declining solidarity, the Dutch government (like many others) resorted to a return to normality using the banner of individual responsibility.

However, such individual responsibility is practically and ethically problematic. Not only is individual responsibility unworkable in light of a highly contagious (and thus *intersubjective*) disease, this policy also presupposes not a clearly definable (but false) distinction between the vulnerable and non-vulnerable, failing to supply citizens with the necessary tools (such as masks and knowledge) to carry out their individual responsibility.[5] And so, a (fatalistic) politics of indifference arose towards COVID that particularly affected Long COVID patients. In contrast to the earlier years of the pandemic, where the numbers of infected patients were closely monitored, the Dutch government refused to register the number of Long COVID patients. In contrast to the earlier years of the pandemic, where many resources were spent on public awareness campaigns, the government refused to spend money on public awareness campaigns. And while there was a lot of investment into the development of vaccines, there was no proper investment into biomedical research and treatment of Long COVID. To make matters worse, the Dutch Minister of Health equated COVID with an ordinary cold or a flu and even publicly ridiculed Long COVID researchers for being scaremongers and stigmatised patients for having unrealistic expectations regarding the timeframe of biomedical research (Matthies-Boon & Sharon, 2024).

The problem for patients was, however, not such research would take a long time, but rather that next to nothing was being started. Long COVID patients suffered a severe political abandonment, characterised by a head-in-sand ostrich discourse that located the pandemic temporally in the past rather than in the continuous temporal present. This political abandonment is traumatic in that it not only fails to recognise the embodied and mental trauma of Long COVID endured by those living with the condition but also makes patients voiceless: unable to speak back at this political injustice. Patients are not able to gather in physical demonstrations because of both physical incapacitation and the threats of COVID reinfection.

But this politics of indifference also directly contributed to the social stigmatisation and isolation of Long COVID patients. With the populace being factually uninformed about both Long COVID and the other chronic health risks that repeated COVID infections pose, patients are frequently told that they should just pull themselves together, as they 'look fine', as well as suggestions that it may be 'a burn out' that is causing their symptoms. Such statements not only fail to recognise the immunological severity of the disease but also the existential suffering it entails. It places the burden of responsibility solely on patients' shoulders. And in a utilitarian fashion, Long COVID becomes regarded as a matter of individual bad luck, rather than an issue of structural injustice in the context of an ongoing pandemic that demands a significant change in medical, political and social responses.

This lack of social understanding combined with a (denialist) societal return to normality means that many Long COVID patients find themselves alienated from the world around them. As I wrote in my diary:

> I now feel like an excrement of the pandemic. A remnant, clutter, junk that can be swept away. And our lives are getting harder and harder. [..] no perspective, no preoccupation, no social contact, nothingness. Furious anger because of powerlessness. Your life in other people's hands while you are already drowning. Constant stress. Unable to sleep. It's all too slow... there is no progress. There is no will. Again, we are stuck, remain suspended because for most people it's over—and so they just let us drown. (personal diary, 27 February 2024)

Or as Anne Vroegindeweij, a fellow patient, wrote in her book on Long COVID (entitled the 'Those who were left behind"), she felt angry at all those people who turned away, who lived on as if nothing happened, and left her behind (Vroegindeweij, 2023, p. 16). 'This', she writes, 'is the loneliest feeling'. Moreover, patients are often cast out or excluded by relatives, friends or acquaintances as they remind them of the pandemic, or are being 'too negative' and 'complain too much' in light of their disabled chronic state (Vroegindeweij, 2023, p. 133). Of course, such social abandonment often happens in chronic illness, as other people carry on with their lives and perhaps do not wish to face the existential realities of fragility, sickness and death (Carel, 2016). However, in Long COVID, this social abandonment is extreme both because the illness affects the entire body (often making patients even unable to send a WhatsApp message or make a phone call) and because it is an ugly reminder that not all is 'normal' in the post-COVID world: a reminder that many people wish to deny or forget.

What hit me particularly hard was not only that society had largely left Long COVID patients behind, but particularly that social activists who are usually so concerned with issues of justice also turned their backs on postviral patients. The activists that I used to hang out with perhaps made a few online comments in 2021, but then mostly carried on as if the COVID pandemic never even happened. It hurt not only that they failed to recognise the social and political injustice of Long COVID, and the lack of relations of care, but also that in conversations around social safety, physical safety from infectious diseases was readily ignored. A lack of COVID-safe spaces significantly contributes to social isolation and the increased (relentless) internalisation of risk. As a Long COVID patient, one has to continuously assess risks. Is there enough ventilation? Do people come too close? Are they sick? Is my mask airtight, and so on. As I noted down in July 2023: 'I live in pandemic time, continuously, every day in and out, with no relief in sight. I am just so tired. So very tired. Every day is a struggle, with other people and with the different reality I live in'.

Long COVID patients thus experience a huge schism, a huge gap, between the lived reality of those that continued to live in a pandemic lifeworld of risk and unsafety, and those that moved into a post-pandemic lifeworld:

> Society, the lack of care, indifference, continuing as if all is normal. I, and my Long COVID groups, live in a parallel world. One could write a seriously dystopian novel about this. It feels like we are a leper colony, cast out by the world. But also, if only we could actually create our own world, then it would not be so bad, as we could create our own world wherein people would be considerate of each other's physical concerns, where we would mask, test and take care. But the problem is that, while we have been de facto banned from the world returned to normality, we cannot even create our own world—we are part and parcel of the 'ableist' world, much to our own physical (and mental) detriment. (personal diary, 5 September 2025)

Admittedly, this boundary between the abled and disabled is (as usual) porous. Hundreds of millions of people, including direct acquaintances, became Long COVID patients in the years after 2022, and the numbers continue to grow as unmitigated COVID infections continue across the world.

Yet the feeling of social abandonment found its worst expression in the experience of mask discrimination, which ranges from cancelling public talks or television interviews or moving my talk online because 'the audience would not want to see a mask' to outright abuse consisting of spitting, kicking, hitting and deliberate coughing in the face as well as swearing. While mask discrimination may occur anywhere, all of my experiences occurred in the Netherlands or by Dutch people in border region of Germany where I live. This is not surprising, as Dutch public health officials themselves downplayed the efficiency of masks while politicians publicly ridiculed them. And since people were told 'not to be afraid' of the COVID virus, those who wear a mask are cast not only as 'Other' but also as 'fearmongers'. Masks were thus never as institutionalised in the early years of the pandemic in the Netherlands as they were in other places, such as Germany. For instance, when I went to pick up my glasses at the opticians, a woman just outside the shop spat at me, insisting that I should take off that 'muzzle'. Or when after having been housebound for weeks due to a flare up, I had finally gathered all my energy to go to a local shop with my daughter to buy her a toy, a Dutch woman swore and shouted at us for wearing a mask. At this point, I was too numb to even argue back. I could not anymore, but when we got back, I broke down in tears.

Mask discrimination adds insult to injury and contributes to the traumatic layering of the post-viral abandonment that Long COVID patients endure every day. This experience led me to conclude that:

> In addition to a broken body, I walk around with such intense sadness. As if my soul has burst into tiny pieces and I am trying my best to glue it together—but every pain, every symptom, as well as every moment of aggression, exclusion and exception creates another crack... I will never be normal again. (personal diary, 17 June 2024)

Conclusion

I have argued in this chapter that Long COVID patients are subject to multilayered traumatic status subordination in the form of bodily, medical, political and social abandonment. Trauma is here not so much regarded as inaccurate brain wiring due to the cognitive overload following a specific event, but rather as a chronic state of abandonment wherein patients are not only un- and misrecognised, but also effectively rendered voiceless. In addition to the severe bodily incapacitation that patients often describe as a form of living death, they are not only directly subject to medical psychologisation, but also other forms of medical neglect that emerge from the long tradition of the psychologisation of post-viral illnesses as well as the cancellation of protective measures in health facilities. To make matters worse, patients are politically abandoned by governments that seek to return to 'normality' under the banner of individual responsibility. Through a lack of investment into biomedical research and treatment as well as the creation of public awareness of the long-term consequences of repeated COVID infections, governments cultivate a politics of indifference that has direct consequences for patients' social interactions. Not only do patients feel left behind, stuck in a pandemic mode of existence while others returned to normal—they are also subject to social stigmatisation, isolation and even aggression. In order to overcome these multilayered traumatic burdens, we need governments and health agencies to prioritise medical, social and political recognition of COVID and Long COVID, rather than an emphasis on individual therapeutic interventions.

Notes

1. Of course, we occupy different roles in different phases of our lives. However, in different situations, these roles might be reversed as they are situationally constituted. Underlying these differentiations is, however, a much more fundamental assumption that as human beings as such we are equal—to deny this is to engage in a performative contradiction.
2. In the context of the psychologisation of postviral illness, it is important to note here that the postviral illnesses such as Long Covid are in terms of their physical manifestions very much a matter for objective biomedical science.
3. In the absence of proper investment and infrastructures, the quality of Long COVID clinics is largely dependent on individual doctors and their willingness to invest time and effort into researching this complex multisystemic organ disorder.

4. Private conversations with medical professionals in Germany, 5 June 2024.
5. It is for this reason that the amended NICE guidelines are so crucial, which state that particularly those with exercise intolerance and PEM should not be submitted to such therapies but abide by a strict PACING regime itself so as to not aggravate their symptoms.
6. Of course, the individual wearing of FFP2 and FFP3 masks helps, but one-way masking remains less effective than collective masking, especially inside crowded indoor spaces.

References

Al-Aly, Z., Davis, H., McCorkell, L., Soares, L., Wulf-Hanson, S., Iwasaki, A., & Topol, E. J. (2024). Long COVID science, research and policy. *Nature Medicine, 30*(8), 2148–2164. https://doi.org/10.1038/s41591-024-03173-6

Alford, C. F. (2016). *Trauma, culture, and PTSD.* Palgrave. https://doi.org/10.1057/978-1-137-57600-2

American Psychiatric Association. (2014). Diagnostic and statistical manual of mental disorders, Fifth Edition—Coding Update. In *American Psychiatric Association.* American Psychiatric Association.

Ärzteblatt, D. Ä. G., & Redaktion Deutsches. (2023, March 31). *Long COVID und die Psycho-Ecke: Wiedergeburt eines reduktionistischen Krankheitsverständnisses.* Deutsches Ärzteblatt. https://www.aerzteblatt.de/archiv/230476/Long-COVID-und-die-Psycho-Ecke-Wiedergeburt-eines-reduktionistischen-Krankheitsverstaendnisses

Carel, H. (2016). *The phenomenology of illness.* Oxford University Press.

Chang, H. (2016). Autoethnography in health research: Growing pains? *Qualitative Health Research, 26*(4). https://doi.org/10.1177/1049732315627432

Chourasia, P., Goyal, L., Kansal, D., Roy, S., Singh, R., Mahata, I., Sheikh, A. B., & Shekhar, R. (2023). Risk of new-onset diabetes mellitus as a post-COVID-19 condition and possible mechanisms: A scoping review. *Journal of Clinical Medicine, 12*(3). https://doi.org/10.3390/JCM12031159/S1

El-Rhermoul, FZ., Fedorowski, A., Eardley, P., Taraborrelli, P., Panagopoulos, D., Sutton, R., Lim, P. B., & Dani, M. (2023). Autoimmunity in Long

COVID and POTS. *Oxford Open Immunology, 4*(1). https://doi.org/10.1093/OXFIMM/IQAD002

Geraghty, K. J., & Blease, C. (2019). Myalgic encephalomyelitis/chronic fatigue syndrome and the biopsychosocial model: A review of patient harm and distress in the medical encounter. *Disability and Rehabilitation, 41*(25), 3092–3102. https://doi.org/10.1080/09638288.2018.1481149

Jason, L. A., & Dorri, J. A. (2022). ME/CFS and post-exertional malaise among patients with Long COVID. *Neurology International, 15*(1), 1–11. https://doi.org/10.3390/NEUROLINT15010001

Kihlstrom, J. F. (2008). Trauma and memory revisited. In B. Uttl, N. Ohta, & AL. Siegenthaler (Eds.), *Memory and emotion: Interdisciplinary perspectives* (pp. 259–291). Blackwell Publishing Ltd.

Kindlon, T. (2011). The PACE trial in chronic fatigue syndrome. *The Lancet, 377*(9780). https://doi.org/10.1016/S0140-6736(11)60684-3

Mannix, L. (2023, January 31). Tracey Spicer's slow road to recovery from the 'living death' of Long COVID. *Sydney Morning Herald*. https://www.smh.com.au/national/tracey-spicer-s-slow-road-to-recovery-from-the-living-death-of-long-COVID-20230131-p5cgoo.html

Matthies-Boon, V. (2022). *Breaking intersubjectivity A critical theory of counter-revolutionary trauma in Egypt*. Rowman & Littlefield.

Matthies-Boon, V., & Sharon, T. (2024). Maatschappelijke meerstemmigheid onder druk. Waarborgen van pluralisme tijdens een gezondheidscrisis. In H. I. M'hamdi, A. Rotteveel, v. Remassi & A. Haverkamp (Eds.), *Long COVID: Een diagnose van exclusie.* Boom Bestuurskunde.

Prater, E. (2024, January 2025). COVID survivors may be at a greater risk of Parkinson's disease–like symptoms in the future, researchers warn. What you need to know to protect your health. *Fortune Well*. https://fortune.com/well/2024/01/24/COVID-survivors-risk-parkinsons-disease-like-symptoms/

Pszczołowska, M., Walczak, K., Misków, W., Antosz, K., Batko, J., Karska, J., & Leszek, J. (2024). Molecular cross-talk between long COVID-19 and Alzheimer's disease. *GeroScience, 46*(3), 2885–2899. https://doi.org/10.1007/S11357-024-01096-1

Ratcliffe, M. (2012). The phenomenology of existential feeling. In J. Fingerhut & S. Marienberg (Eds.), *Feelings of being alive* (pp. 23–54). De Gruyter. https://doi.org/10.1515/9783110246599.23

Ratcliffe, M. (2020). Existential feelings. In T. Szanto & H. Landweer (Eds.), *The Routledge handbook of phenomenology of emotion* (pp. 250–261). https://doi.org/10.4324/9781315180786-25

Regunath, H., Goldstein, N. M., & Guntur, V. P. (2023). Long COVID: Where are we in 2023? *Missouri Medicine, 120*(2). https://www.thelancet.com/jour

Renz-Polster, H., & Scheibenbogen, C. (2022). When COVID does not heal: Post-COVID courses with fatigue and exercise intolerance. *Deutsche Medizinische Wochenschrift, 147*(20). https://doi.org/10.1055/a-1849-8953

Schomerus, G. (2024, September 2). *Is there a stigma of long COVID?* Unite to Fight, Youtube: https://youtu.be/xx8rV2YeIj8. Accessed 6 August 2025.

Smith, J (2024, August 9). *Treatment changes urged after ME patient's death.* BBC. https://www.bbc.com/news/articles/czrgmdv4z0go

Stein, E., Heindrich, C., Wittke, K., Kedor, C., Kim, L., Freitag, H., Krueger, A., Toelle, M., & Scheibenbogen, C. (2023). Observational study of repeat immunoadsorption (RIA) in post-COVID ME/CFS patients with elevated ß2-adrenergic receptor autoantibodies—An interim report. *medRxiv.* https://doi.org/10.1101/2023.08.31.23294813

Thaweethai, T., Jolley, S. E., Karlson, E. W., Levitan, E. B., Levy, B., McComsey, G. A., McCorkell, L., Nadkarni, G. N., Parthasarathy, S., Singh, U., Walker, T. A., Selvaggi, C. A., Shinnick, D. J., Schulte, C. C. M., Atchley-Challenner, R., Horwitz, LI., Foulkes, A. S., Authors, R. C., Consortium, R., … Zisis, S. (2023). Development of a definition of post-acute sequelae of SARS-CoV-2 infection. *JAMA, 329*(22), 1934–1946. https://doi.org/10.1001/JAMA.2023.8823

Vink, M., & Vink-Niese, F. (2022). Is it useful to question the recovery behaviour of patients with ME/CFS or Long COVID? *Healthcare, 10*(2). https://doi.org/10.3390/HEALTHCARE10020392

Volberding, P. A., Chu, B. X., & Spicer, C. M. (2024). *Long term health effects of COVID-19 disability and function following SARS-CoV-2 infection.* Committee on the Long-Term Health Effects Stemming from COVID 19 and Implications for the Social Security Administration.

Vroegindeweij, A. (2023). *De Achterblijvers: Over de vergeten pandemie van Long COVID.* De Geus.

Ware, N. C. (1992). Suffering and the social construction of illness: The delegitimation of illness experience in chronic fatigue syndrome. *Medical Anthropology Quarterly, 6*(4), 347–361. https://doi.org/10.1525/MAQ.1992.6.4.02A00030

Wasonga, J. O. (2014). HIV: A psychosomatic disorder. *Journal of Education and Human Development*, *3*(4). https://doi.org/10.15640/jehd.v3n4a6

Weinstock, L. B., Brook, J. B., Walters, A. S., Goris, A., Afrin, L. B., & Molderings, G. J. (2021). Mast cell activation symptoms are prevalent in Long-COVID. *International Journal of Infectious Diseases, 112.* https://doi.org/10.1016/j.ijid.2021.09.043

11

The Double Bind: Gaslighting, Cultural Violence and the Post COVID Experience

Mary Zournazi

Introduction

After a couple of years of masking up and being cautious about exposure to COVID-19, I contracted the Delta viral variant once the latest pandemic restrictions had been lifted in my hometown of Sydney. The Delta variant had already wrought devastating effects in India, with one of the largest numbers of COVID deaths recorded in the world and the near collapse of its health system (Jha et al., 2022) and yet many of the implications had been largely undocumented and understood. Closer to home, I had read about the Delta experience, and I had assumed that once I 'battled' the virus, it would move out of my body; I had not realised the full severity of it. During the period of my quarantine, I was admitted to hospital as a virtual patient and considered a 'medium' risk even though my own experience felt much more extreme. One night I was convinced I would die, and I started to understand how quickly from

M. Zournazi (✉)
NUspace, University of Newcastle, Newcastle, NSW, Australia
e-mail: mary.zournazi@newcastle.edu.au

D. Lupton (ed.), *Long COVID and Society*,
https://doi.org/10.1007/978-981-96-9168-5_11

the onset of the disease vital organs could shut down. I felt it myself; I was fighting for my life in my own home, in isolation and in fear of what might happen to me. It was terrifying.

Several months passed, and I thought I 'had recovered', but over time a strange manifestation took place: I developed vertigo which was proprioceptive and not the usual inner ear diagnosis. My perceptual field became distorted, which meant my whole bodily movement was compromised. Over time I learnt this was a result of neuro-inflammation due to the COVID virus transgressing my blood-brain barrier and affecting my brain as well as my respiratory system. Elsewhere (Zournazi, 2025), I have termed this experience a 'phenomenology of vertigo' to understand how my visual and bodily experience was compromised. For this chapter, I focus on how the chronicity of bodily and neurological trauma and its 'invisibility' led me to understand the forms of gaslighting that are emergent from the ways chronic health conditions and Long COVID experience are managed and understood.

It is no surprise that when the World Health Organization declared COVID was no longer a 'global health emergency' in May 2023, it may have seemed a relief to some. As COVID protections were removed and the reporting of daily numbers of those dying and contracting the virus waned in the public arena and media, there seemed to be an overwhelming sense that the experience of COVID itself would also magically evaporate: the deaths, the anger, the despair, the mourning and the ill health. It is precisely the interlocking levels of social and cultural impact of bodily trauma of COVID and its full lived experienced that have not been sufficiently understood. Drawing on the anthropologist and philosopher Rene Girard's ([1977] 2008) work on the function of desire and cultural violence, and anthropologist and social scientist Gregory Bateson ([1972] 2000) and his double bind theory, this chapter will provide some critical philosophical understandings on how gaslighting emerges in the context of long COVID and how this gaslighting is symptomatic of different forms of the psychodynamics of cultural violence in daily life and social relationships. The aim of this essay, then, is to explore the cultural violence of gaslighting and how it impacts on the experience of 'COVID', long, short and thereafter—since when does it ever end?

Crazy Making

Gaslighting as a term emerged in the context of popular and everyday language to describe the phenomenon of when the experience of another is reduced to or rather denied its existence, and in this process, the goal is to 'drive the other person' crazy or annihilate their experience. The classic film *Gaslight* (Cukor, 1944), a psychological thriller based on the play of the same name by Patrick Hamilton, brought attention to the interpersonal realm and affective harm of the abuse of power and relationships. In critical terms, the concept of gaslighting developed in a more psychological framing from the 1960s onwards (cf. Barton & Whitehead, 1969; Calef & Weinshel, 1981; Dorpat, 1996) and has now become frequently used in popular culture to describe attempts to challenge people's sense of reality.

In the film, Ingrid Bergman plays Paula Alquist, who is subtly manipulated over time by her husband Gregory Anton (played by Charles Boyer). There is a motive for Gregory's behaviour: he has a double life, implicated in the murder of Paula's aunt for her wealth and jewels. He marries Paula to gain access to the aunt's house (left to Paula) and the treasure he believes is hidden there. The film title refers to the illumination of the house by gaslights in the Victorian era—the standard form of domestic lighting at the time. Night after night, unbeknownst to Paula, Gregory enters the attic and searches for the jewels, and the house gaslights dim and flicker. When Paula confronts him about the noises she hears in the attic and the dimming of the gaslights, he dismisses her and convinces her she must be imagining it. Gregory further tricks Paula into thinking her memory is defective and that she is a thief. He isolates her from others as part of his strategy. In other words, through the structure of their relationship, Gregory maliciously makes Paula doubt her experiences and sanity. Over an extended period and through different forms of recreating a 'fabulation' of the truth, he establishes a power dynamic that confuses and distorts her sense of reality and makes her emotionally dependent on him.

The experience of 'gaslighting' in the film indicates 'interpersonal' gaslighting through manipulative behaviours and it sheds light on the issues that can emerge in the context of gaslighting more broadly. In its contemporary use, the experience of gaslighting refers to how serious doubt about one's sense of self and experience can be manipulated through isolation or the denial of their lived reality, and through a process that leads to the establishment of new sets of 'truth'. In this sense, the film provides a context to pursue one of the key elements of gaslighting: the 'crazy making' framework that often makes the person who is being gaslit question not only themselves, but the very nature of the 'trust' and safety established in different forms of their lived reality. In Paula's case, a pivotal issue is the existence of a letter that proves the duplicity of her husband and implicates him in the murder of her aunt, which he systematically denies. By Gregory continuing to deny the letter's existence and her version of events, there is a strong sense that her evidence and sense of the world are in dispute. That is, Paula's reality of disclosing (or we could say her voice) and understanding her own life world in the context of lived experience are continually called into question by Gregory.

In an early work on different forms of crazy making, psychoanalyst Harold Searle (1959) makes an important observation: that the power dynamics involved in the often-contradictory messaging and actions in relationships reveal the degree to which the annihilation of another person's reality and experience can take emotional hold and consequence. In other words, these crazy making symptoms become the tools to investigate how the 'fabulation' or establishing of different versions of the 'truth' can manifest. It is in this sense that I consider how gaslighting works in terms of the language of Long COVID and other chronic health conditions and lived experience. What is often in dispute in these experiences is the 'evidence': especially when the 'evidence' has yet to be clearly understood in medical terms or diagnosis, or when it is invisible. Taking shape, then, is that the evidence itself, the testimony of the patient or person expressing the symptoms in medical, organisational or other broader medical systems leads to the doubt in the symptoms themselves. That Long COVID might be 'all in the mind' and not real, or in the cultural sense, that COVID did happen, but it is no longer referred to, has real and harsh consequences for people who are still experiencing the impacts of the disease.

Authors such as Sebring (2021), Sweet (2019) and later Abramson (2024) have argued that the different dynamics of gaslighting, the affective and sociological elements of these experiences, and the impacts felt can be morally damaging. They can also operate to socially validate different forms of abuse through the silencing of experience. I would add that in relationship to Long COVID, gaslighting emerges out of the dynamic of interpersonal experience that are shaped by social phenomena insofar as these phenomena exist and are constituted through different types of sociality and experience.

In Abramson's book *On Gaslighting* (2024), she opens out some of the moral issues in the 'denial' of the lived experience of COVID, stating it is not just the denial per se that is the problem, but it is in the formation of how the denial unfolds in a systemic way. Abramson writes,

> At each step, it *looks like* one is being called on to engage in an ordinary exchange of offering evidence and shared reasoning. But the more one proceeds in what in any other context would be the appropriate way to proceed—by reasoning, by offering evidence—the more one will be led by the gaslighter to doubt whether one is even capable of recognizing what qualifies as either good evidence or reasoning. (2024: p. 68, emphasis in the original)

Abramson argues for the intricacy of how gaslighting emerges through a complex web of psychosocial dynamics (although she may not necessarily refer to them as this) and the 'moral' harm that is experienced through the process. There are implications and moral injury to a person when their 'safety' and 'evidence' in disclosing a condition is under scrutiny, and often it has been fraught not only with the 'disbelief' of its chronicity and seriousness but also in the subject's very claim to the illness itself.

As Au et al. (2022) have argued, one of the consequences of Long COVID and chronic health more generally is its 'diagnostic odyssey'. This terminology demarcates precisely the odyssey element of chronic health. At each step of the way, you are dealing with different diagnoses, adapting yourself to the prognosis, and working with the health challenges, and at the same time, finding yourself cast adrift as you enter a new element of the illness journey that is complex and complicated.

As part of this experience, Au et al. (2022) write that the difficulties emerge due to the changes of the narratives around the construction of the illness in the public sphere. Moreover, the legacy of this bind is the often-contentious interactions with medical professionals, organisations, and the broader medical system that constitutes the individual experience of gaslighting. They consider gaslighting as an 'ontological politics' that gives conceptual weight to the often tacit and invisible forms of abuse that can evolve in sociological and affective realms of the experience. In this regard, extending some of these ontological issues and the profound impact on the shaping of the social responses and narratives to Long COVID and other chronic health conditions more broadly can help to disentangle the mechanisms that shape social and cultural silencing.

In the Long COVID context, then, the ontological questions and issues at stake are the forms of cultural forgetting as public health have narratives shifted and changed in relation to the media and political strategising of the virus. In this shift away from the public sphere, the private 'hell' of living through Long COVID can create a further sense of isolation for the person and disbelief in the symptoms of the illness. In other words, 'chronic health' issues often associated with bodily experience and trauma of the COVID virus have retroactively lost much of the public-facing health concerns. The impact has been the social distancing, so to speak, from bodily trauma itself.

The Double Bind of Gaslighting: 'It's Not That We Don't Believe You...'

A friend of mine tells me of her experience in a professional encounter around her Long COVID condition and recalls an episode where she was told 'it's not that we don't believe you' in relationship to her symptoms. The question of belief in this example brings into play the issues of gaslighting that reflect the 'double bind' where individuals often find themselves placed in uncomfortable positions and questioning the very nature of their experience illness. It is in this regard that Rene Girard's work and the Gregory Bateson's double bind theory bring the social, cultural and affective dimensions of a kind of 'doublespeak' and trauma in everyday experience. They help us to understand the double-bind and the philosophical and social questions at stake in the cultural practices of silencing in relation to illness. Specifically, Bateson's idea of double bind theory explores how people's behaviour or language can infer one thing while actively contravening the reality of another person. Most often it is referred to via the example of a mother saying they 'love' their child while at the same time their body language indicates the opposite and therefore causing confusion for the recipient of the gesture. Similarly, as my friend recalls, the very notion that 'it's not that we don't believe you' in its double negative articulation echoes this confusion and sense of doubt for the recipient of the message.

Usually, as noted previously, gaslighting may be understood in the affective and interpersonal realm, and for those people who experience Long COVID and its implications, it involves the negation of meaning and experience. Bateson's work on the double bind theory can be instructive. Although initially correlated in relationship to schizophrenia, double bind theory resonates with the individual and social experience of Long COVID. In this context, the gaslighting experience is caught in language and power structures, and it becomes within the context of language and governance systems a series of coercive power relations and effacement of experience. The idea of the double bind, then, relates to how people's behaviour or language state one realm of the 'truth' while reinforcing and actively deriding the reality of another. In a sense, it is the 'signs' of language and the communicative relation that induces a form of compliance or ignorance that drives the dilemma for people living with Long COVID.

When the reality of lived experienced is denied in the context of illness, then the reality of 'illness' becomes formalised under specific criteria and cultural narratives generated at any given moment. In some ways, Girard's work on mimetic desire that he developed in relation to cultural scapegoating becomes useful here. Although I will not go into detail of the scapegoating, what we can understand are some of the ideas around how desire can be shaped through the struggle or contravening of social codes emergent out of a 'shared' desire for an object, and in this shared desire is where meaning takes place. If the desire itself becomes modelled on differing forms of experience and cultural myth or narrative, then this is where the 'sacrifice' take place. That is, in the shared struggle to enunciate a cultural meaning around different logics is where a double bind occurs. Girard writes,

> If desire is allowed to follow its own bent, its mimetic nature will almost always lead it into a double bind. The unchanneled mimetic impulse hurls itself blindly against the obstacle of a conflicting desire. ([1977] 2008, p. 157)

Long COVID introduces the complexities into the scenario of *desire* and of gaslighting, and the phenomenon lends itself to understanding trauma associated with the silencing of experience. It is in this sacrifice, as Girard might put it, that we can examine some of the implications of the ways in which different forms of silencing such as in medical gaslighting and organisational politics around 'care' and illness can take place. And in this sense, it is because of the 'sharing' of the desire to make sense of experience that the power of the double bind emerges and becomes part of the process of 'crazy making' so poignantly depicted in the film *Gaslight*. That is, it is by the very 'destroying' of difference, or disagreement, that the effects of gaslighting can be most felt. In the context of chronic health conditions such as Long COVID, the very space in which the 'desire' to prove the same object—shaping and reshaping of cultural narratives on health—is where the silencing of the other and doubt takes place.

In other words, as Girard argues, the 'desire for the same thing' has two elements in operation and can relate to the framework of understanding implications of Long COVID on lived experience. On the one hand, there is an attempt that all parties 'share' meaning about an event: that is, how we might understand the long-term experience of COVID. However, as the public discussion around COVID waned, then we enter the second order. The desire for shared meaning becomes in itself conflict, and so what is understood by shared meaning of Long COVID sits strangely in opposition to the experience itself. It is in these moves that the 'normalising' effects of public responses to health issues, and in the most tragic sense, the odyssey of individual journeys through

COVID, become bound up in the narrative of duties of care, of risk management, that deliver more normalising tendencies and structures of silencing of lived realities.

Abramson (2024) discusses how these forms of normalising in the gaslighting experience 'radically' undermine the sense of trust and foundational capacities for relating to others. These practices make an impact by reinforcing a space that contravenes any sense of 'disagreement' over what's at stake in one's lived experience. She argues that facts then become indisputable, and therefore, there is no validity to suggest that there is anything different. That is, 'it's not that we don't believe' asserts precisely that the 'facts' themselves are in doubt, and this is played out in the interpersonal space of the gaslighting experience. According to Abramson:

> To get you to doubt yourself, the gaslighter counts on you having an investment in getting to the truth of the matter, an investment that justifies having and maintaining a working presumption that you might be wrong, which in turn can motivate self-doubt in the face of the gaslighter's counter-claims or purported evidence. (2024, p. 145)

Even more so at the cultural level, the more the experience of COVID is 'repressed' and the more the narratives shift away from public concern or health directives, the more they proliferate in new forms of 'normalising' language around experience. In this gap, the experience of Long COVID can fall. These processes reflect some of the power dynamics in which gaslighting can take place in the interpersonal space, but they also offer some ways to understand the forms of 'fabulation' which enable the reproduction of different kinds of narratives and 'truths'. Ironically, Michel Foucault's (1978) powerful observations in various works, including the *History of Sexuality Vol 1*, are echoed: that once something is denied, it is ever more produced in social discourse. Therefore, the mechanisms that give the gaslighter so much power are ultimately means into which cultural stories and narratives circulate and reinforce by their very nature the annihilation of another's experience.

In the context of Long COVID, gaslighting can manifest when different forms of *authority*, whether medical, judicial, organisational or interpersonal, take hold of the pervading narrative of what constitutes a sick or well body. As Abramson (2024) notes, often what gives 'manipulative leverage' is the acknowledgement of legitimate forms of experience and within the normalcy of the codified norms of acceptable or unacceptable risk and policy. The most important elements in the context are correlative to the gaslighting dynamic, which include isolating, denial of experience and fabrication of reality, which, in turn create the possibility that the gaslighter draws on the cultural sphere around them. That is, the social dynamics that enable the belief systems to take place that enforce their own desire to annihilate not only the other but also the various structures of meaning themselves: 'emptying' out of any real relationship to care and concern. It is through the unravelling of a double bind that we can start to understand what's at stake in forms of gaslighting that can often surround chronic illness, especially Long COVID.

One theme we can see emerging is that the epistemic and non-epistemic wrongs of gaslighting are inextricably tied up with one another. This is true both as a practical matter and analytically. Following Freud, we might say the 'reality testing' aspect of gaslighting is precisely the inability for its pathways and framework to be diagnosed as they move almost through a slipstream of disguise and fabulation within the realms of the language adopted by institutions and public discourses around questions of care and risk management. I will now turn to looking more closely at bodily trauma and Long COVID and the mechanisms of being gaslit.

When Care Becomes Gaslit

The ontological politics of the long COVID experience is precisely the symptoms that have no language or expression in medical diagnosis. Indeed, the neuro-physiotherapist who was treating my vertigo condition said I was the first person and the 'test' case for understanding the type of condition I was experiencing. I wrote in my diary about some of the oddity of the experience, and the manifestations of bodily trauma. For example:

> As the weeks and months progressed, my strange shimmer of the world started to become more pronounced in my bodily movements. My bodily response or 'shimmer' became my biological markers of the state of inflammation of my brain, and it manifested itself while walking or standing. For example, often while walking I would inadvertently lean to the left, and as result of this bodily disposition I found myself bumping into things: household objects, walking into street poles and sometimes walking into door frames. It seemed my body was trying to compensate for what had been traumatised or disturbed in its neural pathways. I also started to get what seemed like short blackouts: I would sit down and place my foot into a position and only to find what seemed like a second later to be somewhere else in space. As this bodily experience progressed, I developed a more profound loss of short-term memory and for the first time in my life I became dyslexic.

Because of the nature of my experience, and being a 'test' case, there has been a space of ontological misrecognition and returning to Searle's point, it can evoke not only the crazy making process of a double bind situation but it also articulates what is important in the power dimension: that is, how to articulate the 'trauma' of illness itself can remain unresolved in the chronicling of different illness experiences. It is the means of the disclosure or 'testimony' of experience—bearing witness to one's own experience—that becomes thwarted for people with Long COVID and how it is ongoingly understood, ignored or rejected. While Abramson argues that the epistemic injustice of gaslighting is more complicated than Fricker's (2007) original accounts of this injustice and testimonial sensitivity, I would argue that there is a form of a larger 'cultural amnesia' that manifests in the trauma of silencing chronic illness experiences. And another significant aspect of this 'trauma' is how different forms of epistemic injustice and silencing cross social, class and cultural lines that disrupt the trust in the ability to convey experience.

As such, this injustice gets played out in the perverse formulation of gaslighting through different gendered, class and racial politics. Most harmfully, gaslighting can be found in the often assumed 'empathetic' relation of understanding illness. As Abrahams notes, there can be an empathetic quality to gaslighting, and in the sphere of gendered violence and illness, not only man to woman but also woman to woman that amplifies how a 'sick' person may be understood. In *Gaslight*, it is in the coercive behaviours that 'are empathetic' to Paula's experience that simultaneously act to reduce her world to delusion and doubt. In my friend's experience, of 'believing' or 'not believing' her condition, it was in the very recognition that a person has some kind of condition and therefore empathetic to it. However, where it comes undone is when empathy, whether consciously or not, becomes the vehicle through which the categorisation or instrumentalisation of illness becomes part of the struggle of meaning. Yes, a medical practitioner, professionals or family members and friends may recognise that Long COVID may exist, but they will not *agree* to the space of difference: that is, how experience itself manifests and is lived.

This insight resonates with the philosopher and physician Paul Komaseroff's (2025) point around empathy: that is often assumed to reflect some kind of universal value, but it is in reality, it is historically and culturally contingent. Further and specific to the topic of gaslighting here, as Abramson writes, power dynamics are a factor in the efficacy of gaslighting that appeals to

> empathy in a very particular ways, with differential impacts on marginalized communities. First there is the simple fact that people with less power have greater need, as a practical matter, to get along with those who have relevantly more power than vice versa. (2024, p. 81)

As Abramson has argued, it must be acknowledged that gaslighting involves a toolkit of various kinds, including the normative structures of what is a stake when a shared belief becomes a struggle for meaning and articulation for those who experience illness, and the mechanisms that make people doubt their own experience and context of evidence shared. As a result of these methods of gaslighting within the context of Long COVID, 'moral injury' can be created, in which the person experiencing the health problems in question may feel they have no recourse to reject the forms of cultural silencing that arise in their individual contexts. Through moral injury, there is a sense of 'loss' that can occur, as well as doubt, which can reconfirm the original trauma, resulting in the gaslit person losing the ability to feel safe and ultimately to heal.

The work of Arthur Frank (1995, 2004) is extremely important to return to in relation to the problems of 'testimony' of experience, especially for chronic illnesses. Over many decades, Frank has emphasised the importance of testimony and the renewal of generosity in creating a space for those silenced through medical or institutional negligence to be heard. Frank speaks of the different forms and possibilities for understanding the process of generosity, which involves the capacity to 'listen' to the wounds of the body and the experience of illness. This approach might be what we could call a 'good mimetic' desire, and in this context, it might be the possibility of articulating shared experience that does not lead to the undermining of the experience of Long COVID.

Conclusions: What's at Stake?

Recently, in one of my classes, a student asked me this pertinent question: 'When can you write about trauma'? She was specifically referring to COVID trauma and silencing, and although still vivid in her mind, she recognised that the worldly upheaval that was globally felt had seemed to disappear from everyday conversation and public discourse. In this 'post-pandemic' climate, this issue is ever more pertinent. What I have addressed in this chapter are some of the forms of violence that can frame responses to Long COVID and to the notion of 'illness' itself. The trauma of the experience can lead to an existential silencing, and that can result in forms of 'moral injury' and effacement of experience. This form of effacement is a growing trend in different types of public discourse around Long COVID, and 'chronic' illness more generally.

To help think through the ontological issues at stake in this cultural effacement, I have drawn on several thinkers to provide a way to explore and examine the implications of gaslighting and how to think about the communicative and social practices that need to be relational rather than operational, and humane rather than dismissive. To put it differently, there needs to be a space in which other articulations of what 'care' might mean in a therapeutic and healing sense are enabled to counter the often-instrumental relationship to chronic illness. As the experience of Long COVID shows, and what might come thereafter, is that chronic illness experiences are varied and wide. The recognition of these stories is essential to post-pandemic worlds and the ways in which these experiences are lived across a wide range of psychosocial, class, labour, gendered, cultural and ethnicity categories. This involves rethinking the parameters of chronic illness. And today reframing chronic illness and its 'invisibility' in the logistics of public discourses of health and ontological politics is vital.

References

Abramson, K. (2024). *On gaslighting*. Princeton University Press.

Au, L., Capostescu, C., Eyal, G. & Finestone, G. (2022). Long COVID and medical gaslighting: Dismissal, delayed diagnosis, and deferred treatment. *SSM—Qualitative Research in Health, 2*. https://doi.org/10.1016/j.ssmqr.2022.100167

Barton, R., & Whitehead, J. A. (1969). The gas-light phenomena. *Mental Health, 293*(76), 1258–1260.

Bateson, G. ([1972] 2000). *Steps toward an ecology of mind.* University of Chicago Press.

Berenstain, N. (2020). White feminist gaslighting. *Hypatia, 35*, 733–758. https://doi.org/10.1017/hyp.2020.31

Calef, V., & Weinshel, E. (1981). Some clinical concepts of introjection: Gaslighting. *The Psychoanalytic Quarterly, 50*(1), 44–66. https://doi.org/10.1080/21674086.1981.11926942

Cukor, G. (1944). *Gaslight*. Metro-Goldwyn-Mayer.

Dorpat, T. (1996). *Gaslighting, the double whammy, interrogation, and other methods of covert control in psychotherapy and analysis.* Jason Aronson Inc.

Girard, R. ([1977] 2008). *Violence and the sacred*. (P. Gregory Trans.). Continuum.

Frank, A. (1995). *The wounded storyteller*. University of Chicago Press.

Frank, A. (2004). *The renewal of generosity*. University of Chicago Press.

Fricker, M. (2007). *Epistemic injustice: Power and ethics of knowing*. Oxford University Press.

Foucault, M. (1978). *The history of sexuality. Volume 1: An introduction* (R. Hurley Trans.). Vintage Books.

Jha, P., Deshmukh, Y., Tumbe, C., Suraweera, W., Bhowmick, A., Sharma, S., Novosad, P., Fu Hang, S., Newcombe, L., Gelband, H., & Brown, P. (2022). COVID mortality in India: National survey data and health facility deaths. *Science, 375*(6181), 667–671. https://doi.org/10.1126/science.abm5154

Komesaroff, P. (2025). Against empathy: History of an error. (Abridged unpublished paper).

Ruiz, E. (2020). Cultural gaslighting. *Hypatia, 35*, 687–713. https://doi.org/10.1017/hyp.2020.33

Searle, H. (1959). The effort to drive the other person crazy—An element in the aetiology and psychotherapy of schizophrenia. *British Journal of Medical Psychology, 32*(1), 1–18.

Sebring, J. (2021). Towards a sociological understanding of medical gaslighting in western health care. *Sociology of Health & Illness, 43*(9), 1951–1964. https://doi.org/10.1111/1467-9566.13367

Sweet, P. (2019). The sociology of gaslighting. *American Sociological Review, 84*(5), 851–875. https://doi.org/10.1177/0003122419874843

Zournazi, M. (2025). 'Phenomenology of vertigo': Trauma, neuroplasticity or how I learnt to juggle (Unpublished paper).

Part VI

Specific Social Groups

12

'I Have Disappeared': Long COVID, ME/CFS and Inclusion in Church Communities

Penny Pullan

Introduction

In 2017, the (then) senior bishop and principal leader of the Church of England, Justin Welby, explained the need to offer love and inclusion in the life of the church to everyone, without exception. He stated:

> No person is a problem, or an issue. People are made in the image of God. All of us, without exception, are loved and called in Christ. There are no 'problems', there are simply people. (Welby, 2017)

In this chapter, I explore how true these ideals of inclusion are for those living with contested, invisible illnesses within the Church of England: especially focusing on those with Long COVID or Myalgic Encephalomyelitis/Chronic Fatigue Syndrome (ME/CFS). Little is known about how many members of church congregations are living

P. Pullan (✉)
St Hild College, Sheffield, UK
e-mail: penny@makingprojectswork.co.uk

D. Lupton (ed.), *Long COVID and Society*,
https://doi.org/10.1007/978-981-96-9168-5_12

with these conditions. What we do know is that the number of those with Long COVID symptoms has been increasing across England and Scotland, exceeding 2 million in early 2024 (Office for National Statistics, 2024).

Invisible illnesses often cause social problems for those who live with them. Vickers (2002, p. 5) explains how most people are unsensitised to these conditions. As a result, they are associated with 'labelling, stereotyping, stigmatisation and/or discrimination'. Invisible conditions often fluctuate in severity, which can lead to others seeing them as 'unproven, contested and doubted', adding to the stigma (Finesilver et al., 2020). Pantelic and colleagues (2022) found that 75% of participants with Long COVID report 'always' experiencing social stigma. Clutterback and colleagues (2024) found that stigma and discrimination are felt particularly keenly by disadvantaged patients with possible Long COVID when trying to access healthcare. Women are more likely than men to suffer from Long COVID (Cohen & van der Meulen Rodgers, 2023) and three times more likely to have ME/CFS (Cortes Rivera et al., 2019). A tendency to minimise and stigmatise conditions with a female bias such as these, fits historical patterns, as women's health complaints have often been disregarded or even labelled as 'hysteria'. Long COVID has similarly been labelled by New Zealand psychiatrists as 'hysteria' (Little et al., 2024).

The symptoms of Long COVID often overlap closely (albeit not completely) with ME/CFS (Komaroff & Lipkin, 2023), an illness that comes with its own history of social stigma. The deeply flawed PACE trial initially appeared to show that ME/CFS could be treated moderately effectively with graded exercise therapy and cognitive behavioural therapy (White et al, 2011). Wilshire and colleagues (2018) showed that the results did not support this finding, following vigorous campaigning by ME/CFS patients and scientists working together to obtain access to the original trial data (Rehmeyer, 2016).

Would this experience of social stigma and stereotyping in wider society also extend into Church of England churches, or would they live out their call to include everyone? In the Hebrew Scriptures, every person is considered made in the image of God (Genesis 1.27).

In the Bible, Saint Paul uses a metaphor of the human body to describe the church as the Body of Christ (1 Corinthians 12), locating members of the church community as equivalent to organs. All people are explained as equal in terms of hierarchy, all belong, and, indeed, weaker people are described as indispensable. If one suffers, all suffer together with them. Conversely, all can share gifts with others. All are important, especially those who suffer or are weaker. This metaphor echoes Jesus' teaching in the Beatitudes, where he directly addresses those on the margins of society. In Luke's version, Jesus declares blessings upon the poor, the hungry, and those who weep, but woe to those who are full, rich and those laughing now. This highlights that the oppressed and vulnerable are to be valued and supported (Luke 6:20–25), flipping the societal norms of the time with Jesus' radical inclusivity. Later, he calls his followers to 'do to others as you would have them do to you' (Luke 6.31), treating others with the dignity and respect that they themselves desire. In both Paul's and Jesus' teachings, each person is valued as integral to the whole community, especially those who are often overlooked.

The implication of all these ideas is that people with invisible illnesses should be fully included in church life, feel that they belong, and they are accepted by others, and be able to share their gifts and ministry with others, free of stigma and discrimination. Before exploring this issue further, I consider the changes that came about since the advent of COVID-19 and how these affected people in church communities, more generally and then those living with illness. This study was undertaken four years after the start of the COVID pandemic in 2020, when lockdowns were introduced in England. In research undertaken during these lockdowns, Baggerley and colleagues (2024) explored the impact on people of faith in the UK. They found that religious coping strategies such as prayer were helpful to communal worshippers' mental health. Village and Francis (2023), focusing on people belonging to Church of England communities, found that improvements in spiritual wellbeing during lockdowns positively correlated with improved mental and also physical health.

Despite not meeting in person during periods of lockdown and other restrictions on physical movements outside the home, churches were able to provide support and comfort to parishioners online. Online church services often replaced in-person community worship, with people joining in from their homes. Baggerley and colleagues (2024) found that some worshippers missed the social interaction that comes from physically being with others. In contrast, those who had previously been unable to be part of their church communities in-person, due to disability or illness, often found lockdowns to be 'a time of freedom and expansion as more opportunities for participation opened up'. They could join services flexibly online, either attending live or joining in asynchronously later, as their health conditions allowed (Jacobs & Richardson, 2022, pp. 217–218). After lockdowns, COVID protections such as the requirement to mask indoors and social distancing meant that clinically vulnerable people could attend in-person churches safely if they were well enough to do so. However, once these protections were ended in England in July 2021, things changed. Jacobs and colleagues (2021) wrote at the time: 'The institutional church has abandoned many of us who are at higher risk from COVID, who will be too afraid to attend unsafe church buildings'. They explained how 'vulnerable' people had been told that they should not attend worship in church buildings. The tide had turned, and exclusion was back once again. To rub salt into the wound, many churches have since stopped or reduced their online service offerings.

The experiences of members of church communities who live with Long COVID, ME/CFS and other invisible illnesses remain largely overlooked by researchers, apart from a mention by Jacobs and Richardson (2022, p. 79) of barriers to involvement in church for some people with ME/CFS, as churches were 'not designed for people' with such illnesses and their needs. My study attempted to close this gap in 2024 by exploring the research question: 'How are people of working age with invisible illnesses and chronic conditions (particularly those with ME/CFS and Long COVID) included in their Church of England church communities, and how much do they feel they really matter and belong?'.

Methodology

My approach to this research question was to invite members of Church of England communities of working age (18–65 years) who were living with an invisible illness such as ME/CFS or Long COVID to complete an online survey in January 2024 and to invite a subset of these respondents to participate in semi-structured interviews later that year. Participants answered questions on demographics and their ratings of inclusion and belonging in church. They also shared comments in response to open-ended questions, often providing long and rich textual descriptions of their experiences.

At first, recruiting participants was challenging. Initial attempts tended to attract those most engaged in church, typically priests or lay ministers. By expanding to patient groups (ME Association, ME Action and Long COVID groups) and social media advocates, the number and range of participants increased, with evidence of snowball sampling, where 'existing study subjects recruit future subjects from among their acquaintances' (Liamputtong, 2006, pp. 48–9). A total of 61 survey responses that met the criteria were received by March 2024. I interviewed 13 participants from this group of respondents. Interviews were semi-structured, with initial questions, plus the opportunity to explore individuals' experiences. Interviews were conducted over Zoom, recorded and then transcribed. This study produced large amounts of quantitative and qualitative data, which I managed using Dedoose software. All data were anonymised before upload, with participants allocated labels with a prefix: survey-only participants (S) and interviewees (I), along with a unique ID number: for example, S36 or I09.

Participant Demographics

The survey sample size is not statistically representative, so these results apply to these participants only. Of the 61 survey participants, 32 live with ME/CFS, nine with Long COVID and 4 live with both. Two have cancer. Others reported different combinations of illness, often including auto-immune conditions.

The age distribution of survey participants shows a greater burden of illness in older people approaching retirement age. Participants' biological sex assigned at birth was overwhelmingly female (56 respondents, compared with 5 assigned male at birth).

Ratings of how included survey participants felt in their church communities spread from 1 (not at all included) to 5 (wholeheartedly included), with slight peaks at 1 and at 5. When focusing only on those who can't attend church in-person anymore, due to the severity of their illness, inclusion scores change to show a peak at 1 (not at all included).

When inclusion scores were plotted for those living with Long COVID, and also for ME/CFS, the peak was also at 1 (not at all included), whereas, when plotted for those living with cancer, the peak was at 5 (wholeheartedly included). This indicates lower levels of inclusion reported by those with Long COVID and ME/CFS, compared with some other invisible illnesses.

Of the 13 interview participants, 5 live with ME/CFS, 4 with Long COVID and 2 have both ME/CFS and Long COVID. Two have other invisible illnesses. Their ratings of belonging in church life were spread evenly from 1 (not at all) to 5 (wholeheartedly). In their interviews, they explained how their illnesses affected them; their illness severity ranged from 2 (mild/moderate) to 7 (very severe) on the Jahanbani ME/CFS Severity Scale (2024). The median was 6 (housebound, unable to undertake any cardiovascular activity or work).

Analysis Approach to Qualitative Data

The chosen approach to analysing the qualitative data was Braun and Clarke's (2022) reflexive thematic analysis, using the researcher as instrument. This popular method for developing, analysing and interpreting patterns across a qualitative dataset involves first becoming very familiar with the data, then coding data systematically, before developing themes. It sees a reflexive, 'subjective, situated, aware and questioning' researcher as of value (Braun & Clarke, 2022, p. 5). This was particularly appropriate because of my experience of caring from my husband with ME/CFS for the last 34 years. As a reflexive researcher, I could critically reflect on both my own lived experience as a carer and having seen my husband's experiences of exclusion from churches. It allowed me to tap into my own experience as a resource, rather than a bias, while exploring deep and nuanced stories from study participants, drawing on their words throughout.

The first step of my analysis was multiple readings of all of the data, both interview transcripts and comments from free-text responses in the online surveys, with a focus on aspects of inclusion and belonging, or the lack of these. Fifty codes were developed to capture the complexity, nuances and dynamics described by the participants. These codes were sorted into meaningful themes, and the data relating to each theme were collected. Themes were reviewed against the entire qualitative data set to ensure a good fit, and then themes were named.

Themes

This section shares eight themes developed from the qualitative survey and interview data, drawing on participants' own words. Five of them are negative, and three are positive, in terms of inclusion and belonging of individuals living with invisible illnesses in their church communities.

Theme A: 'I'm Valued for What I Do, Not Who I Am'

This theme highlights a church culture that values 'doing' over 'being'. When able to do less than expected, participants felt less valued. 'In church it's all about what you can do, what rota you can be on', said interview participant I26. I30 added: 'I feel there's a lot of pressure. You only seem valued if you do stuff'. This pressure is experienced as particularly challenging for study participants with the least energy. Survey participant S14 feels 'of no value to the church as I am not well enough to volunteer for anything'. S36 said 'I do feel valued but only if I can conform to a pattern of activity I can't sustain'.

This pressure applies to those with an official role as clergy too. I09 (a priest) says: 'In ministry, there is a huge emphasis on doing, on achieving, on productivity, on being energetic, being youthful'. I03 (another priest) felt highly valued by their congregation for what they do, not who they are, explaining: 'There's a culture of burnout culture or martyr culture [...] a "real" priest or "real" Christian looks like somebody that is working so hard to be like Jesus. I see that as really problematic: seeing each other as "less than" when we are taking rest or when we are putting in boundaries'.

Theme B: Rotas Are a Nightmare

Rotas are cultural artefacts that allow churches to organise their 'doing'. They allow people to share in ministry across teams, but at particular cost for those with fluctuating symptoms. Inflexible rotas prevent people serving the church community if they can't predict that they will be well enough on the day. S07 explains: 'I never know whether I'm going to feel ok or not so don't like to commit to things. Hence, I don't get as involved as I might otherwise and therefore feel less included'. I26, living with ME/CFS, suggested: 'They need something flexible that takes into account fluctuations'. I20 with Long COVID explained: 'You can rest for a couple of days before, thinking, I've got home communion tomorrow. You wake up and feel like you've been smacked over the head'. I30, living with ME/CFS, explained how people are othered and labelled 'unreliable' if they can't predict when they will be well enough: 'They'll just say, oh well, we won't bother because she's unreliable. She's a bit all over the place'. Others were described as 'unreliable' after letting people down at the last minute. Here, we have out-group stereotyping in action, with people being seen as lazy or unreliable due to illness, rather than character flaws (Burke, 2018, p. 120).

Flexibility and understanding are key with rotas. Two participants lead music and have control of their rotas, which is helpful. I24, with Long COVID, can rely on her organist's backup: 'When I have to drop out suddenly, I could just leave everything in his capable hands'. A flexible approach allows people to step into slots at the last minute. I05 is happy, if well that day, to 'do the reading or read somebody's intercessions that they've written but haven't turned up'. I09 (a priest) asks for awareness and managing of expectations around needed adjustments for her ME/CFS. S53 (also a priest) said: 'The severity of my symptoms differs from day to day meaning I can't commit to rotas and events'. Her church community 'are understanding and will still ask, but without pressure'.

Theme C: Church Harms People Physically, Mentally and Spiritually

This theme covers some shocking experiences of harm from church communities: the opposite of the ideal of inclusion. Some physical harm is due to doing too much (Themes A and B). I05 is pressured to do more than is comfortable: 'Although I explain how unwell I am, they react to what they see'. I34, living with Long COVID, described attending in-person church as: 'beautiful and massively overwhelming. I went to bed for two weeks. Frankly, it's not worth that. It was painful and exhausting'. Others described needing days to recover after church services due to their ME/CFS.

COVID infections also cause harm. I30 was infected in church by someone 'recovering from COVID' and she has new chest pains, less energy and more pain than before with ME/CFS alone. I35 worries that there is 'no safe inclusion for people with chronic illnesses', such as her ME/CFS. Her clergy said, regarding mitigations: 'Everyone just stopped, so we're just not bothering' and 'There's nothing I can do really'. I09, with ME/CFS and other complications, 'got very, very ill. I had to go off sick for ten months' when infected with COVID. She is more accepting: '[COVID] has had a huge impact each time, but it's part of our life now. I'm trying to balance caution with not living in fear'. I17 says: 'I've gone downhill again since [getting COVID]. I am very conscious of getting it again, but I also feel I need to live'. This is a difficult balance in a world where COVID infections are ongoing but all mitigations to help protect people have been dropped. I26 was pressured by the leader of her church to do more than she could manage with ME/CFS. The vicar thought she was making excuses and continued to press her. This led to a mental health crisis, affecting her faith. S49 saw behaviour like this as bullying, describing church as 'not a safe place for an ill person who is suffering, scared and vulnerable'.

Healing too can be handled poorly, causing harm. S28 recounts: 'People disbelieving and continually praying for my healing and telling me to repent. It affected me so much emotionally […] I really believed God hated me'. S61 found the emphasis on healing miracles problematic: 'They stopped communicating with me when I failed to recover from ME'. S60 gets frustrated when people try to pray to cure her, feeling that they're driven by helplessness. Priest I03, living with ME/CFS, finds painful even 'the standard Church of England liturgy where there's a big conflation between health and salvation in the language'.

Theme D—Treated Differently

Many participants experienced different treatment from others. I09 (a priest) explained how, when training, people wondered if she could minister with ME/CFS and said: 'if God healed you, then maybe you could do it?' Priest I03 also referred to challenges with training with ME/CFS: 'if you weren't able to do things […] they wanted to challenge rather than making any reasonable adjustment'. I26 shared how she wasn't well enough to attend a church event to help people discern their gifts, due to her ME/CFS: 'They would not share the materials or anything about it with me. This left me feeling I had no gifts and written off'. I30 shared the challenges of ME/CFS being invisible: 'People find it easier to cope with when they can see some outward sign'. I17, living with ME/CFS and Long COVID sometimes asks to sit down in church and people ask him why? I09 explains: 'if you've been through something yourself, you've got a completely different perspective and understanding as if you haven't been through it. I don't look ill'. I20 described her different treatment with Long COVID compared to visibly disabled people: 'They've been good with them, but terrible with me!'

I30 says those more able are valued: 'They seem to be more in the loop and spoken to more'. She is told she is not a full member of church because she can't join a house group (a small group that meets in person in someone's home one evening each week to study the Bible and pray together). This is impossible for her with her ME/CFS. No accommodations have been offered. I12 with Long COVID misses attending church but can't sustain a whole service. If she had permission to leave partway through, she said: 'I would go because I would feel that I would be welcomed, rather than frowned upon'. I26 mentioned: 'There's also a lot of talk of bringing people in from the margins, expecting them to fit into the mould [...] on their terms'. I30, also living with ME/CFS, found this frustrating: 'There's a way I can do this, but it might look completely different to the way you're doing this. And are you open to that?'. She added: 'Working is easier, because they make reasonable adjustments'.

Inclusive Church is a network of UK churches all of which agree to this statement:

> We believe in **inclusive church** – a church which celebrates and affirms every person and does not discriminate. We will continue to challenge the church where it continues to discriminate against people on grounds of **disability, economicpower, ethnicity, gender, gender identity, learningdisability, mental health, neurodiversity,** or **sexuality**. We believe in a Church which **welcomes and serves all people** in the name of Jesus Christ; which is scripturally faithful; which seeks to proclaim the Gospel afresh for each generation; and which, in the power of the Holy Spirit, allows all people to grasp how wide and long and high and deep is the love of Jesus Christ. (Inclusive Church, 2019, emphasis in the original)

Surely churches in this network would be better at the inclusion of people with invisible illnesses? 'They are very into being inclusive of LGBT', explained I26, but not invisible illness. I35, with ME/CFS, finds the same: 'Inclusion is fine if it's young, vibrant people who can do things. Every service starts with: "We are a fully inclusive Anglican Church." Then I shout at the screen, "No, you're not!" I have been increasingly excluded, as more other people have been included'. I03, a young priest with ME/CFS, wants acceptance as they are, instead of people assuming they have loads of energy: 'sweeping statements from elderly congregants, "when you're this old, you'll know how tired we feel"'. Stigmatising by the church community included people being told off for being late or not attending. S28 was told: 'how sinful I was—as evidenced by being ill—and that I clearly had not sufficiently confessed my sins'. I26 was told: 'Suffering is a temporary thing. God will make it all right'. S36 summed it up: 'When they try to include me, I feel different as it's always a special effort that feels a trouble'.

Theme E—'I Have Disappeared'

The phrase given to Theme E, which came from I26 (ME/CFS), resonated with six interviewees who couldn't attend church in-person. They echoed it: 'Out of sight and out of mind. I feel I've been abandoned'. (I35, ME/CFS), 'You do disappear. When I was well, I felt I belonged' (I12, Long COVID), 'No one contacted me, no one came to visit me' (I30, ME/CFS) and 'Excluded and forgotten' (S47, ME/CFS). It's an extension of Theme D from difference to exclusion.

Participant I34 with Long COVID felt disadvantaged by being working age: 'My church community value and include [housebound] older people but I'm just forgotten about. People say I can't be bothered to try and get to church'. When she asked for home communion, they said they were too busy taking this service to elderly people who 'needed' it. I20 with Long COVID, formerly working for the church explained: 'You do feel like you've just literally been forgotten. I'd like to think I'm still thought of, that it would be rather sad if not. I was completely engaged in church and I sadly feel completely disengaged. You feel forgotten, not really cared for'.

I12 shared her experiences:

> After a year [of Long COVID and being forgotten], I offered to make some special cakes [for a church sale]. They liked them and said, 'Can you do that for our monthly coffee morning?' I take the cakes down once a month. I make and freeze them one day, take them down the next day and then rest and recover for several days.

Did I12 receive anything back? 'No, not at all'. She's valued for baking, but otherwise she feels left out of the church community. Similarly, S51 said: 'I don't feel valued, [instead I'm] completely ignored by others.' She felt that 'having been through so much, I might be used to encourage others, especially those who are hurting and feel in despair and hopeless'. Sometimes secular support was better, safe and more accepting: 'You don't need church, you need friends who'll walk with you', says S28. I12 chooses 'time in the garden' or 'visiting M&S [department store Marks & Spencer]' over attending church, which has forgotten about her since she developed Long COVID.

Many participants felt cut off as church service livestreams stopped. S36 feels this keenly: 'I am not of enough value to have access to church'. I24's Facebook morning prayer community was stopped to focus on advertising events. I35's church now provides a broadcast without interaction. With ME, she feels 'shut [out] with no access to the main events, despite having the technology. We are supposed to be grateful'.

Theme F—Online Helps If...

Participants reported how COVID lockdowns eliminated difference and enabled them to belong, echoing reports by Jacobs (2020). I35, after many years of ME, said: 'Suddenly there was a level playing field. Everything was on Zoom and I could take part!' Many lamented how things have reverted to in-person participation in church life. For some participants, however, these online services were still available, allowing them to continue to be active members of the church. I05 describes her Zoom church: 'We all feel equally included. We each have one box on a screen, the same size, and same access to the microphone. If I'm feeling really bad, I can turn off the video, stick my head down on the desk and just listen'. This flexibility allows people to 'participate at the level you are able'. Community is formed and people belong: it's 'a good in itself, not just as a poor cousin for those who can't get the "real thing"'.

Leaders sometimes worry Zoom church might detract from in-person church but I30 said: 'It's a powerful tool. I'm not sure if [leaders] realise that'. After being cut off with ME/CFS and unable to attend for years prior to the COVID pandemic, she described how 'feeling part of it and knowing what's going on is the most wonderful thing!'. I24 explained how 'designed for online' services are better. I20 watches such well-designed, peaceful Cathedral Evensongs, which fit her Long COVID symptoms better than her own church's rather chaotic family service.

Participants suggested that a livestreamed service doesn't provide the same community as interactive services. S31 agreed: 'I want a church community, but I ended up feeling absurdly grateful for just being able to watch'. I30 shared how valuable a group for 'discussions online' was, but this has since been discontinued. Such a group could support others too, such as parents and those who travel for work. Hybrid church meetings facilitate I24's attendance with Long COVID, but she doesn't know what's going on as much as she used to.

Online Zoom church brings new ministry opportunities. I34 leads a Christian community online, despite her Long COVID: 'We do art, we do Bible studies, we pray. It's just lovely. Lots of online chatting. It seems to really bless people'. I26 attends another online church for disabled people, 'Disability and Jesus', where she enjoys 'their preaching. They do it in a short time. It's not as long. They *get* disability', she says, including her ME/CFS.

Theme G—Supportive Leadership

Supportive church leadership was significant for participants feeling included, valued and belonging. This was both through leader's language and interactions, as well as the culture and processes they put into place.

S46's vicar says: 'Stand if you can—God doesn't mind if you don't'. This use of language is really helpful for many. Priest participants shared their own ways of including others through modelling embrace, demonstrating pacing and bringing disability theology to their congregations. Several described supportive leaders with family experience of invisible illnesses. I30 shared that: 'ministers who have ME themselves bring that perspective, it's helpful'. I17's vicar, 'fortunately' for him, used to have ME/CFS. He said: 'It makes such a difference!'. His previous vicar dismissed anyone with illness. I17 said: 'I felt I couldn't tell him. I saw how he treated [others with ME/CFS]'. I26's leader tried to shame people back from 'TV church': 'Stop lounging around at home with a coffee'.

She said that hearing this while living with ME/CFS: 'It made me feel unwelcome and like I didn't belong'. I30's previously unsupportive vicar changed perspective as a family member developed Long COVID. She says: 'I've been able to give them helpful advice'. While it's not changing church practice yet, 'he's got that little bit more understanding that my energy doesn't go as far'.

Theme H, Church Could and Should Be...

Participants shared many ideas how church could provide appropriate welcome, inclusion, valuing and belonging to those with invisible illnesses, bringing together ideas from across the other themes. I26 said church would be 'more welcoming, more joyful, more like Jesus' where people could come as they are, without judgement of their illness. I09 shared how it would provide a sense of community, where people are known and feel they belong, which I06 said would be 'very healing'. I24 suggested that pain and fatigue would be accommodated with kindness. S42 said this would give people the freedom to be open and honest about their struggles. S02 would feel free to turn down requests. Several people said that this ideal supportive church would pray for people. I06 explained how members would be sensitive to invisible illnesses, noticing flares and pain. Language would be chosen carefully, adds I09, such as: 'stand if you are able or comfortable'. I24 shares the idea that church members could model not standing. I17 suggests having sofas and arms on chairs (providing support to sit down or stand up) for accessibility for all.

I20 suggests gentle, more relaxed, less noisy, shorter services, without tiring interaction, so people can come with no expectations. I30 would like a café style so people can pop in and out. I17 wants 'bite-size', accessible preaching, and I30 suggests bullet points for limited attention spans. Preaching explores invisible illness among other life experiences, acknowledging that suffering is real for many. Several participants emphasise the importance of disability and liberation theologies, along with disability awareness training. Questioning should be welcomed.

I03 suggests that people could be more open about loss, supported by liturgy and worship. I24 finds Psalms bring lament and difficulty helpfully into worship. I30 would like people to sit and listen with those going through tough times. I06 suggests good pastoral care, noticing missing people, and calling them to check in and offer help, and I35 wants visits and prayer with homebound church members. S29 suggests messages of support and I20 suggests email updates, to keep housebound members in touch. In our world with the risk of COVID infections ever present, I35 explains that church should create an environment safe for all, with good air quality, encouraging people to stay away if sick. A dedicated space for wearing masks should be offered for those who want to protect themselves, with interactive online services for those who can't attend in-person.

All people should be encouraged to bring their gifts, S55 says, with roles appropriate to their fluctuating abilities. S32 suggests congregations check in and pray for ministers who are ill and offer practical help. S55 describes her church which models 'strength in weakness, beauty from brokenness, growth from suffering, great capacity from incapacity: the upside-down kingdom'. S68 imagines how the church can be 'wounded, but also wonderful'. Whatever the tradition of the church, people should feel valued and loved, and that everyone genuinely cares, in whatever ways they attend church and contribute to the church community.

Discussion

These powerful themes show participants have a variety of experiences of their Church of England communities, which often fall short of the Christian ideal of all congregation members being fully included in church, feeling that they belong and being able to share their gifts with others. As the interviews demonstrated, valuing 'doing' over 'being' was common, and the expression of this through rotas was problematic due to fluctuating symptoms. This work ethic culture of 'we are defined by what we do' reveals ableism (Rothman, 2018, p. 94) and goes against inclusion of all, but appears unnoticed and unexamined by church leaders. Volf's (1996, pp. 36–37) ideas apply here: 'Our [church's] coziness with the surrounding culture has made us so blind to many of its evils that, instead of calling them into question, we offer our own versions of them in God's name and with a good conscience'. Volf further suggests the necessity of 'cultivating the proper relation between distance from the culture and belonging to it'.

Participants shared how churches cause harm to people with Long COVID and other invisible illnesses in many different ways: physically, mentally and spiritually. This is the complete opposite of inclusion, belonging and interdependence suggested by Christian teachings and ideals. It seems that many of these harms are not inflicted intentionally but instead are due to lack of awareness or lack of care. One such example is COVID reinfection. Clergy's lack of action and apparent helplessness in the face of this risk to their congregations seems typical of the individualism of public health in the West, ignoring the possibilities of masking and clean air (Lupton, 2022).

Many participants felt othered and treated differently because of their invisible illnesses, which were minimised or misunderstood. So-called inclusive churches focused inclusion on other marginalised groups, over people with ME/CFS or Long COVID. Some people conflated illness with sin. Practices of othering left participants marginalised, stigmatised or even excluded. Six of those interviewed had disappeared from their church communities entirely. Once again, marginalising and exclusion are not intentional, stemming rather from a lack of care or noticing when others are absent, described by Volf as the 'havoc wreaked by indifference' (1996, p. 77). Here, the Western individualistic culture is at play, described by Hofstede (2010, p. 92) as where 'ties between individual are loose: everyone is expected to look after him- or herself and his or her immediate family', rather than others.

More positively, online church services and groups can be part of the solution, enabling people to belong and even to minister to others from home, when done well and in an interactive and inclusive way. Supportive, empathetic leadership makes a difference to participants with Long COVID and ME/CFS, encouraging them to feel valued and that they belong. Such leaders often have lived experience of their own or family illness. They use inclusive language, putting relationships first, encouraging all to play their part in the church, as members of the metaphorical the Body of Christ. Other aspects of a more inclusive and accessible Church of England were shared by the participants, describing a church where each person is valued and listened to, and they and their needs are noticed, seen and taken into account. People are honest, open and kind and take disability seriously. Outside cultural influences such as individualism and ableism should be replaced by inclusion of all people, whatever their disability, visible or invisible.

Conclusion

This study is the first to seek to explore inclusion of people with invisible illnesses such as Long COVID and ME/CFS in Church of England communities. In doing so, it offers many windows of insight into lives of people who are often not noticed, not included and sometimes completely disappear from their communities. The themes developed show many opportunities to improve inclusion for those with invisible illnesses in the Church of England, by moving towards Christian ideals of the church fully including every member, and moving away from cultures of ableism, individualism and indifference.

There are limits to this qualitative study, which aims to share nuanced stories of complex experiences from a small number of people. The use of an online survey for intake and Zoom interviews presents issues of accessibility, as only those with technological access and enough energy can take part. Interview participants were all White British. Only one participant identified as male and one as non-binary, so the work could extend into a broader range of racial and ethnic backgrounds and with more participants who identify as other than female, as well as into Christian denominations beyond the Church of England or to other faith communities. It would be helpful to hear the perspectives of church leaders too.

Acknowledgements This chapter is drawn from the author's Durham University MA thesis, conducted through St Hild College in 2024. The author thanks the participants for sharing their experiences, Reverend Dr Sally Nelson for supervision, and Dr. Malcolm Pullan for inspiring this study. He has lived with ME/CFS since 1990, and his experience in churches includes times of exclusion (Pullan & Pullan, 2021).

Ethics Approval Ethics approval for this study was given by the Yorkshire Theological Education Partnership, of which St Hild College is a part. Informed consent was provided by each participant.

References

Archbishops' Council. (2009). *Celebrating diversity in the Church of England: National parish diversity monitoring 2007*. Church of England. https://www.churchofengland.org/sites/default/files/2017-10/celebratingdiversitygsmisc938_0.pdf

Baggaley, R. F., Ho, K. M. A., Maltby, J. et al. (2024). Impact of the COVID-19 pandemic on communal religious worshippers' mental health and the benefits of positive religious coping. *Heliyon, 10*(21). https://doi.org/10.1016/j.heliyon.2024.e39093.

Braun, V., & Clarke, V. (2022). *Thematic analysis: A practical guide.*Sage.

Burke, P. (2018). *Contemporary social psychological theories*. Stanford University Press.

Clutterbuck, D., Ramasawmy, M., Pantelic et al. STIMULATE-ICP Consortium. (2024). Barriers to healthcare access and experiences of stigma: Findings from a coproduced Long COVID case-finding study. *Health Expectations, 27*(2). https://doi.org/10.1111/hex.14037

Cohen, J., & van der Meulen Rodgers, Y. (2023). An intersectional analysis of Long COVID prevalence, *International Journal for Equity in Health, 22*. https://doi.org/10.1186/s12939-023-02072-5

Cortes Rivera, M., Mastronardi, C., Silva-Aldana, C. T. et al. (2019) Myalgic encephalomyelitis/chronic fatigue syndrome: A comprehensive review. *Diagnostics, 9*(3). https://doi.org/10.3390/diagnostics9030091

Dou, D. R., Zhao, Y., Belk, J. A. et al. (2024). Xist ribonucleoproteins promote female sex-biased autoimmunity. *Cell, 187*(3), 733–749. https://doi.org/10.1016/j.cell.2023.12.037

Finesilver, C. et al. (2020). Invisible disability, unacknowledged diversity. In J. Leigh & N. Brown (Eds). *Ableism in academia: Theorising experiences of disabilities and chronic illnesses in higher education.* (pp. 143–60). UCL Press https://doi.org/10.2307/j.ctv13xprjr.14.

Hofstede, G.H. (2010) *Culture and organisations: Software of the mind. Intercultural cooperation and its importance for survival* (3rd ed.). McGraw-Hill.

Inclusive Church. (2019). *Inclusive Church vision statement.* https://www.inclusive-church.org/

Jacobs, N. L. (2020, May 21). Disabled people say welcome to our world. *Church Times.* https://www.churchtimes.co.uk/articles/2020/1-may/features/features/disabled-people-say-welcome-to-our-world

Jacobs, N. L., Major, E. & Tupling, K. (2021, July). *Statement on the Church of England's COVID guidance to churches.* https://naomilawsonjacobs.com/statement-on-the-church-of-englands-covid-guidance-to-churches-july-2021/

Jacobs, N. L., & Richardson, E. (2022). *At the gates: Disability, justice and the churches.* Darton, Longman and Todd.

Jahanbani, F., Sing, J. C., Maynard, R. D., Jahanbani, S., Dafoe, J., Dafoe, W., Jones, N., Wallace, K. J., Rastan, A., Maecker, H. T., Röst, H. L., Snyder, M. P. & Davis, R.W. (2024). Longitudinal cytokine and multi-modal health data of an extremely severe ME/CFS patient with HSD reveals insights into immunopathology, and disease severity. *Frontiers in Immunology Autoimmune and Auto inflammatory Disorders: Auto inflammatory Disorders, 15.* https://doi.org/10.3389/fimmu.2024.1369295

Komaroff, A. L., & Lipkin, W. I. (2023). ME/CFS and Long COVID share similar symptoms and biological abnormalities: road map to the literature. *Frontiers in Medicine, 10.* https://doi.org/10.3389/fmed.2023.1187163

Little, J., Higgins, M., & Palepu, R. (2024). Long COVID—Can we deny a diagnosis without denying a person's reality? *Australasian Psychiatry, 32*(1), 44–46. https://doi.org/10.1177/10398562231222809

Liamputtong, P. (2006). *Researching the vulnerable.* SAGE.

Lupton, D. (2022). *COVID societies: Theorising the coronavirus crisis.* Routledge.

Office for National Statistics. (2024). *Self-reported coronavirus (COVID-19) infections and associated symptoms, England and Scotland: November 2023 to March 2024.* https://www.ons.gov.uk/peoplepopulationandcommunity/healthandsocialcare/conditionsanddiseases/articles/selfreportedcoronaviruscovid19infectionsandassociatedsymptomsenglandandscotland/november2023tomarch2024

Pantelic, M., Ziauddeen, N., Boyes, M. et al. (2022) Long Covid stigma: Estimating burden and validating scale in a UK-based sample. *PLoS One, 17*(11). https://doi.org/10.1371/journal.pone.0277317

Pullan, P., & Pullan M. (2021, October 15). Health: Surely things will get better? *Church Times*. https://www.churchtimes.co.uk/articles/2021/15-october/features/features/health-surely-things-will-get-better

Rehmeyer, J. (2016, September 21). *Bad science misled millions with chronic fatigue syndrome. Here's how we fought back*. Stat. https://www.statnews.com/2016/09/21/chronic-fatigue-syndrome-pace-trial/

Rothman, J., (2018). *Social work practice across disability* (2nd ed.). Routledge.

Vickers, M. (2002). *Work and unseen chronic illness*. Routledge.

Village, A., & Francis, L. J. (2023). The effects of spiritual wellbeing on self-perceived health changes among members of the Church of England during the COVID-19 pandemic in England. *Journal of Religion and Health, 62*, 2899–2915. https://doi.org/10.1007/s10943-023-01790-y

Volf, M. (1996). *Exclusion and embrace: A theological exploration of identity, otherness, and reconciliation*. Abingdon Press.

Wang., Y, Hunt, K., Nazareth, I., et al. (2013). Do men consult less than women? An analysis of routinely collected UK general practice data. *BMJ Open, 3*. https://doi.org/10.1136/bmjopen-2013-003320

Welby, J. (2017, February 15). *Statement from the Archbishop of Canterbury following today's General Synod*. Archbishop of Canterbury. https://www.archbishopofcanterbury.org/statement-archbishop-canterbury-following-todays-general-synod

White, P. D., Goldsmith, K. A., Johnson, A. L., et al. (2011). Comparison of adaptive pacing therapy, cognitive behaviour therapy, graded exercise therapy, and specialist medical care for chronic fatigue syndrome (PACE): A randomised trial. *The Lancet, 377*, 823–836. https://doi.org/10.1186/1745-6215-14-386

Wilshire, C.E., Kindlon, T., Courtney, R. et al. (2018). Rethinking the treatment of chronic fatigue syndrome-a reanalysis and evaluation of findings from a recent major trial of graded exercise and CBT. *BMC Psychology, 6*(1). https://doi.org/10.1186/s40359-018-0218-3

13

The Debilitating Discourses of Long COVID: The Public Pedagogies of Sporting Bodies

Matt Ventresca and Mary McDonald

Introduction

Sporting organisers worldwide memorably responded to the COVID-19 pandemic's onset by cancelling or postponing events. The absence of sporting events through much of 2020 came to symbolise how much COVID-19 was disrupting social life. As societies gradually reopened, athletes' bodies became prominent sites of scientific intervention as many competitors masked, were routinely tested for the novel coronavirus, and most accepted mandated vaccinations so that they could continue playing. However, much the same as with other aspects of social life globally, sports organisations gradually shed these protective strategies, further exposing athletes to COVID illness. We have traced the sociocultural implications of such trajectories through the creation of the *COVID*

M. Ventresca (✉) · M. McDonald
School of History and Sociology, Georgia Institute of Technology, Atlanta, GA, USA
e-mail: mventresca3@gatech.edu

D. Lupton (ed.), *Long COVID and Society*,
https://doi.org/10.1007/978-981-96-9168-5_13

Sports Project (https://covidsportsproject.hsoc.gatech.edu/), a website of multimedia resources exploring the COVID-sport nexus.

This chapter examines media representations of three professional athletes with Long COVID playing in major North American leagues: Women's National Basketball Association (WNBA) player AD Durr and National Hockey League (NHL) players Jonathon Toews and Brandon Sutter. Durr, a Black, non-binary athlete, was the second overall pick in the 2019 WNBA draft and experienced Long COVID early in the pandemic while a member of the New York Liberty team. Toews, who is White, was a four-time all-star and long-time captain of the Chicago Blackhawks. He announced in February 2023 that Long COVID was forcing him to pause his career. Sutter, who is also White, played over a decade in the NHL and was among the 21 Vancouver Canuck players to contract COVID during a 2021 team outbreak. Durr, Toews, and Sutter are some of the most prominent North American athletes to publicly acknowledge their experiences with Long COVID: an important status given Long COVID's broader invisibility within sport and other cultural spaces.

To better understand the formation of Long COVID narratives in elite sport, we examined over 130 news stories about these players' illnesses. We secured these stories through the Nexis Uni database, searching for the keyword 'Long COVID' and each athlete's name. We then eliminated duplicate articles to arrive at our final sample. We analysed the articles following Foucauldian theories of discourse analysis (Foucault, 1972, 1991; Khan & MacEachen, 2021), investigating how these narratives produce conceptions of 'truth' about Long COVID that are represented as universal and self-evident despite being shaped by social relations of power. We evaluated how these discourses (re-)produced and/or resisted the dominant socio-cultural, economic, and political dynamics of elite sports. We were especially attentive to how these athletes' stories informed broader understandings of health, illness, and recovery in the context of a pandemic that had affected every country across the globe. We also noted significant absences within these discourses and considered how these exclusions constrained possibilities for more nuanced conceptions of Long COVID.

Our analysis synthesises three main themes: (i) athletes' symptoms and suffering; (ii) militarised metaphors of 'battling' illness; and (iii) uncertainty in returning to the (sport) workplace. At first glance, these representations highlight how young, able-bodied individuals are not immune from the debilitating consequences of COVID and seemingly counter dominant pandemic risk narratives primarily focused on the 'vulnerable' elderly, disabled or those with pre-existing medical conditions. Yet these narratives stop short of examining the social and political conditions in which Long COVID occurs and erroneously suggest that individuals are responsible for their own health. These storylines gloss over the social inequities shaping Long COVID experiences and fail to confront broader pandemic discourses of ableism.

This analysis demonstrates how sports media discourses are important, although underappreciated, sites of public pedagogy infused with competing meanings around (un)healthy bodies in pandemic times. The concept of public pedagogy acknowledges that popular culture forms are important communicative sites through which people learn about issues of social, political and economic importance: in this case, Long COVID. As such, this analysis helps illuminate 'the broader educational force' of popular culture (Giroux, 2004, p. 60) with an emphasis on sports and athletes as vehicles for ideological messages. In what follows, we first discuss how sport's economic and cultural power has helped cultivate meanings around health and COVID. We then elaborate on the three analytical themes of athlete suffering, illness 'battles' and uncertainty. We conclude by considering why athlete narratives have failed to sustain meaningful public discussion about the debilitating effects of Long COVID and explain the need for critical counter-narratives highlighting the pandemic's broader sociocultural dynamics.

Elite Sports in a COVID-19 World

There is no escaping the social and economic power of the global sports industry. Much of sports' reach as a site of public pedagogy is facilitated through a media/promotional complex with mutual economic benefits to elite sports organisations, media and advertisers. While always challenged and resisted, historically dominant sporting representations too frequently reproduce normative discourses related to race, class, gender, ability, and capital with an emphasis on the supposed exceptionalism of young, able, masculine bodies.

Elite sports' capacity for public pedagogy impacts conceptions of health (Magdalinski, 2009; Waddington, 2000). High-ranking athletes are often celebrated as exemplifying ideal health and ability, representing the maximum potentials of physical strength and endurance. Yet scholars have traced contradictions within this 'sport-health ideology' (Waddington, 2000), explaining how athletes are regularly subject to injury risks and strenuous physical demands that damage their bodies (Magdalinski, 2009). An athlete's health is commonly framed as the capacity to compete rather than a state of well-being. An extensive medical infrastructure has therefore developed around elite sport, tasked with keeping athletes 'healthy' and able to perform. Athletes who cannot 'stay healthy' and remain productive, then, are typically deemed to be expendable (Magdalinski, 2009). As such, elite sports are typically sites for the cultural reification of able-bodiedness as the epitome of good health (Magdalinski, 2009; Silva & Howe, 2019).

Sports media's influence on ideas about health extended into the COVID pandemic. Early on, however, health discourses were intertwined with—and often overshadowed by—other societal concerns. While uncertainty reigned amidst game and event stoppages in March 2020, American sports coverage represented themes of loss: both the immense economic losses across the global sports industry and the perceived cultural impact of a world without elite sporting competitions (Bell, 2021). Although media regularly reported the names of athletes who tested positive for COVID, health-related stories were minimal in early coverage (Bell, 2021; Narcotta-Welp & Cavalier, 2023). By May 2020, many professional sports leagues announced plans to resume their seasons. These developments were at the forefront of discourses celebrating societies' supposed return to normal (Rowe, 2020).

Much like global society more broadly, capitalistic claims around economic stability and profit-making helped accelerate the reopening of elite sports (Profitt et al., 2021). Media coverage reinforced these dynamics with stories fluctuating between concern for athletes' safety and openness to health risks as an acceptable cost of re-starting the sports economy (Hindman et al., 2021). Given that athletes are valuable commodities, sports organisations developed medical protocols to limit COVID spread and maintain a 'healthy' workforce.

Narratives celebrating scientific and health expertise were especially extensive around the construction of sequestered bio-secure 'bubbles' to enable sporting events restart in July 2020 (Baggaley, 2020; Previtte, 2020; Wetsman, 2020). These bubble environments were sites of continuous medical surveillance and technological intervention to eliminate risk of COVID infection. Athletes were regularly tested for the novel coronavirus, masking protocols were enforced, and facilities were routinely sanitised (Mack et al., 2023; Salazar & Katz, 2021). The overall effectiveness of such protocols in mitigating COVID spread attested to the importance of investing in public health interventions while making the logics of public health measures visible to media audiences.

However, this visibility simultaneously obscured how structural inequalities contribute to and exacerbate disease processes. Elite athletes were certainly subject to medical surveillance and often 'confined' to isolated spaces; yet they were also privileged in having access to the latest safety and mitigation technologies (Pavlidis & Rowe, 2021). The medical infrastructure of elite sports was extended to include COVID protections largely unavailable outside of these environments. The privileges bestowed on athletes to help restart the global sports economy contrasted with the pandemic's broader health disparities. Indeed, ableist ideologies, along with 'preexisting social and economic precarity', meant that some bodies, including older individuals, those with disabilities, racialised minorities and essential workers, were considered expendable and made even more vulnerable to the pandemic's deadly and disabling effects (Abrams & Orsini, 2022, p. 166).

These pandemic discourses inform representations of Long COVID among athletes; yet an important tension pervades these forms of public pedagogy. While audiences could witness athletes' struggles, increasing awareness that could inspire broader advocacy (McGannon et al., 2024), Long COVID portrayals remain situated in dominant sports discourses. Athletes are typically portrayed as having resilient, healthy and able bodies, as well as being embodiments of competitiveness, self-responsibility and productivity (Andrews & Silk, 2018). Our investigation illuminates how athlete narratives occupy this contradictory space and how they inform—and constrain—understandings of Long COVID.

Somatic Suffering: Narrating Long COVID Symptoms

The Durr, Sutter, and Toews cases each articulate different stories regarding the early stages of their COVID illnesses, helping establish the heterogeneity of Long COVID and its effects. Diagnosed in June 2020, Durr was often bed-ridden and lost 32 pounds/15 kgs in 6 months while experiencing extreme fatigue and severe lung pains. They were finally cleared to resume playing basketball 18 months after their initial infection (Amour, 2021; Beer, 2021; Lee, 2021). Sutter caught COVID in March 2021 and later recounted that, after feeling recovered from his initial infection, he started 'having a couple of issues of being short of breath' in May and June (quoted in Canadian Press, 2021; Kuzma, 2022). Sutter reported worsening symptoms through the northern summer of 2021, including elevated heart rate and severe shortness of breath: his laboured breathing made it feel like 'someone was sitting on my chest' (quoted in Johnston, 2022). Media accounts of Durr and Sutter's struggles with COVID are similar, as both players are quoted describing how harsh symptoms impacted their quality of life. In contrast, stories about Toews are much less detailed, although some mention his symptoms of lethargy, fatigue and pain (Lazerus, 2021). Interestingly, Toews' illness was most often narrated through a concurrent diagnosis of chronic immune response syndrome, a somewhat ambiguous condition whereby exposure to biotoxins such as mould generates an overactive inflammatory response to bodily stressors.

Collectively, these accounts serve a pedagogical function in highlighting common markers of Long COVID: fatigue, vomiting, nausea, lung pain, shortness of breath, persistent cough, cognitive impairment, gastrointestinal distress, confusion, headaches and coughing up blood—to mention but a few manifestations. Descriptions of each athlete's symptoms were frequently accompanied by elaboration on the seriousness of Long COVID or statistics estimating the prevalence of Long COVID within the general population, thus suggesting that these athletes' stories are not isolated cases. For instance, some stories cite American Medical Association estimates 'that anywhere from 10 to 30 per cent of people who contract COVID-19 may experience symptoms at some time after they recovered from their initial infection' (Johnston, 2022; Guardian Sport, 2022) or explain that Long COVID is associated with over 200 symptoms (Guardian Sport, 2022). Additional storylines emphasised the non-linear and unpredictable nature of Long COVID. One story conveyed how 'common symptoms linger. New ones develop' (Lee, 2021) with another describing players 'working through physical and emotional peaks and valleys' (Johnston, 2022).

Discussions of the athletes' symptoms served contradictory ends. At first glance, they appear to counter commonsense perspectives that COVID overwhelmingly has an impact on those who are older, have preexisting medical conditions or are immunocompromised. This ableist narrative emerged early in the pandemic not simply as an assessment of medical risk, but as a method whereby governments sought to assure their citizens that the pandemic posed little danger to 'healthy' people (Abrams & Orsini, 2022). The cases of Durr, Sutter, and Toews convey a more complicated picture and challenge what journalist Nancy Armour (2021) characterises as a 'dangerous misperception'. As Durr relates, 'People say all the time, "You're young, you're an athlete, you're in great shape." Obviously, that doesn't matter when it comes to COVID' (quoted in Armour, 2021). These stories communicate that anybody, including elite athletes who presumably epitomise health and fitness, might be vulnerable to debilitating Long COVID symptoms.

In some examples, this susceptibility is portrayed through the athlete's inability to return to fitness routines or any level of athletic performance. Durr reveals 7 months after their initial COVID infection that they 'still [couldn't] even shoot a free throw'. At one point, Sutter suggested that 'with my lungs and my breathing and any exertion, I just can't do it. I stop and feel like I have to cough something out and just feel like

I can't get oxygen into my body' (quoted in Kuzma, 2022). Sutter also recounts in 2022 that despite feeling '100 percent better than a year ago', he couldn't train or workout. Sutter said, 'When I take it easier, I'm ok; but when I work out, it just crushes me' (quoted in Kuzma, 2022). In other instances, these athletes explain how their difficult symptoms have impacted their lives beyond sport. Durr said in 2021, 'there are days I feel great. I can go out, like go to the store, clean the house, and others I just want to stay in bed, I feel like I have been hit by a bus' (quoted in Seven Months, 2021). According to Toews, there were 'times when it was hard not to feel sorry for myself, because it became so repetitive—just waking up in the morning and just feeling that dead weight of no desire, no excitement, no inspiration to do anything at all. It was mentally tough' (quoted in Lazerus, 2021).

In briefly capturing what Cheston and colleagues characterise as the 'somatic suffering' of Long COVID, these athletes' accounts 'attempt to make visible what others cannot know, cannot understand, and very often, are unable to see' (Cheston et. al., 2023, p. 9). As also experienced by other patients, athletes with Long COVID thus inhabit a 'third space' in between the binary outcomes constructed through dominant governmental and media narratives: that COVID is either mild and results in full recovery or severe enough to result in hospitalisation and death (Cheston et. al., 2023). As such, these athlete storylines serve a pedagogical function in taking Long COVID across the 'threshold of invisibility' (Cheston et al., 2023, p. 13) and detailing some of the bodily effects of a still poorly understood disease. The ways in which these stories are narrated, however, focus on individual struggles, thus drawing attention away from the inadequacy of public health infrastructures within and beyond sport.

Individualising Illness Battles

Amidst vivid language documenting Long COVID's physical and mental toll, media representations frequently depicted the athletes through a familiar trope of an individual battling illness: a discourse that has been well-documented in discussions of cancer and HIV/AIDS (Lupton,

2012; Sontag, 2013). For instance, one headline proclaimed that Sutter was launching a comeback 'after a two-year battle with COVID' (Tychkowski, 2023). Durr's Long COVID experience is characterised as a 'complicated and arduous battle' (Basketball-Liberty, 2020). Another report asserted that for 'three years now Jonathan Toews' body has been at war with his mind, his heart, with his desire. But he wanted to play again. He had to play again' (Lazerus, 2023).

Importantly, this militarised narrative of battle articulates with another common framing within sport: athletes fighting on and off the field to overcome barriers to success (Hughes & Coakley, 1991). This dominant 'overcoming the odds' narrative, where athletes are encouraged to achieve success and strive for distinction no matter the obstacles, is perhaps most problematic when athletes accept bodily risks to play through pain, injury and illness (Coakley, 2021). Given that high performance sports culture has long normalised the adage of 'toughing it out', it is not surprising that sports storylines continue to reify this portrayal where health is sacrificed in the 'battle' to get back into the game.

This framing is evident in portrayals of Durr, Sutter and Toews, where their recoveries were narrated as 'fights', demonstrating determination and toughness. For example, after Durr missed the 2020 WNBA season, they expressed the desire to return to play in 2021, saying: 'I'm not a quitter. I definitely fight [...] No matter where I am right now, I know every day is important to my recovery process, so I just try to keep going' (quoted in Lee, 2021). Jonathan Kolb, Liberty General Manager echoes this sentiment, suggesting that Durr 'hasn't given up [...] doesn't give up and wants to prove to everyone that [they are] a fighter' (quoted in The Second Overall, 2021). Similarly, Toews is represented as having the determination 'to continue fighting through the fatigue and pain and emotional struggle that come with his dual diagnosis of Long COVID and chronic immune response syndrome' (Lazerus, 2023).

These militarised metaphors are aligned with language used early in the pandemic suggesting that nations were at war with a submicroscopic enemy in the form of the COVID virus (Isaacs & Priesz, 2020). War metaphors were commonly used by government officials and medical practitioners to mobilise nations' public health resources (for example, ventilators, masks, personal protective equipment) as well as a sense of collective responsibility for containing the pandemic. Yet war-based conceptualisations of the COVID pandemic have their shortcomings. They can promote fear and anxiety around illness and reduce complex ethical dilemmas to simplistic matters of good versus evil. Such metaphors can stigmatise those who become ill as traitors in the battle against COVID rather than people impacted by gaps in public health infrastructures (Isaacs & Priesz, 2020). This was indeed demonstrated in early representations of athletes who tested positive for COVID (Narcotta-Welp & Cavalier, 2023).

The Durr, Toews and Sutter storylines link such militarised meanings to preexisting sport discourses by focusing on individual battles to return to play. These individualised narratives reproduce sports discourses of pushing through pain and injury without interrogating the often-debilitating consequences of such athletic norms. Importantly, these narrow storylines gloss over the 'infrastructures of harm' within elite sports cultures: the environments, systems and practices through which athletes' bodies are managed, commodified, and put at continuous injury risk in the name of performance and productivity (Ventresca, 2020). Such infrastructures are most evident in the underpinnings of sport's concussion crisis, but they extend to broader organisational, medical, and economic systems that normalise harm to athletes' bodies as an inevitable part of elite sports. The COVID pandemic added new dimensions to these infrastructures. While athletes had privileged access to COVID protections in the pandemic's early stages, the push to 'return to normal' involved relaxing health measures across sports workplaces and increased rates of athlete infection, including teamwide outbreaks as seen in 2021 with Sutter's Canucks team.

The conventional trope of the athlete comeback story further constrains meaningful recognition of the sociopolitical specificities of COVID-19 and Long COVID. These individualistic framings serve to insulate sport industry leaders from accountability for managing and redressing the systems that produce athlete harm. The lack of critical attention to the systems surrounding athletes' Long COVID experiences parallels the gradual decline of public concern for addressing broader pandemic infrastructures of harm. Such infrastructures in the COVID era include (but are not limited to): poor building ventilation that facilitates the spread of airborne diseases, muddled public heath messaging, insufficient funding for COVID research and monitoring, inadequate sick leave policies for most workers, anti-mask sentiments, minimal mitigation efforts in schools, healthcare settings, and many other essential workplaces (Feldman & Bassett, 2024; Galvão, 2023). Early discussions of these infrastructures soon faded due to high remediation costs and a capitalistic devaluing of labour amidst calls to 'get back to business'. Devoid of such context, militarised framings articulate a familiar sensibility that individuals are responsible their own health, even when disparities in protections and resources persist.

Uncertainty and Privilege: Working Out and Out of Work

Representations of the illness experiences of Durr, Sutter and Toews highlighted how the variability and unpredictability of Long COVID symptoms posed challenges for establishing a clear path to recovery and getting back to work. Navigating these issues 'is a grind' (Sutter quoted in Johnston, 2022) as these athletes, like most with Long Covid, sought answers amidst uncertainty (Koffman et al, 2020). Like many others with Long COVID, 'the hardest part' for these athletes might have been 'trying to figure out for the longest time what was wrong' (Sutter quoted in Tychkowski, 2023). Sutter further elaborates on how his Long COVID experience clashed with typical trajectories of injury rehabilitation:

> You break a bone, you have a broken leg or a knee problem, or a shoulder or something, you go 'OK we got six weeks, we got eight weeks, and we're back to normal.' This has just been dragging on and on. (Johnston, 2022)

Durr similarly expressed frustration with the lack of certainty around their illness: 'I always had a positive mindset, but I just got used to being sick for so long and doctors not being able to give me any type of response, answer, anything' (quoted in Negley, 2021). Near the end of his hockey career, Toews lamented that 'it just got to the point where I just wasn't recovering and was just progressively getting worse [...] and I was getting pretty alarmed. Something that we're clearly not getting to the bottom of" (quoted in Friesen, 2023).

Despite this uncertainty, news reporting affirmed that these athletes had clear social and economic advantages compared to the majority of those living with Long COVID. As elite athletes and valuable commodities, these players had access to exceptional medical care. For example, the New York Liberty connected Durr with the Mount Sinai Health System, the first American clinic dedicated to Long COVID. Durr was subsequently treated by specialised, sympathetic doctors who prescribed medications to help manage their symptoms (Armour, 2021). In July 2022, Sutter visited Calgary's Hoffman Clinic to receive 'intravenous treatments to fight protein inflammation' (Kuzma, 2022). Toews worked 'with doctors to figure out why his body—his temple, his instrument, his entire life—was betraying him' (Lazerus, 2021).

These athletes' ability to receive ground-breaking therapies and high-level care contrasts with the broad inaccessibility of specialists and treatment across healthcare systems. As celebrities within well-connected sports organisations, the athletes had material advantages in navigating often-fragmented healthcare systems that were politicised and weakened during the pandemic (Au et al 2022). Unlike many Long COVID and other patients in the US healthcare system who often need to stop treatments due to associated costs and inadequate health insurance, these athletes were helped to persist in pursuing their recoveries. Additionally, Long COVID patients, as with others living with chronic illnesses, are subject to 'gaslighting' by doctors who downplay or dismiss patients' illness experiences (Au et al., 2022). We found no suggestion in the stories we surveyed that Durr, Sutter, or Toews experienced such a dismissive dynamic; if they did, it was not a matter of public record.

Ultimately, the material advantages that come with being a professional athlete enabled each athlete to exit their sports workplaces to focus on their recovery or transition into related jobs, a privilege not afforded most workers. Toews stepped away from hockey after the 2023–2024 season at the end of an 8-year $84 million USD contract. He then journeyed to India seeking alternative healing therapies. Long COVID kept

Sutter from playing the 2021–2022 and 2022–2023 seasons. He retired in 2023 after being released by the Edmonton Oilers after earning over $31 million USD throughout his career. Durr sat out the 2020 and 2021 seasons but returned to the WNBA in 2022. After averaging only 10 minutes a game with the Atlanta Dream in 2023, they went unsigned for the 2024 season. Durr was subsequently hired as an assistant basketball coach at the University of North Carolina at Charlotte. Even when each athlete's comeback attempt proved unsuccessful or unsustainable, the details comprising their stories, and what is left out, communicate simplistic, underdeveloped conceptions of Long COVID that reproduce problematic pandemic narratives.

Concluding Thoughts

The news stories about these elite athletes' Long COVID experiences analysed in this chapter appeared while both the US and Canadian governments increasingly promoted a narrative of collective restitution. This narrative suggests that each nation had successfully overcome the disenabling circumstances wrought by the pandemic, despite continuing persistently high rates of COVID infection, hospitalisation and mortality (McCoy, 2023). Sports stories were important for encouraging acceptance of this restitution narrative (Atkinson, 2023). As elite sports returned 'triumphantly and defiantly' to routines resembling pre-2020 'normality', they communicated the message that the 'war against COVID-19' had surely concluded (Atkinson, 2023, p. 792). Indeed, major North American sports organisations began eliminating COVID protocols in 2022 (Ventras, 2022).

The power of this restitution storyline is demonstrated in how elite athletes' experiences of Long COVID are minimised and even erased. Post-retirement portrayals of Sutter and Toews failed to specify why their careers ended. An article conveying Sutter's analysis of a recent NHL coaching change only states that he 'announced his retirement from the NHL last fall after attempting a comeback with the Edmonton Oilers' (Garioch, 2024). When Toews posted on social media about his India trip, a subsequent story outlining his medical recovery describes his ailment as 'some health issues that kept him away from the NHL since the 2022–2023 season ended' (Parise, 2024). Other coverage of Toews' India trip mentions Long COVID in a manner similar to any other sports injury. For example, one article states, 'Now a free agent, Toews was limited to 53 games during the 2022–2023 season as he missed significant periods of time due to the effects of Long COVID and chronic immune response syndrome. He recorded 15 goals and 16 assists' (TSN.ca Staff). Thorpe et al. (2023) explain how pandemic sporting spaces can be marked by missing bodies, their absences creating unsettling atmospheres of loss, dread, and uncertainty. Yet sports discourses mitigate these affective disruptions by making the absence of COVID-stricken athletic bodies appear routine. Long COVID is therefore reduced to simply another 'health issue' within an athlete's career cycle of performance, injury, substitution, and inevitable replacement.

Militarised narratives also continue to pervade discussions of Long COVID among athletes. Coverage of Durr's hiring as an assistant coach mentioned that their 'professional career came with a fair share of adversity' since they missed two WNBA seasons while 'suffering from the effects of COVID-19' (Cubit, 2024). This framing of Long COVID as personal adversity again aligns with broader individualised sports injury narratives. Similar coverage of 2024 medal wins by Australian Olympic sailor Matt Wearn and British Paralympic triathlete Lauren Steadman focused on how their determination and hard work allowed them to prevail despite the devastating effects of Long COVID (Dutch, 2024; Pengilly, 2024).

These storylines reveal the limitations of athlete narratives as forms of public pedagogy around Long COVID. Initial portrayals of athletes' somatic suffering generated space for public recognition of Long COVID experiences when such acknowledgement was mostly lacking in mainstream media. Yet, while challenging the notion that young healthy people could not be impacted by Long COVID, these representations offered only momentary disruptions of society's dismissal of COVID illness. Too often the decontextualised, individualistic and militarised framings of these stories characterise Long COVID as a personal trouble rather than a social or public health concern. Moreover, athletes' Long COVID experiences tend to get swallowed up by familiar discourses of sports injury constructed around individual journeys of adversity, rehabilitation and hard work. As such, these narratives did little to displace the systemic 'othering' of disabled bodies cast as already infirmed and therefore expendable (Abrams & Orsini, 2022). The attention given to medicalised attempts to 'cure' these athletes similarly reproduces ableist discourses that obscure how structural inequities shape illness experiences.

The ideological trappings of elite sports leave little space for critical interrogation or more complex Long COVID narratives. The routine portrayals of athletes undergoing medical procedures normalise their privileged access to specialised COVID care. And while clinicians' refusal to take Long COVID seriously is a well-documented aspect of online illness narratives (Russell et al., 2022), its absence from the discourses we examined might reflect athletes' embeddedness within medical infrastructures. However, the story of British National Team rower Oonagh Cousins is a rare exception to this trend. Cousins missed the 2020 Tokyo Olympics due to Long COVID and still experiences symptoms. She has been outspoken about her difficulties navigating the medical system where practitioners frequently dismissed her physical ailments as manifestations of psychological problems (Schraer & Grant, 2024).

The dismissal of Cousins' experiences helps explain why athlete narratives have not contributed to establishing Long COVID as an urgent public health concern: especially when other sports issues have done just that. For example, representations of brain injury among elite athletes have informed framings of concussion as a public health crisis (Ventresca, 2019). While neuroscientific evidence has functioned as 'proof' of the severity of the concussion crisis, Long COVID remains under-appreciated and under-theorised in formal medical and scientific spaces.

The high-profile world of elite sport could be a context to promote broader public acknowledgement and medical recognition of Long COVID. Yet capitalising on this potential would require sports media to disrupt individualised and militarised framings of athlete injury, better explain athletes' privileged access to medical treatment and contextualise athlete experiences within broader social inequalities. These commitments would facilitate connections between attention-grabbing stories about elite athletes and online narratives that illuminate how experiences of Long COVID are influenced by economic disparities, medical negligence and the impacts of ableism, racism, and sexism (Miller, 2024). Some portrayals of Durr, for example, focus on how their Long COVID diagnosis overlapped with their journey as a non-binary athlete (for example, Togethxr/Uninterruped, 2022). Yet these representations are generally framed as stories of personal struggle and triumph without explicitly mentioning how Black and non-binary people might experience Long COVID differently from White or cisgender people. Making such connections would afford broader public visibility into the complexities of Long COVID and into the pandemic's intersecting inequalities.

References

Abrams, T. & Orsini, M. (2022). Waves of ableism: Affective arrangements in the time of COVID-19. *Canadian Journal of Disability Studies, 11*(3), 154–180. https://cjds.uwaterloo.ca/index.php/cjds/article/view/930

Andrews, D. L., & Silk, M. (2018). Sport and neoliberalism: An affective-ideological articulation. *Journal of Popular Culture, 51*(2), 511–533. https://doi.org/10.1111/jpcu.12660

Armour, N. (2021, December 15). Long-haul COVID cost WNBA star two seasons; Durr: "I just got used to being sick." *USA Today.* https://www.usatoday.com/story/sports/wnba/2021/12/14/asia-durr-looking-forward-return-wnba-after-bout-long-covid/8892583002/?gnt-cfr=1&gca-cat=p

Atkinson, M. (2023). Interview (s) with the vampire: Research opportunism during a global catastrophe. In Andrews, D.L., Thorpe, H. & J.I. Newman (Eds.). *Sport and physical culture in global pandemic times: COVID assemblages* (pp. 771–795). Palgrave Macmillan.

Au, L., Capotescu, C., Esyal, G. & Finestone, G. (2022). Long COVID and medical gaslighting: Dismissal, delayed diagnosis and deferred treatment. *SSM-Qualitative Research in Health, 2.* https://www.sciencedirect.com/science/article/pii/S2667321522001299

Baggaley, K. (2020, October 15). The NBA bubble was a one-of-a-kind COVID-19 success story: Masks and social distancing were crucial.

Popular Science. https://www.popsci.com/story/health/nba-coronavirus-bubble-success-science/

Bell, T. R. (2021). SportsCenter: A case study of media framing US sport as the COVID-19 epicenter. *International Journal of Sport Communication, 14*(2), 298–317. https://doi.org/10.1123/ijsc.2020-0258

Beer, T. (2021, April 14). Jayson Tatum, still dealing with long-term COVID effects, reveals he uses an inhaler before games. *Forbes.com*. https://www.forbes.com/sites/tommybeer/2021/04/14/jayson-tatum-still-dealing-with-long-term-covid-effects-reveals-he-uses-inhaler-before-games/

Cheston, K., Cenedese, M. L., & Woods, A. (2023). The long or the post of it? Temporality, suffering, and uncertainty in narratives following COVID-19. *Journal of Medical Humanities, 46*(1), 3–20. https://doi.org/10.1007/s10912-023-09824-y

Coakley, J. (2021). *Sport in society: Issues and controversies* (13th ed.). McGraw Hill.

Cubit, A. (2024, September 16). Former Louisville women's basketball star Asia 'AD' Durr joins Charlotte coaching staff. *Yahoo! Sports*. https://sports.yahoo.com/former-louisville-womens-basketball-star-190033446.html

Dutch, T. (2024, September 5). Paralympian Lauren Steadman had 'zero expectations' before winning bronze while managing Long COVID. *Self Magazine*. "https://www.self.com/story/lauren-steadman-long-covid-2024

Feldman, J. M., & Bassett, M. T. (2024). US public health after COVID-19: Learning from the failures of the hollow state and racial capitalism. *British Medical Journal, 384*. https://doi.org/10.1136/bmj-2023-076969

Foucault M. (1972). *The archaeology of knowledge* (Translated from French by A. M. Sheridan Smith). Pantheon Books.

Foucault, M. (1991). Questions of method. In G. Burchell, C. Gordon, & P. Miller (Eds.), *The Foucault effect: Studies in governmentality* (pp. 73–86). Harvester Wheatsheaf.

Friesen, P. (2023, March 28). One last skate? Jonathan Toews fighting off Long COVID for a proper Chicago goodbye. *Edmonton Sun*. https://winnipegsun.com/sports/hockey/nhl/toews-fighting-off-covid-for-proper-chicago-goodbye

Galvão, J. (2023). COVID-19: Forgetting a pandemic that is not over. *The Lancet, 401*(10386), 1422–1423. https://doi.org/10.1016/S0140-6736(23)00637-2

Garioch, B. (2024, May 9). Former Canucks winger Brandon Sutter believes Travis Green will have success with senators. *Ottawa Citizen.* https://ottawacitizen.com/ottawa-senators/former-canucks-winger-brandon-sutter-believes-travis-green-will-have-success-with-senators

Giroux, H. (2004). Cultural Studies, public pedagogy, and the responsibilities of intellectuals. *Communication and Critical/cultural Studies, 1*(1), 59–79. https://doi.org/10.1080/1479142042000180926

Guardian Sport (2022, April 27). NHL's Brandon Sutter says Long COVID has sidelined him for entire season. *The Guardian.* https://www.theguardian.com/sport/2022/apr/27/brandon-sutter-long-covid-nhl-ice-hockey-vancouver-canucks

Hindman, L. C., Walker, N. A., & Agyemang, K. J. A. (2021). Bounded rationality or bounded morality? The National Basketball Association response to COVID-19. *European Sport Management Quarterly, 21*(3), 333–349. https://doi.org/10.1080/16184742.2021.1879191

Hughes, R., & Coakley, J. (1991). Positive deviance among athletes: The implications of overconformity to the sport ethic. *Sociology of Sport Journal, 8*(4), 307–325.

Isaacs, D., & Priesz, M. A. (2020). COVID-19 and the metaphor of war. *Journal of Paediatrics and Child Health, 57*(1), 6–8. https://doi.org/10.1111/jpc.15164

Johnston, P. (2022, April 27). Canucks: Brandon Sutter's Long COVID has taken an emotional and physical toll. *Postmedia Breaking News.* https://theprovince.com/sports/hockey/nhl/vancouver-canucks/canucks-brandon-sutters-long-covid-has-taken-an-emotional-and-physical-toll

Khan, T. H., & MacEachen, E. (2021). Foucauldian discourse analysis: Moving beyond a social constructionist analytic. *International Journal of Qualitative Methods, 20.* https://doi.org/10.1177/16094069211018009

Koffman, J., Gross, J., Etkind, S. N., & Selman, L. (2020). Uncertainty and COVID-19: How are we to respond? *Journal of the Royal Society of Medicine, 113*(6), 211–216. https://doi.org/10.1177/0141076820930665

Kuzma, B. (2022, July 27). "It just crushes me": Sutter still battling Long COVID. *Vancouver Sun.* https://theprovince.com/sports/hockey/nhl/vancouver-canucks/canucks-brandon-sutter-still-stuck-in-covid-19-long-hauler-maze

Lazerus, M. (2021, June 30). Blackhawks' Jonathan Toews opens up about the longest year of his life: "The best worst thing that's ever happened to me." *The Athletic*. https://www.nytimes.com/athletic/2682532/2021/06/30/blackhawks-jonathan-toews-opens-up-about-the-longest-year-of-his-life-the-best-worst-thing-thats-ever-happened-to-me/

Lazerus, M. (2023, April 6, 2023). Jonathan Toews on his NHL playing future: "If it's not hell yeah, it's a hell no." *The Athletic*. https://www.nytimes.com/athletic/4388410/2023/04/06/chicago-blackhawks-jonathan-toews-future/

Lee. M. (2021, April 21). Down for the long haul; For some athletes, debilitating COVID symptoms linger for months, threatening their careers. *The Washington Post*. https://www.washingtonpost.com/sports/2021/04/19/athletes-long-haul-covid-justin-foster/

Lupton, D. (2012). *Medicine as culture: Illness, disease and the body*. Sage. https://doi.org/10.4135/9781446254530

Mack, C. D., Merson, M. H., Sims, L., Maragakis, L. L., Davis, R., Tai, C. G., & DiFiori, J. (2023). The "bubble": What can be learned from the National Basketball Association (NBA)'s 2019–20 season restart in Orlando during the COVID-19 pandemic. *The Journal of Applied Laboratory Medicine, 8*(6), 1017–1027. https://doi.org/10.1093/jalm/jfad073

Magdalinski, T. (2009). *Sport, technology and the body: The nature of performance*. Routledge.

McCoy, C. A. (2023). How does the pandemic end? Losing control of the COVID-19 pandemic illness narrative. *Global Public Health, 18*(1), 1–12. https://doi.org/10.1080/17441692.2023.2195918

McGannon, K. R., Hladun, W., Kulkarni, S., Bundon, A., & Pegoraro, A. (2024). From birth to rebirth: Comeback meanings in media stories of Canadian athlete mothers' sporting journeys. *Sport, Education and Society, Online First*. https://doi.org/10.1080/13573322.2024.2376249

Miller, S. C. (2024). Long COVID and disability justice: Critiquing the present, forming the future. In J. M. Reynolds & M. E. Gary (Eds.), *Disability justice in public health emergencies* (pp. 107–119). Routledge.

Narcotta-Welp, E., & Cavalier, E. S. (2023). A Community of athletic pariahs?: Guilt, shame, and social control in the COVID-19 Pandemic. In D. L. Andrews, H. Thorpe, & J. I. Newman (Eds.), *Sport and physical culture in global pandemic times: COVID assemblages* (pp. 295–319). Palgrave Macmillan.

Negley, C. (2021, December 15). Cleared to play, Asia Durr still dealing with flare-ups after "worst case" of long-haul COVID. *AOL.com*. https://www.aol.com/cleared-play-asia-durr-still-170553978.html

Parise, V. (2024, November 21). Jonathan Toews provides health update via Instagram. *Yahoo! Sports*. https://sports.yahoo.com/jonathan-toews-provides-health-via-183247370.html

Pavlidis, A., & Rowe, D. (2021). The sporting bubble as gilded cage. *M/C Journal*, *24*(1). https://doi.org/10.5204/mcj.2736

Pengilly, A. (2024, July 6). 'It was taken away from me': The Olympic champion who spent a year battling long COVID. *Sydney Morning Herald*. https://www.smh.com.au/sport/sailing/it-was-taken-away-from-me-the-olympic-champion-who-spent-a-year-battling-long-covid-20240705-p5jrcl.html

Previtte, S. (2020, June 19). NBA to use 'smart rings,' big data to fight coronavirus in Disney bubble. *New York Post*. https://nypost.com/2020/06/19/nba-to-use-smart-rings-to-detect-coronavirus-within-bubble/

Profitt, J., Salazar, N. E., Cortese, J., & Merle, P. (2021). The rush to return to live sports: A political-economic analysis of sports entertainment in the time of COVID-19. *The Political Economy of Communication*, *9*(1), 22–40. http://polecom.org/index.php/polecom/article/view/135

Reuters. (2020, July 7). *National Post*. Liberty's Durr to miss WNBA season due to coronavirus. https://www.reuters.com/article/us-health-coronavirus-basketball-wnba-idUSKBN2482NG/

Rowe, D. (2020). Subjecting pandemic sport to a sociological procedure. *Journal of Sociology*, *56*(4), 704–713. https://doi.org/10.1177/1440783320941284

Russell, D., Spence, N. J., Chase, J. A. D., Schwartz, T., Tumminello, C. M., & Bouldin, E. (2022). Support amid uncertainty: Long COVID illness experiences and the role of online communities. *SSM-Qualitative Research in Health, 2*,. https://doi.org/10.1016/j.ssmqr.2022.100177

Salazar, J. W., & Katz, M. H. (2021). COVID-19 lessons from the National Basketball Association bubble—Can persistently SARS-CoV-2–positive individuals transmit infection to others? *JAMA Internal Medicine, 181*(7), 967–967. https://doi.org/10.1001/jamainternmed.2021.2121

Schraer, R. & Grant, P. (2024, May 21). Long COVID course is 'exploiting people', says ex-GB rower. *BBC*. https://www.bbc.com/news/health-69040592

Anonymous. (2021, January 28) Seven months after testing COVID-19 positive: "As if I had been hit by a bus,". *CE Noticias Financiarias English*.

Silva, C. F., & Howe, P. D. (2019). Sliding to reverse ableism: An ethnographic exploration of (dis)ability in sitting volleyball. *Societies*, *9*(2). https://doi.org/10.3390/soc9020041

Sontag, S. (2013). *Illness as metaphor and AIDS and its metaphors*. Farrar.

The Canadian Press. (2021, October 12). Canucks forward Brandon Sutter still experiencing COVID-19 symptoms: GM. *Sportsnet*. https://www.sportsnet.ca/nhl/article/canucks-forward-brandon-sutter-still-experiencing-covid-19-symptoms/

The COVID Sports Project. https://covidsportsproject.hsoc.gatech.edu/

Anonymous. (2021, January 28). The second overall drama of the draft eight months after coming back positive for COVID. *CE Noticias Financieras English*.

Thorpe, H., Jeffrey, A., & Fullagar, S. (2023). Re-turning to fitness 'riskscapes' post lockdown: Feminist materialisms, wellbeing and affective respondings in Aotearoa New Zealand. *Gender, Place & Culture, 31*(1), 102–123. https://doi.org/10.1080/0966369X.2023.2195132

Togethxr/Uninterrupted (2022, August 24). Never knocked down: The AD story. *Togethxr*. https://www.togethxr.com/blogs/films/never-knocked-down-the-ad-story

TSN.ca Staff (2024, November 21). Ex-Blackhawks captain Toews reveals 'healing journey' in India. *TSN*. https://www.tsn.ca/nhl/ex-chicago-blackhawks-captain-toews-reveals-healing-journey-in-india-1.2208032

Tychkowski, R. (2023, September). After two-year battle with COVID, Sutter launching comeback with Edmonton Oilers. *Edmonton Sun*. https://edmontonsun.com/sports/hockey/nhl/edmonton-oilers/after-two-year-battle-with-covid-sutter-launching-comeback-with-edmonton-oilers

Ventresca, M. (2019). The curious case of CTE: Mediating materialities of traumatic brain injury. *Communication & Sport, 7*(2), 135–156. https://doi.org/10.1177/2167479518761636

Ventresca, M. (2020). The tangled multiplicities of CTE: Scientific uncertainty and infrastructures of traumatic brain injury. In J. Sterling & M. G. McDonald (Eds.), *Sports, society, and technology: Bodies, practices, and knowledge production* (pp. 73–98). Palgrave Macmillan.

Ventras, J. (2022, March 3). NFL becomes first major American sports league to drop COVID-19 protocols. *New York Times*. https://www.nytimes.com/2022/03/03/sports/football/nfl-covid-protocol.html

Waddington, I. (2000). *Sport, health and drugs: A critical sociological investigation*. Routledge.

Wetsman, N. (2020, July 7). Sports bubbles are good places to study COVID-19. *The Verge*. https://www.theverge.com/21311885/sports-bubble-covid-research-nba-oura-saliva-test-symptom-monitoring

14

Long COVID in Children, Young People and Families

Alice MacLean, Cervantée Wild, Sarah Nettleton, Sue Ziebland, and Kate Hunt

Introduction

Long COVID is a novel condition which only first attracted any attention amongst medical circles and the general population after patient-led efforts in 2020 to raise awareness of persisting symptoms many weeks or months after initial infection with COVID-19 (Callard & Perego, 2021).

A. MacLean (✉) · K. Hunt
Institute for Social Marketing and Health, University of Stirling, Stirling, UK
e-mail: alice.maclean@stir.ac.uk

C. Wild · S. Ziebland
Nuffield Department of Primary Care Health Sciences, University of Oxford, Oxford, UK

C. Wild
Faculty of Medical and Health Sciences, Department of Paediatrics: Child and Youth Health, School of Medicine, University of Auckland, Auckland, New Zealand

S. Nettleton
Department of Sociology, University of York, York, UK

D. Lupton (ed.), *Long COVID and Society*,
https://doi.org/10.1007/978-981-96-9168-5_14

Long COVID defied collective representations ('narratives') (Wild et al., 2024) of COVID in the early stages of the pandemic in 2020/1: namely that infection resulted either in relatively inconsequential illness (like 'mild' flu) which resolved within two weeks in the vast majority of the population, or caused an acutely serious and potentially life-threatening illness in vulnerable members of the population (defined as older people and those with pre-existing chronic illness). A burgeoning literature, including our own UK-based study of adults' experiences of Long COVID (Anderson et al., 2024; MacLean et al., 2023a), has documented not only the severity of people's symptoms, and the profound impact of Long COVID on their daily lives, but also many people's longstanding struggles to have their illness recognised and validated by medical professionals and people beyond their immediate household, including colleagues, friends and family.

Our research found that 'vanguard patients' (MacLean et al., 2023a)—those experiencing Long COVID earliest in the pandemic—both had to bear the burden and impacts of their symptoms and the additional emotional work of collectively and individually working to have their illness recognised. While patients found some initial validation in their emerging realisation (usually through digital media and sources) that they were not alone in experiencing 'often bewildering, disabling life-changing and fluctuating but persistent constellations of symptoms' (MacLean et al., 2023a, p. 9), most had to fight for recognition of their condition by healthcare professionals. We argued that vanguard patients commonly experienced 'rejected' candidacy ('feeling disbelieved, discounted/uncounted, and abandoned and that their suffering was invisible to the medical gaze and society' (MacLean et al., 2023a, p. 1)) or 'diverted' candidacy (usually by the apparent presumption by doctors they encountered that their symptoms were attributable to underlying psychological morbidity). The minority whose candidacy was 'validated' in medical encounters were the only ones with more positive experiences to relate, even in the face of the dearth of effective treatments for Long COVID (MacLean et al., 2023a).

While many of these challenges are known to have persisted for adults experiencing Long COVID, very few studies have focused on the experiences of children, young adults and families. In this chapter, we address this gap, drawing on narrative interviews conducted in the UK with children, young adults and parents and other family members caring for people with Long COVID. The data are from in-depth narrative interviews (n = 77) from linked UK qualitative studies about COVID experiences, which used identical methods of data collection and overlapping teams, as reported in more detail elsewhere (Anderson et al., 2024; MacLean et al., 2023a; Wild et al., 2024). These studies included interviews with 22 children and adolescents aged 10 years or older with Long COVID, 39 parents/caregivers (21 of whom had Long COVID themselves, 12 who were caring for a child or young person with Long COVID and six who both had Long COVID themselves and were caring for their child with Long COVID), one young person caring for a parent and 15 young adults who first contracted COVID in their 20 s. In terms of ethnicity, 48 participants were white British or white 'other', 15 were Pakistani British and 13 were from a range of other ethnic minority groups. We included participants from all countries within the UK (England, Scotland, Wales and Northern Ireland) and from urban and more rural areas. Interviews were conducted between February 2021 and July 2022.

In what follows, we provide an overview of the wide-ranging impacts of Long COVID on these groups, across multiple facets of their lives, such as school, relationships, mental health, family life and help-seeking. Moreover, we explore the ways in which participants' illness experiences are expressed in the context of complex family environments, intersecting or colliding with financial difficulties, job insecurity and self-care at home. Further analyses as well as hundreds of selected extracts from the interviews in written, video and audio formats, are available on the public facing websites covering various aspects of COVID on hexi.ox.ac.uk (see Family Experiences of Long COVID, Long COVID in Adults, and COVID-19: Intensive Care Experiences).

Experiences of Long COVID in Children

While we (MacLean et al., 2023a) and many others have reported on the way that people with Long COVID have so often felt overlooked, invisible and unheard, our interviews with children and adolescents with Long COVID, and with parents caring for these young people, suggest that the dismissal of their lived experience has been even more profound. We have argued elsewhere (Wild et al., 2024) that they have faced a 'double invisibility'. This centres around three assumptions: (i) that for the vast majority, COVID is mild and (almost) everyone recovers; (ii) that children are not vulnerable to or badly affected by COVID; and (iii) that by 2022 the pandemic was essentially 'over'.

These collective representations ('narratives') of the pandemic, as interpreted by our participants, have been reflected in an analysis of UK media characterisation of Long COVID in children and young people. This analysis found that children's voices were silent in media coverage. Furthermore, when parents' voices featured, the reporting highlighted 'minimisation of Long COVID [in children and young people], barriers to care, and experiences of personal attacks [...] Health care professionals emphasised the rarity of Long COVID in [children and young people] and overemphasised psychological components' (Connor et al., 2024, p. 1). Connor and colleagues concluded that:

> Media characterisations contributed to epistemic injustice [for children and young people and the] disempowering portrayal of parents promotes stigma and barriers to care ... [contributing] to negative healthcare experiences and enacted testimonial injustice, where [children and young people's] and parents' credibility was diminished due to unfair identity prejudice, in their invalidation of Long COVID. (Connor et al., p. 1)

We illustrate below how strongly these findings chime with the children and young people and their parents' accounts included in our study.

In relation to the collective representation that COVID-19 is mild and (almost) everyone recovers after a short illness, Sara, a mother of an 8-year-old with Long COVID said 'everybody tells you COVID is [over] in two weeks, unless you're elderly and then you are in the A&E, in the ICU. That's it, there are the options'. Beth, another mother of an 8-year-old, said that when she spoke about her child's illness, people asked questions such as: '"Does Long COVID even exist? Is it even a thing?" you know, "Is it not just that she would have been poorly anyway?"'. Beth felt that there was no real understanding that a child might suffer long-term debilitating symptoms following COVID infection. Rather, it was suggested that 'maybe I'm overreacting, you know'. Richard, a GP whose 13-year-old son had Long COVID, encapsulated his frustration about the lack of willingness to believe that children get Long COVID, by saying, 'The whole British public don't get [understand] it'. This fuelled the common and confident assertion by health care professionals and others, that 'children don't get COVID'. For example, Richard reported being told by other medical professionals: 'Well look [Richard], kids don't get [it], chances are it's just another virus and you're just anxious, go home', before his son was discharged with no follow-up.

The lack of definitive biomarkers and diagnostic medical tests in relation to Long COVID, and the unpredictable, changing and episodic nature of people's symptoms left people with little ammunition to counter charges of 'overreacting'. Richard also reported the pain clinic team that saw his teenage son infantilised him in their dismissal of his experience:

> They were really condescending, they talked to him like he was, like, a 7- or 8-year-old, in baby language. And it just made things worse, I mean, it basically made him suicidal. My son [said], 'I hate talking to that woman, she just makes me feel like a baby, treats me like a child'. And they did nothing but make him a million times worse.

Others reported similar feelings of being totally dismissed. Joanna, a 16-year-old with Long COVID, for example, was told her symptoms were 'in her head'. Her mother reported that the doctor had suggested that she herself was pushing 'nut job sort of crazy stuff that [she had] learned from [patient support website]'. Leah, a 14-year-old, was accused of being 'dramatic'. Catherine, a parent, said:

> instead of looking at a patient [her son] and wondering why suddenly this 16-year-old's gone from sprinting up mountains on a bike to not being able to get up the stairs, they are being told that he needs to see a psychologist [...] The symptoms don't fit into an easy box. And doctors tend to put it into whatever box they know that seems to fit, which might be anxiety or chronic fatigue syndrome or something like that.

Other parents had reportedly been accused of jumping on a bandwagon or indulging a 'fad', or as Beth reported, 'an overreaction ... like everyone's talking about Long COVID, let's jump on their Long COVID train'. They worried that their competence as a parent was being totally undermined by the medical professionals they consulted:

> I was getting worried, over the whole of last year—'Am I going to be investigated by the social services for Munchausen by proxy?'. Fortunately [my son] was in a hospital in agony and with all these symptoms that [the paediatrician] could see that, you know, that we weren't making it up. But you just start having these strange thoughts when you're at home because you're not working, and you start worrying that 'Am I coming across as that as a parent?' (Richard)

This treatment from the medical profession and healthcare system left many parents feeling abandoned, anxious that they were not able to do enough to garner the care that their very sick child needed, as encapsulated by the poignant account below from Sasha, the mother of a 10-year-old girl. Sasha's daughter had been very unwell with a range of symptoms, including chest pain, left arm weakness, extreme sensory sensitivity, a rash, brain fog, loss of taste and smell and inability to eat. Sasha had been providing 24-hour care for her daughter over several months, but still worried that she was not able to do enough:

> So I think we've just felt rather belittled and fobbed off for the whole journey with a very, very sick child, and we've been given some diagnoses which have been sort of full stops, like 'functional pain', full stop [...] I managed to secure some contacts through people I know, doctors who have children with Long COVID, and those have been extremely supportive and they're echoing things that we have said. So, it's really

> been down to us to navigate her care. And that's been the major stress: are we doing enough to nurse a sick child day and night? You know, a sense of not being believed that she was ill, that I was being an over-reactive mother, that she wasn't that sick, when she was, and she's described as one of the most severe Long COVID cases by the doctors I'm speaking to who have Long COVID children.

In addition to what was often experienced as blanket disbelief about children's experiences of Long COVID, or their parents' accounts on their behalf, people interviewed in 2021–22 also encountered a collective weariness with the pandemic as a whole, which served to undermine their lived experience even further. As one mother of a very young child with Long COVID said, '[Long COVID is] an underlying issue that no-one wants to face, and [they hope] that it will just go away—people will get better and it will go away' (Lindsey, mother of 4-year-old with Long COVID and whose partner also had Long COVID). Francesca, a mother of a 6-year-old with Long COVID said the common view was that 'Most people are absolutely fine, so why should we consider the freaks who don't get better within a few [days]?'.

Thus, as we have argued elsewhere, in the face of these collective representations of COVID, which seemed invested in denying in particular that Long COVID could affect children, 'children and adolescents, and their parents struggled to signal the severity of their condition and elicit care in the manner expected for other debilitating illnesses', condemning them to a 'double invisibility' (Wild et al., 2024, p. 1) founded on widespread scepticism about the existence of Long COVID per se and a deep-rooted belief that children and young people absolutely would not be affected. It is likely that this double invisibility has slowed progress towards effective treatments for children and young people with Long COVID, as well as being highly detrimental to their mental health and well-being and that of their parents.

As well as often encountering reported dismissal of children's experience of having Long COVID in medical encounters, children and their parents also had to contend with the reactions of the education system, and of their peers (MacLean et al., 2023b). Many of the adolescents we spoke to spoke of yearning to be able to go back to school, both to try to get back on track with their education and to regain a sense of normality. Lily (a 14-year-old who had had Long COVID for 6 months) said, 'I just want to go back to school. Right, I know a lot of kids can't say that, but [I want to] just go back to my normal routine'. Maggie (aged 11) said, 'Sometimes I have really bad meltdowns where I just want to be back to normal [...] I do half days at school [...] go in at like 11am, and I come home and I just, I'm crying and I'm like, "I just want to be normal again"'. Joanna (aged 16), who had had Long COVID for over 18 months, described the hardest part as

> not being able to go to school or like see people my age, socialise and everything. It's all like online for me now over, like, social media or [text] messages [...] seeing other people [...] my age that are going out in school or doing all their exams [and] doing lots of things throughout the summer that I would like to be able to do, but I just can't. I think is that's quite hard.

While their education was seen as a normal and valued part of their lives, many children and young people and their parents were demoralised by their inability to bridge the chasm between their day-to-day experiences of debilitating fatigue, headaches and brain fog alongside other debilitating symptoms and the energy and stamina that they needed to sustain any return to normal school life. According to Emma, the parent of an 11-year-old girl with Long COVID: 'my daughter would struggle, do a day [at school] and then she'd be in bed for two days. She'd crash, she couldn't get out of bed, she felt dizzy, nausea. [It was like being] on a roller coaster'.

If they were able to get back into school, children and young people described how their interactions with their peers were jeopardised. Hugo, a 13-year-old with Long COVID, reported that: 'I couldn't really do anything [with friends] at break. I was just resting. I struggled going up the stairs. I can't do PE. Yeah, I just feel tired after every lesson'. On top of these struggles, children and young people described feelings of distress about the total uncertainty about how long their illness may last, disrupting their lives, friendships and their education. As Billy (aged 14) put it: 'it's never ending—you're in a maze and you turn around the corner and "Oh, is this going to be the end," but it's a dead end, that's what it feels like'.

Emilia, aged 15, who said she had always enjoyed learning and never really struggled at school before, described the challenges of trying to concentrate on learning:

> Something's just blocking my thoughts. I can't take in English, I can't analyse anything. It's like your sort of chain of thoughts is just completely, you know, broken, like I can't have more than one thought that leads to another one. It's just like my brain is just a cement block and it's just all messed up. It's so bad not being able to fully focus in class and struggling with the work and then not having the energy to do the homework. [I've been] just feeling really, like, stupid. I couldn't do the work even if it was work that I could do before. [So] then in that way it impacts [...] your self-esteem and things like that.

Young people and their parents reported their interactions with schools and teachers as being a 'mixed bag' (Billy, 14-year-old with Long COVID), often reflecting the scepticism encountered in medical interactions. Some commented that teachers have been understanding and accommodating, whilst others experienced a complete lack of understanding of Long COVID amongst school staff. The complexities of school systems, physical structures and timetabling raised some problems (for example, young people being unable to climb stairs to an upstairs classroom), and many were unable to manage online learning from home. All in all, many of these children and young people experienced their life as on hold. Their physical inability to do the things they enjoyed, including going to school, seeing their friends and taking part in family life, negatively impacted their mental health, their self-esteem and their sense of identity, as Emilia also described:

> I can't do the things that I love, and I can't do the things that make me feel like me. Long COVID has been the only thing I've really thought about for the last six months because it impacts every single part of my life. Whether it's the fatigue, or whether it's not being able to taste anything and not feeling motivated to eat, not feeling like I have the energy to be out with my friends, you know, it's like the only things I think about.

> The chronic fatigue and the mind fog I would say has had the biggest impact on my day-to-day life because, you know, I can't do the things that I used to be able to do. And then it obviously has an impact on my mental health and it's like a spiral of just not feeling great.

Experiences of Long COVID in Young Adults

For the young people who were in the first decade or so of their adulthood, Long COVID was also experienced as a profound disruption to daily life, threatening or destroying their identity and presumed future. For them, the pandemic and their illness came at a pivotal stage in establishing their independence as adults, an independence which rapidly became more tenuous. Their accounts resonated with poignant descriptions of the suspension of life as they knew it before contracting COVID, alongside deep uncertainty about whether, when or to what extent they might recover, physically and in relation to returning to their relatively newly established adult lives. Other researchers (for example, Callan et al., 2022; Kingstone et al., 2020; Rushforth et al., 2021) have noted the pertinence of the concept of biographical disruption (Bury, 1982) to understanding the experiences of people with Long COVID, but not specifically in relation to young adults. The curtailment of daily life necessitated by these young adults' symptoms led to a bewildering loss of self ('my whole image of myself is basically destroyed' (Felix); 'a part of you dies a bit' (Kathryn); 'I don't' feel like I am that me who I was before' (Charlotte) and a heightened state of liminality ('you're not that same person that you were and you're also not any other person as well' (Faatimah).

These young adults rapidly went from being fit and healthy before contracting COVID—'well and healthy, active, living a normal life' (Ben); 'I've never been ill' (Charlotte); 'a 22-year-old with no prior illness, who is fit and has really a healthy life' (Felix)—to becoming totally unable to continue their lives as before. Michael described Long COVID's impact on him as 'really extreme—the loss of my [university] course and the vision of what life kind of should be like for me; that, that's the most difficult thing'. Others described the difficulties of managing basic aspects of daily life (for example, dressing, showering, working, making food for themselves) and long periods of being bed-ridden, wheelchair-bound or lying on the sofa, while trying to manage their pain, extreme fatigue and other debilitating symptoms, feeling unable to concentrate or think clearly.

The impacts on every aspect of their lives meant those who were students had to suspend or extend their studies and those who were working had to give up, or take long absences from, work, thus threatening their financial independence as well as their identity. This led many to return to their parental home which was interpreted as a 'difficult', 'backwards' step, reflecting 'both their own expectations about the biographical direction of travel (transition) towards full independence, alongside perceived societal expectations about life course trajectories, which often failed to keep pace with increasing trends for young people to live at home for longer' (Hunt et al., 2024, p. 1534). Charles said:

> I would joke at the start, as if I'd regressed back to being 12 years old again, in terms of what my parents were doing for me. [I] was very reluctant to move back in because I had just left. I'd just flown the nest, and I didn't really want to be boomerang kid and come back, again.

Kathryn described how she had 'gone from living by myself, working by myself, travelling by myself, to literally needing help to, like, get into a shower' and Michael described almost returning to his adolescence:

> I don't want to be at home. I want to be at university and progressing. [It's] difficult to see those around you progress and you're kind of static, almost kind of living like you did when you didn't, like secondary school—you know, at home with your parents.

These young people's limited energy and other symptoms also left them unable to resume a social life as COVID restrictions began to ease. Taken together, these changes opened a chasm between them and their friends.

> I was very much the instigator and the organiser of my friendship group and now I'm not, because I just don't have the capacity. So, it's really

hard, because our lives are so different now. They've all got their own homes and some of them have children, whereas I've been back home. So the gap is just so huge. (Lucy)

We have previously argued that the core identities of these young adults had been fractured. They felt 'out of step' with peers and out of time, 'simultaneously both older than their peers (in their reduced physical capacity), yet also younger (in their need for basic care from parents and others)' (Hunt et al., 2024, p. 1536) and they found themselves 'in an unexpected place in their adult lives: not progressing; dependent; unable to work, study, be physically active and have a "normal" social life; and unable to care for themselves or others' (p. 1537). The language used ('moving back', 'regressing back', 'putting back') conveyed a strong sense of reverting to earlier life-stages. We concluded that existing adaptations of the concept of biographical disruption were problematic for this group, instead suggesting that 'biographical retrogression' may more accurately reflect their experiences (Hunt et al., 2024). The absence of medical and societal understanding about potential pathways to, and timeframes for, recovery for Long COVID perhaps explains why their experiences differed in key respects from other forms of biographical disruption described for people in early adulthood (for example, Polidano et al., 2020; Webb, 1998).

Some of these young adults also articulated their concerns about the impact of their illness on their families. Lucy raised practical issues which many families faced, whilst Felix talked about the uncertainties that his illness brought as his parents contemplated a more uncertain future:

So then to come home really relying on everybody around me, you know, everybody had to kind of come together in order to support me. My mum and my brothers had to step in and take me to hospital appointments—everybody had to step up. I'm very much used to supporting my brothers and now, everybody having to support me whilst still trying to run the house but with somebody that's bedbound. So, logistically, the family really have to step up and pull together. (Lucy)

It's stressful for both of us because for [my parents], emotionally, they don't know. I'm here [at home], can't finish my studies, no idea what the future is going to look like. My parents don't know if they have to care

> for me. They have saved enough money for both of them [but] they don't know if I'm able to work or do anything in the future. They may need to care for me. The long-term issue it's like the big elephant in the room. (Felix)

Impacts on Family Life

The disruptive influence on most aspects of family life was also all too apparent when parents who were caring for young children spoke of their experiences, or parents who had Long COVID themselves discussed how their place in the family and ways of being as a parent had been changed. Catherine was one of the parents who described a period of 'really crazy juggling' of work and her son's multiple hospital appointments. Many parents discussed the financial implications of needing to take time off work to care for a sick child, or of being unable to sustain a job because of their own illness. As Maryam, a parent, commented:

> There are food prices going up. Electric, gas, going up. Everything going up. You know, the children, they need everything. We are struggling. Sometimes hands to mouth [...] it's not easy. Sometimes you get the stress, anxiety and it's like, how we going to manage everything?

Relationships were disrupted or put under strain—between partners, with parents and a sick child—and feelings of guilt or sadness that their other children might be missing out because so much attention had to be focused on the needs of child who was so seriously unwell. Parents described how the existence of Long COVID within the family had led to the redistribution of household tasks and the renegotiation of caring roles. These changes were experienced within the existing precarity of the family as a complex, fluid and dynamic environment, sometimes introducing acute anxieties about whether the family unit and relationships within it could survive. Some parents who themselves had Long COVID found it difficult to care for their children and felt like they were absent from their children's lives, even when families as a unit had been able to accommodate and adapt to the new realities of chronic illness:

> I'm well aware of all the developmental things I'm missing with my daughter that she is getting from other places like nursery, or my wife, or when my daughter goes out with my wife and my friends. It's deeply saddening seeing a picture of her on our friend's shoulders out at a farm [rather] than mine. So I've had to learn to accept my limitation. I mean, of course I would like to be who I was before I had Long COVID, very much be the father I envisioned I would be. Whether I'm hopeful? To be honest, I try not to think about it because I don't know how hopeful I am. (Christian)
>
> It was very hard. It's like, I felt so useless, because I wasn't well myself, I couldn't be there for my children. I just felt so bad as well that, you know, and my kids are sick as well and I'm not able to look after them. Because I think for a mother, she always puts—we put our kids first. (Sharifa)
>
> If they need somebody in the night, they don't shout Mummy anymore, they shout Daddy. They don't rely on me the same, which is really sad. I'll just tell you one more thing what's been really, the children's birthdays. My son's third birthday was while I were really poorly at the beginning, and I were just in bed the whole day and not part of his day at all. So, he didn't have the party. He didn't have anybody visit the house, just his grandparents. Whereas, normally, we'd have a party, and their friends come and I'd make a really big occasion of their birthdays. (Charlotte)

One woman described the pressure of caring for a child and partner with Long COVID as 'just constant'. She said the lack of a 'support network for me' had made things 'really hard, it's been quite challenging at times, and it's really tested our relationship to the absolute limit and it continues to do that' (Lindsey). A man described the changed dynamics in his household by saying:

> My wife's described it as, you know, kind of, sometimes she effectively has to be a single parent, but then more actually, because she also feels like she has to look after me as well. So it's, sort of, like a single parent and carer on these days. She'll say, 'I feel resentful or cross because I have to do the cooking and the washing up, and then do my work'. And, you know, it's fair enough really. (Christian)

Concluding Comments

In this chapter, we have drawn on interviews with children and young people, young adults and parents to illustrate some of the profound impact of Long COVID on families. Recent decades have seen major shifts in family roles and expectations alongside increasing pressures on domestic life. Chronic illness is mainly experienced in the domestic 'family' space, and therefore the ways they are experienced and managed needs to be understood within the context of household and family care dynamics. Long COVID has presented particular challenges, not least because it is new, without accepted diagnosis or treatment and very uncertain in its future trajectories. We have shown how families' experiences of Long COVID, including the lack of understanding and support they encountered, frequently left them in an uncertain, open-ended place. Morgan (2020) argued that 'family practices' (the everyday routines and interactions in which families participate) are continually reconfigured. Gregory (2005) demonstrated the impact that chronic illness can have on families, by disturbing the routines, relationships and settings linked to family practices. We have illustrated here how family households and family practices have had to be reassembled to accommodate the illness of one or more family member with Long COVID and what our findings illuminate about the essential valued components of domestic relationships beyond the (potentially substituted) tasks of caring.

Acknowledgements We would like to thank the children, young people and family members who generously gave their time to participate in the interviews, especially as many had limited energy due to their Long COVID. We also thank the funders of the studies: UK National Institute for Health and Care Research (COV-LT2-0005) and Scotland's Chief Scientist Office (COV/LTE/20/04). CW was supported by a Girdlers' New Zealand Health Research Council Fellowship. The views expressed are those of the authors and not necessarily those of the NIHR or the Department of Health and Social Care.

References

Anderson, E., Hunt, K., Wild, C., Netleton, S., Zielbland, S., & MacLean, A. (2024). Episodic disability and adjustments for work: The 'rehabilitative work' of returning to employment with Long Covid. *Disability and Society, 1–23*. https://doi.org/10.1080/09687599.2024.2331722

Bury, M. (1982). Chronic illness as biographical disruption. *Sociology of Health & Illness, 4*(2), 167–182. https://doi.org/10.1111/1467-9566.ep11339939

Callan, C., Ladds, E., Husain, L., Pattinson, K., & Greenhalgh, T. (2022). 'I can't cope with multiple inputs': A qualitative study of the lived experience of 'brain fog' after COVID-19. *British Medical Journal Open, 12*(2). https://doi.org/10.1136/bmjopen-2021-056366

Callard, F., & Perego, E. (2021). How and why patients made Long Covid. *Social Science and Medicine, 268*. https://doi.org/10.1016/j.socscimed.2020.113426

Connor, C., Kranert, M., McKelvie, S., Clutterbuck, D., McFarland, S., & Alwan, N. A. (2024). A critical analysis of UK media characterisations of Long COVID in children and young people. *PLOS Global Public Health, 4*(11). https://doi.org/10.1371/journal.pgph.0003126

Gregory, S. (2005). Living with chronic illness in the family setting. *Sociology of Health & Illness, 27*(3), 372–392. https://doi.org/10.1111/j.1467-9566.2005.00447.x

Hunt, K., Maclean, A., Locock, L., O'Dwyer, C., Nettleton, S., Ziebland, S., & Wild, C. (2024). Young adults' experiences of biographical retrogression whilst living with long COVID. *Sociology of Health & Illness, 46*(8), 1526–1546. https://doi.org/10.1111/1467-9566.13798

Kingstone, T., Taylor, A. K., O'Donnell, C. A., Atherton, H., Blane, D. N., & Chew-Graham, C. A. (2020). Finding the 'right' GP: A qualitative study of the experiences of people with long-COVID. *British Journal of General Practice Open, 4*(5). https://doi.org/10.3399/bjgpopen20X101143

MacLean, A., Hunt, K., Brown, A., Evered, J. A., Dowrick, A., Fokkens, A.,…Wild, C. (2023). Negotiation of collective and individual candidacy for Long COVID healthcare in the early phases of the Covid-19 pandemic: Validated, diverted and rejected candidacy. *Social Science and Medicine—Qualitative Research in Health, 3*. https://doi.org/10.1016/j.ssmqr.2022.100207

MacLean, A., Wild, C., Hunt, K., Nettleton, S., Skea, Z. C., & Ziebland, S. (2023). Impact of Long COVID on the school experiences of children and young people: a qualitative study. *British Medical Journal Open, 13*(9). https://doi.org/10.1136/bmjopen-2023-075756

Morgan, D. H. (2020). Family practices in time and space. *Gender, Place & Culture, 27*(5), 733–743.

Polidano, K., Chew-Graham, C. A., Bartlam, B., Farmer, A. D., & Saunders, B. (2020). Embracing a 'new normal': The construction of biographical renewal in young adults' narratives of living with a stoma. *Sociology of Health & Illness, 42*(2), 342–358. https://doi.org/10.1111/1467-9566.13005

Rushforth, A., Ladds, E., Wieringa, S., Taylor, S., Husain, L., & Greenhalgh, T. (2021). Long COVID—The illness narratives. *Social Science and Medicine, 286*. https://doi.org/10.1016/j.socscimed.2021.114326

Webb, D. (1998). A 'revenge' on modern times: Notes on traumatic brain injury. *Sociology, 32*, 541–555.

Wild, C., MacLean, A., Nettleton, S., Hunt, K., & Ziebland, S. (2024). The double invisibility of Long COVID in children. *Social Science and Medicine, 347*. https://doi.org/10.1016/j.socscimed.2024.116770

Part VII

Coda

15

My Strange Revelations from Grief and Long COVID: How Caring for My Wife Showed Me the Horror and Beauty of Loss from Disease

Ben O'Mara

As I took the bucket of vomit from Gem, her arms pale, cheeks gaunt, hair matted and wet, and she asked me to call the ambulance, I could not help but feel my brilliant, beautiful wife had finally given up. I gave the emergency line operator our address, and Gem dragged her failing body from the floor back onto the bed to wait for the paramedics. My hands trembled in shock from knowing I might lose her in hospital. A shock felt by far too many caring for those, or suffering with, illness since the beginning of the COVID-19 pandemic.

What scared me the most, however, what shook me to my core, was something I could not fully comprehend during another medical emergency for my family. It was the thought of Gem being unable to summon the desire for making it through another day with vaccine-induced Long COVID. Of being unable to push herself through the unrelenting nausea, dehydration, dizziness, pain and low mood without,

B. O'Mara (✉)
School of Social Sciences, Media, Film and Education, Faculty of Health, Arts and Design, Swinburne University, Hawthorn, VIC, Australia
e-mail: bomara@swin.edu.au

D. Lupton (ed.), *Long COVID and Society*,
https://doi.org/10.1007/978-981-96-9168-5_15

from my perspective, comprehensive and effective medical support. To tolerate the reduced salary while away from work. To cope with the increasing medical bills, a lack of a relevant social safety net and the loneliness and the shrinking circle of family and friends as the rest of world relaxed COVID prevention measures and tried to move on. To withstand the horrific pain and suffering that defined much of her life since being administered the AstraZeneca vaccine in 2021 (Carey, 2021), even with her son and me by her side. A vaccine that helped so many people and an important public health measure early in the pandemic, yet left Gem, and my family, feeling like each day might be our last together.

That afternoon, we were lucky. The paramedics were kind and swift. Gem was taken outside into the sunny afternoon and lifted into the ambulance, and I followed, our toddler son in my arms, tears soaking my face. I remember him saying, 'Mum mum's going to hospital'. He sounded happy, as toddlers sometimes do in unusual situations, as if we were about to embark on some kind of adventure. With monumental effort, Gem raised her head, gave us a cheeky smile and a little wave. We both waved back. It was an act so small and hard fought, yet so beautiful and loving, it now feels forever lodged in my mind. An act that gave me hope her spirit was not broken as the ambulance drove to hospital. That she would live another day for us to spend time with her.

Two months later, in November 2024, we were not so lucky. Gem died from a terrible complication associated with Long COVID. My son and I will never be the same.

* * *

I know of other friends and families, online and in person, who have struggled with caring for loved ones trying to deal with Long COVID. In this context, I refer to carers as 'family members or friends who provide day-to-day living support for individual/s who may have significant and substantive health needs' (Coe et al., 2023). Providing care, while important and rewarding, can be very difficult. Parents, for example, can become stressed and exhausted from looking after children and performing additional care work. Picking up medicines, preparing food and drinks, booking doctor appointments, washing bedding and simply listening to their partners express very understandable doubts and concerns take their toll.

Those working may suffer ongoing worry from having to ask for time off from paid employment and having less income. It can feel stigmatising, too, when workplaces are less flexible with family health needs, and one cannot attend work meetings or similar social events due to care duties. Feeling like one is unable to participate on the job while still being a skilled professional can be disheartening.

I've also noticed the impact on siblings, elderly parents and friends. They often provide great love and support and do what they can. But many end up feeling frustrated and angry. Not with their loved ones dealing with Long COVID, but for some, frustration with a health system and society that can sometimes feel so unhelpful, so cruel, so unwilling to listen. Or just angry that something so terrible and debilitating has happened to someone they care about.

I am relieved that caring for my wife helped me and my son spend a few more precious years with her. Providing care made me realise though that it can also be tortuous; a haunting experience that, in my case, was borne from a chronic condition that remains poorly understood, treated and supported. And, from knowing that those suffering with Long COVID are mums, dads, brothers, sisters, aunties, uncles or friends and others just like everybody else. People with unique talents and skills. Who have careers and ambitions. People who matter.

Despite the urgent need for much greater kindness and support, I believe the situation for a lot of carers of those with Long COVID and those suffering with the condition has only become harder. In Australia and similar countries, health policy has focused more on trying to address the acute phase of COVID infection and prevent hospitalisations and death, rather than Long COVID (Costantino et al., 2024). Furthermore, there is a significant gap in understanding about the prevalence of Long COVID, its associated impacts and how to manage them, including how this affects carers. A recent estimate suggests, however, that hundreds of thousands of Australians are likely to be living with Long COVID after a single infection (Costantino et al., 2024). The estimate also suggests there are likely to be many carers who face significant challenges in supporting those suffering from the condition, but with little attention paid to what may help.

Research shows that carers of diverse experiences and backgrounds may benefit from being involved in the design and development of programs and activities aimed at reducing their stress and other difficult emotions (Coe et al., 2023). Use of participatory approaches that draw on the voices and lived experience of being a carer shows great promise. Additionally, it may help to use specific techniques such as trained facilitators, provision of respite for carers and technical assistance, flexibility in participation, enabling connection with other carers and self and creating time and space for reflection and self-care practices (Coe et al., 2023; Mylek & Schirmer, 2023).

Beyond specific programs, and for carers supporting for those dealing with Long COVID, it is critical that future research and practice find ways of increasing social and financial support (Grant et al., 2024; Kennelly et al., 2023). More robust data are required but existing research suggests that contracting Long COVID during employment or being unable to work from fatigue, joint pain and other symptoms can have serious consequences such as reduced pay and job loss and associated financial insecurity (Angeles et al., 2024; Rhead et al., 2024). Carers may find themselves with increased pressure to perform more paid employment in addition to looking after those with Long COVID, even as the care needs become high.

I also know after working as an Information Resources Manager in the Motor Neurone Disease (MND) community for several years, and MND being a life-limiting illness with no cure, that grief and bereavement can be major challenges for carers who have lost loved ones to disease (Motor Neurone Disease Australia, 2021). Such grief can feel intense, stressful and overwhelming (Trucco et al., 2024). I believe the difficulties in grieving are experienced by many carers of those with Long COVID. The disease can cause great uncertainty and feelings of self-criticism and guilt. Grief is one of the biggest challenges I face now as my son and I attempt to rebuild our lives without our beloved Gem.

* * *

I took my son swimming a lot this past summer. He seemed to enjoy the water and having fun and building confidence and skills in a such popular form of recreation, particularly in Australia. But I also knew that swimming with him was a powerful connection to memories of his mum. Gem was a keen and talented swimmer. She often found solace gliding through the water of the Olympic size pools in the town where we lived, or catching big, dumpy waves as we bodysurfed at the beach (O'Mara, 2018). We loved to spend time in the water as a family.

I love to surf and swim but my skills are average at best. I have a short and muscular body that is more suited to the rough and tumble of Australian Rules Football rather than the ordered lines of a swimming pool. My swimming style tends to be a little chaotic and awkward: those stubby arms and legs of mine too impatient, if good at making the water splash.

Sometimes, before Gem had Long COVID, we spent quiet nights at the pool when it was empty. She would sit on its edge and smile at me as I struggled with my clumsy strokes and losing my breath, and she would sometimes giggle. Then, she gently suggested changes to my stroke and breathing technique before effortlessly propelling herself through the water. Her advice always helped. Over the years, I like to think my improvements in swimming skill were significant, but she probably saw me as a cheerful and earnest work in progress. Either way, for the most part, we finished our sessions feeling relaxed, even elated. They were some of my sweetest moments with her and of my life.

Gem shared her joy and sense of play in the water with her son, too. On the days when fatigue was not as bad, or she wasn't overwhelmed by crippling nausea and pain, I helped her make it to the pool, enter the water, and lift our son into her arms. The water's buoyancy made it easier to hold him. Once settled, she liked to zoom him up and down through the water, him squealing with delight. When he was too tired to keep playing, I would help him out, change his clothes, and she did slow walks up and down the pool. I believe walking in the gentle water helped to wake up her muscles and nervous system. She was like that: even through some our toughest times, she remained committed to healing, to getting better.

Gem's persistence reached well beyond the pool. As a family, we were able to support her to keep bouncing back as best she could from illness and disability. I believe she was able to foster enormous courage in continuing her writing and research as one of Australia's leading academics in the fields of public policy and health. It was her courage and tenacity that helped her achieve promotion to full professor in recognition of her research and policy impact, at just 37 years of age (Dickinson et al., 2025). She was a prolific writer and published more than 100 journal articles, four books and many other papers and reports. Her memoir, *No Matter Our Wreckage* (Carey, 2020), was an uncompromising and visceral story about intergenerational trauma, grooming, and consent. A keen collaborator, she was also very generous and supported and inspired so many people in their work, particularly those early in their careers. She continued to defy expectations as she became so unwell and still wrote and published even after some of her darkest, most painful days with Long COVID. Some days, when she was able to stomach it, floating in water restored a clarity that she cherished for her work.

Now, without Gem, I find swimming with our son to be bittersweet. Twice a week I take him to a swimming program at nights for children in a local primary school. Like his mum, he is a spirited and independent soul. He is always keen to pull on his own bathers or get down from the car by himself, even at such an early age. But after I help him get ready, we walk up the school's path and head inside the pool building, a small and well-kept facility for early childhood swimmers that somehow feels both familiar and strange. It is one of the many emotional and weird moments we encounter while adjusting to our new weekly routine.

Most nights in the pool I find to be similar. The odd vibes increase as I lower myself and my son into the water. Its temperature is relatively pleasant yet seems too cool with just the two of us, even a little unsettling. Then, others enter the pool. We are surrounded by friendly mums and dads with their kids, families like my son and me, but they appear different, more relaxed and confident, less drained by loss, as if from another world. I feel ghost-like and out of place with the living as my son and I drift towards the trainers. Then, there is that sharp smell of chlorine. Memories sweep into my mind, as a kid and jumping with glee into the deep end, then, carrying my wife from the pool, her eyes closed, exhausted, too sick to keep swimming. The memory feels both sickening and bursting with energy and life.

Soon, though, my son kicks his legs to explore the pool and finds his way over to one of the instructors who welcomes him with open arms. She swings him around in slow circles and he cries out for more and they both laugh. He seems so happy in the arms of a stranger. I start to cry. But my son splashes me, and the tears disappear in the bubbles and laughter. It is hard to stay sad with him having fun. The pool lessons continue, and for a while, I feel a little better.

In one of Gem's last memoir pieces, she wrote about her weird experience of 're-learning' to speak and read again after the loss of these abilities due to neurological damage stemming from the vaccine injury (Carey, 2025). She described her experience as strange and overwhelming. For someone who lived so much of her life through words, she worried her brain was damaged, and that she would not get control of her words again.

> Relearning is akin to focus. Skills and abilities come in and out of focus. One day you wake up and you can speed read again. Another day, you open your mouth to speak, and speaking has become impossibly hard. It is no longer automatic, and your words are stilted and slow. You never know what you will have on any given day, and just because you have regained or relearned it once is no guarantee it will stay. You are still you, but pieces are missing, and the pieces change each day.

Reading her piece now, her experience resonates with me in sad as well as beautiful ways. I feel the eeriness of everyday life, often imagined through fiction (VanderMeer & VanderMeer, 2010), and as I attempt to grieve and look after our son and myself without her. I am 're-learning' the bizarre art and science of having a family with memories and fragments of her from another time. Of both remembering her and coming to terms with a new reality of parenting alone. And in being a single dad, seeing our son continue his love of swimming with others. Preparing myself to help him through kindergarten and primary school. Discover new passions and challenges in high school. Become a young man who hopefully enters adulthood brimming with intelligence and talent, just like his mum, but with only his dad by his side.

What my son and I do have though, as we try to survive after the devastating loss of Gem and the awful experience of Long COVID, is each other. In the pool, at home, after work, late at night, early in the morning and everywhere and anytime that the pain and uncertainty of grief arrives, I do my best to care for him, and our relationship. He does his best as a fast-growing son with his dad. We are trying to share those uncanny moments of bliss and loss in the pool and the rest of daily life. To rest easy at nights in our beds while knowing it will be just the two of us having breakfast in the morning.

I know Gem would take comfort in us learning how to keep going again as a family. And proud that her son and husband still find courage and relief in the water during such a strange chapter of our lives. It is a process that is not easy, but one still full of beauty and joy, and that we can endure, together.

References

Angeles, M. R., Dinh, T. T. N., Zhao, T., de Graaff, B., & Hensher, M. (2024). The economic burden of long COVID in Australia: More noise than signal? *The Medical Journal of Australia, 221*(Suppl 9), S31–S39. https://doi.org/10.5694/mja2.52468

Carey, G. (2020). *No matter our wreckage: A memoir about grooming, betrayal, trauma and love.* Allen & Unwin.

Carey, G. (2021, June 8). Vaccines are risky for me, but I don't regret getting my COVID jab. *The Guardian.* https://www.theguardian.com/commentisfree/2021/jun/08/vaccines-are-risky-for-me-but-i-dont-regret-getting-my-covid-jab

Carey, G. (2025, April 1). Slow violence, a weird delirium. *Lost Souls, 1.* https://lostsouls.net.au/

Coe, A., Bibb, J., Kritharidis, R., O'Mara, M., Lautman, R., Densley, K., Kovarik, S., Kaylor-Hughes, C., Lewis, M., & Palmer, V. J. (2023). A mixed-methods evaluation of the impacts of an online carer wellbeing and connection program. *PEC Innovation, 3*. https://doi.org/10.1016/j.pecinn.2023.100218

Costantino, V., Grafton, Q., Kompas, T., Chu, L., Honeyman, D., Notaras, A., & MacIntyre, C. R. (2024). The public health and economic burden of long COVID in Australia, 2022–24: A modelling study. *The Medical Journal of Australia, 221*(4), 217–223. https://doi.org/10.5694/mja2.52400

Dickinson, H., Yates, S., Brown, J., & Malbon, E. (2025). Vale Gemma Carey: Warrior, scholar, friend. *Australian Journal of Public Administration, 84*(1), 3–5. https://doi.org/10.1111/1467-8500.70001

Grant, A., Stage, E., Blane, D., Goss, H., Ormerod, J., McIver, S., Duncan, E., Patel, G., Campbell, A., Manson, P., Subramanian, G., & Cooper, K. (2024). Four years in, what are the research priorities for Long COVID? A research priority-setting partnership between people with lived experience, carers, clinicians and researchers. *Health Expectations, 27*(5). https://doi.org/10.1111/hex.70072

Kennelly, C. E., Nguyen, A. T. P., Sheikhan, N. Y., Strudwick, G., Ski, C. F., Thompson, D. R., Bartram, M., Soklaridis, S., Rossell, S. L., Castle, D., & Hawke, L. D. (2023). The lived experience of long COVID: A qualitative study of mental health, quality of life, and coping. *PloS One, 18*(10) https://doi.org/10.1371/journal.pone.0292630

Motor Neurone Disease Australia. (2021). *End of life care: A guide for people living with MND*. Motor Neurone Disease Australia. https://www.mndaustralia.org.au/getmedia/eeaabc08-8c23-41ca-bae9-1e4927a757f3/MNDAus_EndofLifeGuide_digital-version.pdf

Mylek, M., & Schirmer, J. (2023). *Caring for others and yourself: The 2023 carer wellbeing survey*. University of Canberra and Carers Australia. https://www.carersaustralia.com.au/report/caring-for-others-and-yourself-the-2023-carer-wellbeing-survey/

O'Mara, B. (2018, November 2). My partner couldn't walk because of chronic pain. Now we hit the surf together. *The Guardian*. https://www.theguardian.com/commentisfree/2018/nov/02/my-partner-couldnt-walk-because-of-chronic-pain-now-we-hit-the-surf-together

Rhead, R., Wels, J., Moltrecht, B., Shaw, R. J., Silverwood, R., Zhu, J., Hughes, A., Chaturvedi, N., Demou, E., Katikireddi, S. V., & Ploubidis, G. (2024). Long COVID and financial outcomes: Evidence from four longitudinal population surveys. *Journal of Epidemiology and Community Health, 78*(7), 458–465. https://doi.org/10.1136/jech-2023-221059

Trucco, A. P., Backhouse, T., Mioshi, E., & Kishita, N. (2024). Factors associated with grief in informal carers of people living with Motor Neuron

Disease: A mixed methods systematic review. *Death Studies, 48*(2), 103–117. https://doi.org/10.1080/07481187.2023.2191351
VanderMeer, A., & VanderMeer, J. (2010). *The weird: A compendium of strange and dark stories.* Atlantic Books.

Index

A
ableism 6, 17, 282, 284, 291, 304
activism. *See* patient activism
athletes 10, 16, 289–293, 295–303
autoethnography 19

B
Bateson, Gregory 19, 250, 254, 255
Berlant, Lauren 21
biographical disruption 15, 16, 60, 62–64, 67–69, 71–73, 320, 322
biographical retrogression 16, 322
biopolitics 7–9, 132, 134, 144
Bury, Michael 15, 60, 62, 63, 67, 72, 320

C
children 10, 18, 49, 94, 110, 162–166, 168, 186, 193, 235, 237, 312, 314–319, 322–325, 332, 336
chronic fatigue syndrome. *See* myalgic encephalomyelitis/chronic fatigue syndrome (ME/CFS)
church. *See* religion
Church of England 17, 267–271, 276, 282, 284
cognitive behavioural therapy 20, 212, 235, 268
consumer movement. *See* patient consumerism
contested illnesses 10, 11, 14, 86, 99, 100
COVID-19 pandemic 249
  emergence of 6, 43, 121

D. Lupton (ed.), *Long COVID and Society*,
https://doi.org/10.1007/978-981-96-9168-5

mitigations 8, 21, 275
political dimensions 9
crip studies 8
crip time 15

D

death 8, 20, 21, 62, 135, 164, 232, 235, 240, 243, 296, 333
diagnosis 6, 11, 48, 63, 98, 100, 111, 113, 123, 124, 142, 160, 183, 187, 190, 210, 212, 218, 229, 250, 252, 258, 294, 297, 304, 325
disability 6, 8, 9, 15, 36, 52, 76, 111, 122, 159, 165, 167, 186, 189, 190, 207, 270, 277, 280, 281, 284, 336. *See also* crip studies
discrimination 8, 17, 241, 242, 268, 269
double-bind theory 250, 254, 255

E

economic impacts 122, 183, 208
educational settings 9, 163
employment 6, 7, 10, 152, 155–157, 160, 186, 205, 211, 333, 334
epistemic injustice 6, 10–12, 18, 96, 133, 206, 207, 216, 217, 221, 235, 259, 314
ethnicity 8, 160, 262, 277, 313
evidence-based medicine (EBM) 89

F

Facebook 38, 46, 49, 51, 75, 191, 206, 208, 219, 279
families 10, 166, 189, 312, 322, 323, 325, 332, 336
fatigue 4, 11, 16, 39, 50, 61, 64, 69, 85, 88, 91, 94, 96, 98, 114, 139, 152, 154, 156, 160–164, 188, 190, 207, 209, 235, 281, 294, 297, 316, 318, 319, 321, 334, 335
Fleck, Ludwik 14, 86, 87, 93
Foucault, Michel 8, 136, 257, 290
Frank, Arthur 19, 66, 134, 261

G

Gaslight (film) 251, 256, 260
gaslighting 19, 21, 250–261, 300
gender 8, 154, 160, 161, 277, 292
Girard, Rene 19, 250, 254–256
government failures 220
government inquiries 16, 207, 220
graded exercise therapy 20, 212, 235, 268
Great Barrington Declaration 139

H

hashtags 13, 37, 39–42, 45, 49–51, 69, 76
healthcare 4, 6, 7, 9, 12, 14, 15, 18, 19, 43–45, 61, 71, 74–76, 86, 89, 95, 111, 118, 122, 133, 153–157, 159–162, 165–167, 181–183, 185–187, 190, 191, 196, 217, 268, 299, 300, 312, 314, 316
Health Equity Framework 9, 182
hermeneutical injustice 12, 14, 138, 141

I

immunity 134, 138–141, 145
inequalities 7–9, 11, 153, 168, 293, 303
internet 62, 89, 110. *See also* social media

J

John Snow Memorandum 139

L

Lefebvre, Henri 17, 59, 61, 72
Libertarianism 155
Long COVID
  definitions of 4, 142
  hashtags 13, 37, 39–42, 45, 49, 51, 69, 76
  mental health impacts 153
  symptoms 3–5, 13, 14, 35, 37, 39, 41, 59, 60, 65, 66, 68–71, 133, 140, 152, 156, 161, 164, 183, 209, 210, 216, 268, 280, 294, 295
  treatments 59, 124, 132, 214, 312, 317
Long hauler 38, 63, 65–68, 70–72, 132

M

marginalisation 6, 7, 187–190, 194
medical care. *See* healthcare
medical knowledge 14, 91, 123
medical power 6
medical professionals 7, 11, 88, 99, 212, 235, 244, 312, 315, 316
  with Long COVID 12, 13, 18, 98, 215, 254
mental health 16, 153, 158, 164, 165, 196, 216, 269, 275, 277, 313, 317, 319, 320
myalgic encephalomyelitis/chronic fatigue syndrome (ME/CFS) 11, 85, 139, 207, 267

N

narrative 6, 15, 19, 20, 62, 63, 65, 69, 109, 133–135, 144, 217, 229, 254–258, 290, 291, 294–298, 301–304, 312–314
narrative theory 6
necropolitics 8
neoliberalism 7

P

PACE trial 235, 268
pacing 14, 60, 63, 65–72, 74, 109, 114, 115, 120, 214, 280
parents 10, 280, 313, 314, 316–319, 321–323, 325, 333
patient activism 41, 235
patient autonomy 8, 90
patient communities 6, 13, 35, 52, 116, 237
patient consumerism 187
patient expertise 6, 13
patient rights 90
people of colour 8, 17
policy 6, 39, 75, 95, 134, 135, 154, 155, 166, 184, 185, 187, 191, 193–196, 217, 218, 220, 221, 238, 258, 333, 336
political economy 6, 7, 165
post-exertional malaise (PEM) 4, 60, 64, 88, 113, 209, 232

power dynamics 89, 100, 252, 257, 260
prejudice 12, 100, 314
psychosocial perspectives 6

R
religion 269
rhythmanalysis 6, 17, 59, 61, 72, 74
rituals 14, 15, 107, 108, 123

S
self-tracking 13, 60, 61, 70–74
sexual identity 8
slow death 20, 21
social construction of knowledge 6, 14, 86
social determinants of health 6, 7, 153, 155, 161, 187
social justice 6
social media 6, 12, 35, 37, 38, 45, 51, 60, 62, 73, 75, 89, 96, 132, 213, 271, 301, 318. *See also* Facebook; X/Twitter
spoonies 67–72, 75
spoons theory 67, 69
sport 117, 289–293, 296–298, 300–303
stigma 6–8, 15, 17, 68, 88, 188, 189, 192, 195, 268, 269, 314

T
temporality 6, 16, 17, 21, 59–61, 64, 68, 69, 122
testimonial injustice 12, 144, 207, 314
this autoethnography 228
thought collective 14, 86, 87, 98, 101
thought style 14, 86, 87, 91, 93, 97, 99–101
trauma 6, 19, 228–231, 238, 239, 250, 254, 256, 258–261, 336

V
vaccines 137, 209, 239

W
Workplaces. *See* employment
wounded storyteller 19

X
X/Twitter 13, 17, 35–42, 47–49, 51, 52, 67, 68, 70–72

FSC
www.fsc.org
MIX
Papier | Fördert
gute Waldnutzung
FSC® C083411

Kolibri 360 GmbH
Ferdinand-Jühlke-Straße 7
99095 Erfurt, Deutschland
produktsicherheit@kolibri360.de